EIRE £1.33 (inc VAT) USA 2.50 GERMANY 6DM FRANCE

FEBRUARY 1986 No.38 80p

BLITZ

WELL RED!

THE KRAYS
Ronnie & Reggie behind bars

CANNON & BALL
Comic Heroes

DEE SNIDER
Showing signs of Metal fatigue

The return of **Floy Joy**
Fish *— one in a Marillion*
Michael Winner *— director with a Death Wish*
Hollywood Babylon II *: replenished Anger*
Fashion *: Red Hat — No Knickers!*

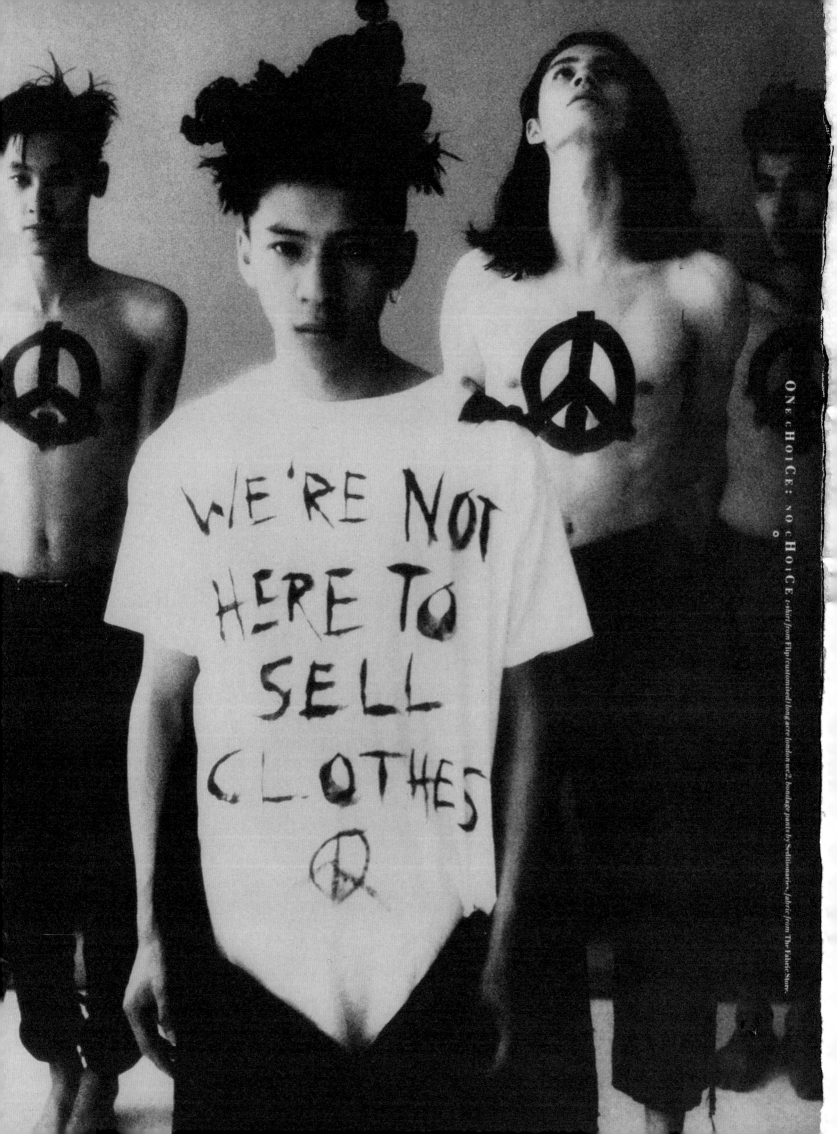

ONE CHOICE: NO CHOICE. t-shirt from Flip/customised long acre london wc2. bondage pants by Seditionaries / fabric from The Fabric Store.

BLITZ

As seen in BLITZ — Fashioning '80s Style
IAIN R. WEBB

Cover: BLITZ #34
September 1985
Photographer: David Hiscock
Details on page 83

Left: BLITZ #45
September 1986
Photographer: Mark Lewis
Details on page 167

ISBN: 978 1 85149 723 2

British Library Cataloguing-
in-Publication Data.
A catalogue record for
this book is available from
the British Library.

Publication designed and
typeset by Northbank, Bath.
northbankdesign.co.uk

Printed and bound in China.

———

Published in England by
ACC Editions, a division
of The Antique Collectors'
Club Ltd, Woodbridge,
Suffolk.

———

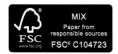

Opposite: *BLITZ* Fashion Manifesto
written by Iain R. Webb c.1985

BLITZ

FASHION:

As Fashion Editor of BLITZ magazine it is my intention to present the most representative of modern fashion trends, alongside pictures which are simply inspired by what I may see around me. It is not my intention to DICTATE, or advocate any one particular trend or designer label, or even to persuade the reader to begin dressing in such a way.
I WOULD HOPE that the pictures are seen as reflections of the multi-faceted society within which we live. They are intended to INSPIRE, DELIGHT, or even, at times, ANGER. They are essentially photographs which just happen to have clothes within their boundaries. These pictures should be used as a springboard for creativity on the part of the reader.

AS FOR PREDICTIONS: My only joy in life is that one can NEVER be certain WHAT, or indeed WHO, will happen next. It would be pointless for me to set myself up as a latter day prophet, and tell you the way to go.

If you do not FEEL it in your heart, then it will NEVER hang correctly from your shoulder.

If you limit your life by the length of your skirt, then your sensibilities will reveal such.

DO NOT ask my opinion - instead feel fabric against your skin, and
DRESS ACCORDINGLY......

Iain R. Webb - Fashion Editor BLITZ.

1 Lower James Street London W1R 3PN 734 8311

Sally Boon, photographer:
When we worked together, I remember there was a lot of time spent researching the shoot as the images were often very cinematic in nature. I watched many films, seeing *Blade Runner* at least five times and spending many evenings wandering around Chinatown, eating wonton noodle soup and just observing the mood there while looking for locations. It was this story that for me seamlessly encompassed your philosophy, by bringing to life so beautifully an elusive and enigmatic mood. You were able to forget the details of the clothes.

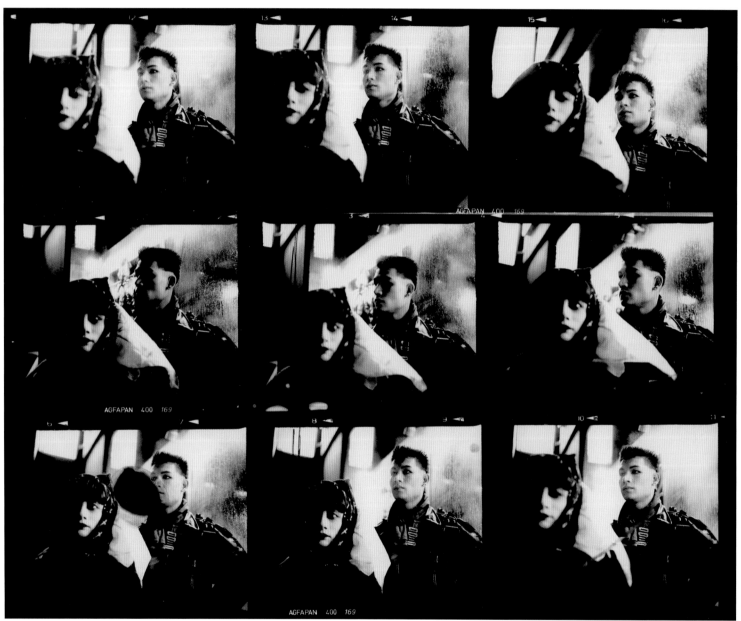

L to R: Labi, David

Photographer: Sally Boon

Models: David Ball, Labi

Make-up: Helen Whiting

Hair: Not Listed

Clothes: Nostalgia of Mud, Kansai Yamamoto, Kitsch, Gregory Davis, Rachel Auburn, Bernstock Speirs

CONTENTS

The memories in this book all
come from original interviews and
correspondence with the author.

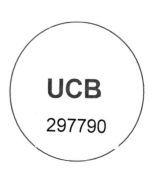

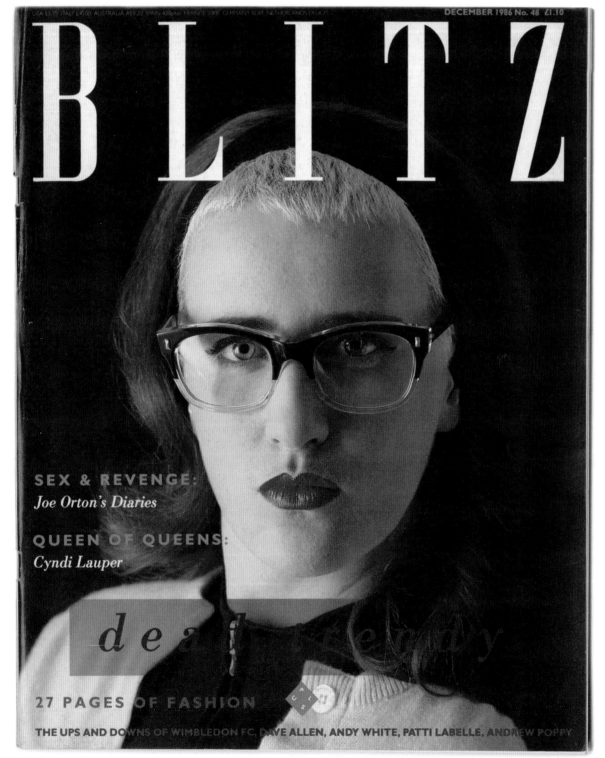

USA $3.95 ITALY L4500 AUSTRALIA A$5.20 SPAIN 420ptas FRANCE 20FR GERMANY 8DM NETHERLANDS DFL6.25 DECEMBER 1986 No. 48 £1.10

BLITZ

SEX & REVENGE:
Joe Orton's Diaries

QUEEN OF QUEENS:
Cyndi Lauper

dead friendly

27 PAGES OF FASHION

THE UPS AND DOWNS OF WIMBLEDON FC, DAVE ALLEN, ANDY WHITE, PATTI LABELLE, ANDREW POPPY

Photographer: Gill Campbell, Model: Martine Houghton

I always wanted to be a stylist because I collected *BLITZ*, and wanted to grow up and be you!

In the early 1980s magazines were hugely important and influential, so one bought everything. It was exciting to have different points of view. For me, *BLITZ* was always the most glamorous of the three, at that point. *i-D* was always apologetic in covering fashion – the people had to be real – and the early editions of *The Face* magazine were all about music types in fashion. *BLITZ*, as I recall, was about fashion and clubs. Wasn't it named after the club? I always liked the end of year round-ups in *BLITZ*, where you were fashionable if you had stripey tights, a Westwood mini crini, a bleached crop, braces, Dr. Martens ... and maybe there was an armour jacket in there too – Richard Torry, not Westwood, obviously!

Am I the only person who has their copies of *BLITZ* bound?

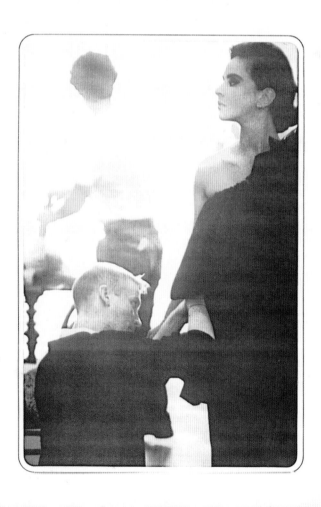

In October 1980 Steve Strange's famous New Romantic nightclub at Blitz wine bar in London's Covent Garden closed its doors for the last time. The previous month, the first issue of a new magazine called *BLITZ* had hit the streets.

Although these two iconic moments of '80s culture are unrelated (*BLITZ* publisher Carey Labovitch says she chose the name because she liked how it sounded and had not actually heard of the club), there is a compelling and stylish thread that links them. Along with many of the photographers, designers, models and the like that featured regularly in *BLITZ* magazine, I was one of the original Blitz Kids (so called by the press) who attended the notorious Tuesday night soirées hosted by Strange. Many of us were fashion students attending nearby St Martin's School of Art, and from the club's opening night onwards we would spend our waking hours focused on putting together a *look* to wear each week. This was mostly pulled together from second-hand shops and army and navy surplus finds, or knocked-up on a sewing machine between (or sometimes during) classes at St Martin's. The *look* could be inspired by an old movie, a classic novel, an historical figure or even a futureworld superhero.

Every week at the Blitz club, as Kraftwerk sang, 'For every camera she gives the best she can', we posed as the flashbulbs popped. "I wanted to look like a black and white photograph", says sartorial co-conspirator Scarlett Cannon. In *BLITZ* magazine, and on the cover of this book, she got her wish.

The Blitz club was full of bright young things wishing to overthrow the establishment with their alternative vision of the world: part nostalgic and rose-tinted, part broken and dystopic post-punk. It was the energy of these would-be fashion designers, writers, artists, make-up artists, filmmakers and photographers that needed a stage on which to perform. In 1980 three magazines were born that would turn the spotlight on this new army of dreamers: *BLITZ*, *i-D* and *The Face*.

I left St Martin's in the summer of 1980, first in my class. Within a week I was last in the dole queue. After working for a year or so as an assistant for designer Zandra Rhodes I jumped into the scary world of the self-employed. I stitched up one-off designs for friends and was featured in an arts magazine called *VIZ* as an 'image maker'. "The dress does not need to be sexy if the woman wearing it is irresistible", I proclaimed somewhat self-consciously.

I made stage clothes for goth rockers Bauhaus and funk band Freeez while penning features for middle-of-the-road women's magazines, and even a music review for *The Face*. I worked part-time in a fancy shoe shop in South Molton Street, a job I was eventually sacked from because my *look* (muslin petti-drawers worn over ripped jeans, Scottish ghillie shoes and a bleached, permed *and* crimped hairdo) was too way-out for ladies shopping for a conical heeled court shoe.

Yet it was this *look* that led to a phone call from photographer Mike Owen, who asked if I would style a shoot for a glossy, large-format Japanese hair magazine. "I remember being very impressed with your enthusiasm and personal style", says Owen, who, pleased with the results, asked if I would like to contribute to a new magazine he was working for called *BLITZ*. I was excited to get the chance and constructed a fashion story inspired by war, with a slew of stylish references including *The Deer Hunter* and

Don McCullin. All went well and the pictures were a hit with publisher Carey Labovitch and editor Simon Tesler, who not only used one of the images on the cover but were also intrigued enough by my accompanying text to ask me to pitch some more feature and fashion ideas. As the magazine was a showcase for new and disparate talent (it originally billed itself as a magazine carrying a mix of art, film, fashion, politics and music) I welcomed the opportunity to write about my friends who, like myself, were attempting to create an alternative scene. Although fashion was my first love, having grown up on a media diet of *The Sunday Times* colour supplement, *Interview* and *RITZ* magazines, I was keenly interested and inspired by creative and stylish people.

So that was exactly what I wrote about in a column called 'People', first appearing in the contributors list in issue 8, dated December/January 1982/83. My first column, on the back page, included Miss Binnie (a neo-naturist cabaret performer whom I had collaborated with at the Blitz club); Alix Sharkey and his new band called Out; and Zwei, a newly launched fashion label by best friend, flatmate, fellow St Martin's graduate and seasoned clubber, Fiona Dealey.

The fashion story 'At War' appeared in the next issue, along with mini-features on set designer and window dresser Mick Hurd and retailer P.W. Forte. My 'People' column (now covering a double page spread) was dedicated to fabulous siblings Mark and James Lebon, Jayne and Lesley Chilkes and a quartet of McGanns (Joe, Paul, Mark and Stephen).

The diversity of subjects reflected my inspirations – from film school graduates Isaac Julien, Sophie Muller and Holly Warburton to models, actors, musicians and writers. I corralled together Pat Cleveland, Eve Ferret, Nick Egan, Kate Garner, Karen O'Connor, Greg Hayman, Sally Brampton, Bodymap and even Barbara Cartland.

By issue no. 11 in May 1983, my name appeared under a separate heading of Fashion. I was given 'Style' pages to edit, which crammed four or sometimes five stories (all with accompanying shoots – if you can call one or two pictures a shoot) onto a double-page spread. Along with photographer and eager conspirator Sally Boon, we cobbled together styled stories inspired by things that took our fancy. In one issue there was a shoot referencing *Liquid Sky*, a trippy independent film by Slava Tsukerman that was a new wave paean to androgyny, aliens, drugs and downtown New York. Our version featured model Linda Millard posing in Zandra Rhodes ballgowns and Johnson's pink pegs. Across the page I interrogated Barking-born Billy Bragg about his personal style. (At this time I was also profiling pop stars from Morrissey to Smeggy of King Kurt for the *NME*, who wanted a bit of this new style to rub off on their readers. That column did not last long!) Bragg's entire shoe collection numbered four almost-identical pairs. Although this mix may have seemed incongruous, I believe it was this diversity that, encouraged by Tesler and Labovitch, would go on to define the *BLITZ* fashion pages.

While the magazine's editorial policy was to welcome fashion stories presented on an *ad hoc* basis (these were being created on next-to-no funds by little teams of creative types running wild across the capital), I somehow managed to be offered the job of Fashion Editor, after ranting in the office that the magazine's fashion pages needed a singular vision if they were to be taken seriously. Suddenly I was responsible for twenty or more pages a month, with an open-ended brief and no budget. In February 1985, I appeared on the masthead as Fashion Editor along with the wonderful Hellen Campbell, who was credited as Fashion Assistant. Hellen had tremendous style with a radical Louise Brooks bob and a penchant for black loafers. We made a peculiar sight together at fancy fashion events. When Hellen left to pursue her career the baton was passed to Darryl Black, who became a wicked co-conspirator. "When I came to work for you it was like getting a little doorway into your crazy mind", she says. We shared many crazy times.

Soon our tiny first-floor office in Soho was filled with photographers wanting to show their work and models parading by or just hanging out for fun. There was a cupboard full of clothes and notebooks overflowing with ideas – be it a Jewish boy modelling Lonsdale sportswear, a Victorian *ingénue* on ice-skates in fake Yamamoto, or jeans found at the back of my wardrobe alongside spanking new Jean Paul Gaultier. There were brides and bag ladies, Amish and Buddhists. No one was left out in our in-crowd. "The work you were doing was really powerful in giving us misfits and vagabonds a home", recalls model Amanda Cazalet.

The impact of this was spreading. Around this time an article in the *International Herald Tribune* entitled 'Fashion's Subculture Goes Way Out In Print' focused on the 'culture shock' being pushed by the trio of new British magazines, *BLITZ*, *The Face* and *i-D*. In the article the doyenne writer, Hebe Dorsey, described the new approach as 'blissfully liberated with a lot of fun-poking at the Establishment.' She noted how the magazines promoted the idea that 'fashion is a happening' and 'no longer for those that can afford it'. She also observed that the styled shoots made *Vogue* look like 'a string quartet next to a punk band'.

The 'We're Not Here to Sell Clothes' image (see frontispiece) is from a story I created that was inspired by my ongoing love/hate relationship with the fashion industry. This shoot epitomised my ethos for the fashion pages. It was not about selling a *look*, it was about saying something. For me, it is a powerful image that has resonated throughout my career and I often return to it to refuel my soul.

No matter the path trodden, from the alternative counter-culture of *BLITZ* and *i-D* to the establishment grip during my tenure as Fashion Editor at the *Evening Standard* or *The Times*, I have always tried to weave other such messages within the fashion images I have produced. I hope that they might move people beyond merely flashing the cash. The purpose has always been to inspire or provoke, engage or enrage.

For me, the concept will always be king. How great it was to have the opportunity to turn those concepts into a reality by styling the fashion stories* that appear in this book. How great were the amazing people I got to work with to make those pictures? And everyone, it appeared, was sharing a common aim: to create an alternative landscape fuelled by the simple desire to put together a *look*. Wearable or otherwise.

*All except one, 'Foreign Affairs' (page 203), which was styled by Darryl Black.

Simon Tesler, Carey Labovitch & Iain R. Webb

What originally prompted you to start a magazine? What were you doing at the time?

Simon Tesler: It was Carey's idea. It was in May 1980 and we were both coming to the end of our first year at university. We met at a party at someone's house, and she said she was thinking of starting her own magazine.

Carey Labovitch: There was a genuine gap in the market for a magazine like BLITZ. Magazines were in my blood. I had previously produced various magazines at school on an old fashioned Roneo machine. But now I was nineteen and found myself desperate to create something a bit more sophisticated, a magazine that I wanted to read that covered all the areas that my generation was interested in, from fashion to music, film, theatre, photography, design. In those days, teenagers were limited by such narrow choices: music newspapers such as NME, or girls' magazines such as Jackie. There just had to be more to life than this!

ST _ Remember that the media industry then was prehistoric compared to now. This was literally the age before computers, before digital cameras, music videos, CDs or mobile phones. In the magazine industry, everything was done on typewriters and with glue. There didn't seem to be any other magazines for our age group. The only colour monthlies were bland titles like 19, Honey or Over 21. There was Cosmo, yes, but no Elle, no Marie Claire, no Glamour, no Q. And virtually none of the hundreds of different supplements you now get with newspapers. All of that came much later, in 1985 or 1986.

CL _ The time was right. Through word of mouth, would-be young journalists and photographers came forward, wanting to contribute and help create something new and exciting. 'Young people' like us were turning their hobbies or interests – such as photography or writing or styling or performance art – into professions because they just couldn't get jobs, and BLITZ aimed to provide just that platform for young creative talent. The music and fashion scenes of the seventies were giving way to a more serious and ambitious generation of the eighties. People like us, hungry for a new creative dawn.

ST _ The big problem was that none of the existing magazines seemed to be interested in commissioning inexperienced writers and photographers. So our idea was something along the lines of, 'Well, if we can't get our stuff in their magazines, let's publish our own'.

Why the name BLITZ?

CL _ BLITZ seemed a catchy name. Somewhere I have a list of all the other short and snappy words that I thought would stand out on the newsstand, but BLITZ just stuck. I liked the zing in the Z, imagined how it would sound if people asked for a copy – 'Hey, have you got a copy of this month's BLITZ?' Sounded exciting, but I had no idea about the club at the time...

ST _ The Blitz club thing was entirely coincidental – I don't think any of us had been to the Blitz club nights when we did the first issue. Blitz was just a wine bar in Covent Garden. We even sold the owners a quarter-page ad. in the back of the first issue!

How did you produce the first issue?

CL _ Literally on a shoestring. I put together the first issue more or less by myself on the kitchen table during the summer of 1980 – cutting up galley type proofs by hand and sticking them down with Cow Gum – and got the magazine out at the beginning of September just before the beginning of the new college term. I had found the printer and typesetter through the Yellow Pages, phoning round from the college payphone. We had sold some pages to a few local advertisers which funded the printing.

We sold copies of the first issue on market stalls in Covent Garden, Portobello Road, Brick Lane and a few newsagents, and the buzz just gradually developed. In was a snowball effect: people who bought it got in touch and said they wanted to contribute, and by the third issue we'd been accepted for national distribution through WH Smith. That was also when we won our first award, The Guardian Student Media Award for Best New Magazine...

The big decision was what to do when we finished university. Most people we knew went off to try to get 'proper' jobs, but we thought we'd take a chance with doing the magazine professionally and see if we could make it work... We came down to London and started with a one-room office in Soho...

What were your roles at the magazine? I seem to remember they kept changing?

ST _ At first our roles were just to do whatever needed to be done, however we needed to do it. In 1980, we were just a couple of kids aged eighteen and nineteen with no experience at all of how magazines worked. We literally picked it up as we went along by talking to people: printers, distributors, advertisers ... anyone who was willing to give us good advice for free.

On the first issue, Carey did virtually everything apart from the writing and photography, and certainly all of the business, design, advertising sales and production side. Gradually over the next few issues as we became partners we split our responsibilities, with Carey taking charge of advertising, promotion and distribution and me running editorial and production.

What was your mission statement? How did you sell BLITZ to advertisers and investors?

CL _ As an independent publication, we had to sell advertising pages up front to pay for the printing, we had no big publishing company behind us for funding. So advertising was a priority. But we felt that they had to be the right ads, pitched to the emerging 'youth' market. We wanted stylish images that would attract our audience and fit with the image of the magazine as a whole, something that hadn't really been done in magazines in those days.

I remember going into what was then a new ad agency called Bartle Bogle Hegarty and trying to sell them a page in BLITZ. The guy had his feet up on the table, and said, "Right, you've got five minutes, amuse me!" So I told him how BLITZ was cool and exciting, full of young creative talent, filling a vital gap in the magazine market for young people in their late teens and early twenties, and he booked a year's worth of specially commissioned Levi's ads on the spot, with BLITZ in the strap line. His name? John Hegarty...

Was it your aim to make BLITZ a broader remit than other style titles?

ST _ I'm not sure it was a conscious thing, especially in the early days. The idea was quite simply to put together the sort of magazine we wanted to read. The magazine started with an 'arts' bias – movies, books, design, art as well as music and fashion – so we kept that going throughout. Certainly we liked the fact that we were perceived as being a little more highbrow than the other titles...

Looking at reader research, the predominantly male readership surprises me – especially as there was so much fashion in the magazine?

ST _ You have to remember how badly served men were by magazines back then. *Smash Hits* and the other pop magazines covered the teen market, but there were no glossy magazines covering music or other forms of what you could call 'youth culture'. We'd been going for six years by the time *Q* came along in 1986. And there was literally nowhere apart from the three style magazines where you'd find men's fashion – especially more affordable men's fashion.

Do you remember how we first met?

ST _ Like everyone else it was through someone who knew someone who knew someone. A photographer who did some fashion pictures for issue no. 6 introduced Carey and me to the make-up artist Debbie Bunn, who introduced us to another photographer, Mike Owen, who knew you. That must have been October or November 1982.

One of my first commissions were the 'People' pages – profiles of several people usually connected by a theme. What made you think I was the man for this job?

ST _ You volunteered! No, actually, after that first fashion shoot, you suggested doing little profile pieces on up-and-coming people – many of them your own friends I think. We thought that was a great idea and it fitted in perfectly with the idea of the magazine. You were part of a really exciting and vibrant group in London and the pieces you did were brilliant.

You soon gave me a 'Style' section to edit that featured several mini-fashion stories. I think some things worked better than others but I guess we were all learning on the job. Do you remember originally offering me the role of Fashion Editor? I won't say 'job', as that implies being paid...

ST _ Well, the 'Style' section grew out of those 'People' profiles, and then the Fashion Editor role developed from that. You certainly deserved it and it seemed right at the time to build upon your creative talents. I remember you said that being the 'Fashion Editor' would make life easier when you were borrowing clothes from Brown's ... and it was my suggestion that the same Fashion Editor should stop storing those clothes in black bin bags in between shoots, after £5,000 worth of garments were accidentally put out with the

day's rubbish! Before long we had rails and tags and daily visits from models.

Looking through the back issues now I am shocked by the actual amount of fashion in each issue, especially as we did pretty much everything on little or no budget. I think that is why most of the shoots were done at night or at weekends so we could get studios free... What did you think of the fashion stories I produced?

ST _ Everything you did seemed fresh and different from anything else in other magazines, and as you got more experienced and more confident about the ideas you were producing, the stories got better and better. I honestly don't think there was another fashion editor at the time producing such a wide variety of different stories. And so many ideas! It wasn't just a case of you bringing in one or two six-page stories each month, but literally five or six separate stories. It's amazing how varied and challenging they were.

The high standard of your work was obviously also appreciated by the designers themselves, so you moved on from merely styling or conceiving a shoot to full-blown interviews with the leading figures in the industry. Not just the up-and-coming stars but legends like Calvin Klein, Jean Paul Gaultier, Jean Muir...

There were a couple of issues in 1986 where you were responsible for well over a third of the editorial pages, either in the form of straight fashion spreads or interviews with designers. The quality of your stories was always so strong, that we were delighted to give them all the space they deserved.

CL _ I remember you were a very handsome boy, with a cheeky sparkle in your eye. You had a way with people, of gently persuading them. Designers trusted you and your judgment, and were prepared to let their clothes be styled in a completely new and unconventional way for *BLITZ*.

Do you have any favourites? Any favourite images?

ST _ Too many to list. But some that spring to mind are David Hiscock's black and white, hand-emulsioned images, especially the one with the stripy tights; the Mark Lewis anti-war spread with 'We're not here to sell clothes'; the Gaultier fishbowl birthday helmet. And of course the Levi's jackets...

CL _ I loved the way you juxtaposed high fashion and mood shoots, street style and glamour. The Hermès scarf was one of my favourites, as was the down and out guy on a park bench in an expensive suit. And the baby

wrapped up in adult clothes. Your images all had a message, a touch of humour or the ironic, and were unlike anything in other fashion pages at the time.

What did you make of my idea to get designers to customise a classic Levi's denim jacket? When did you realise it was more than a few editorial spreads in the magazine?

CL _ I thought the idea was fabulous. I was amazed at how many names agreed – no – were excited to create the garments for *BLITZ*, and for you. It was a tribute to the success of the exciting and unusual fashion pages in *BLITZ*. When I heard that you had commissioned Vivienne Westwood, Jasper Conran, John Galliano, Paul Smith, Hermès, Katharine Hamnett, Richmond Cornejo, who else??? ... I realised immediately that we had to take advantage of this to publicise the issue, and sell as many copies as possible. The spreads in the magazine were amazing, but the '*BLITZ* Designer Collection of Customised Levi's Jackets' had to be SEEN by the general public.

So the first port of call was the London West End theatre scene, and I managed to persuade the Albery theatre to give us the venue free for a one night show featuring a cast of celebrities, which you orchestrated brilliantly along with show producer Mikel Rosen. The house was packed and the performances (filmed by MTV) were all brilliant – Boy George, Nick Heyward, Curiosity Killed The Cat, Leigh Bowery and all the other big names from the period all took to the stage, modelled, sang, performed – it was an incredible night! I remember the roar from the audience when you came out on-stage with Darryl!

But that wasn't enough, I had to stretch it out, and so I approached the Victoria and Albert Museum [V&A] for a room and a date to auction off the jackets to a celebrity audience for charity. Sotheby's conducted the auction in the Raphael Cartoon Court, and, under the direction of Sir Roy Strong, the V&A's young curators were so excited about the idea of attracting a younger audience into a rather old-fashioned museum, that they gave the *BLITZ* Collection a three-month Summer Exhibition in 1987, which you styled with Kevin Arpino. I remember Adel Rootstein donated the mannequins, and Bang & Olufsen donated banks of stacked TVs to show the live stage performances on a loop – all very futuristic in those days!

But we were on a roll, it didn't stop there. The *BLITZ* Designer Collection toured to the Musée des Arts Décoratifs at the Louvre in Paris, and to Barney's in New York. Thanks to you, *BLITZ* was certainly on the international fashion map, and by now was selling all over the world, even as far as the Fiji Isles. Parties were thrown in our honour, such as in New York by the Danceteria, and *BLITZ* fashion and portrait photography exhibitions were held in various galleries and museums, and the magazine won a series of awards... The *BLITZ* photography book *Exposure* was published by Ebury Press, which featured many of your best fashion shoots. It was a whirlwind of exciting parties in the fashion and music scenes. Fun times!

We did get complaints that readers could not see the clothes clearly. Did this ever concern you?

ST _ No. It never came up as far as the business side of the magazine was concerned, and I think the readers loved it. We always considered that the main function of the fashion pages was to inspire artistically, not to serve as a shopping guide. Many of the best images you produced for the magazine worked as art as much as they were pure fashion, and the photographers you chose responded brilliantly to that challenge.

You pretty much gave me a free brief. Was there anything that ever worried you or that you thought went too far?

ST _ Perhaps the only time we went too far was with the spread you did of a black Christ on the cross, complete with a Band-Aid across his abdomen. You'd shot it as an inside spread, but the images were so great that we took the decision to use one as the cover of the Christmas 1985 issue, with the banner headline 'Immaculate!'. The distributors threw a fit.

If I analyse them, I think the fashion pages of *BLITZ* celebrated difference – beauty, ethnicity, sexuality, gender – and challenged accepted notions of cool, taste and status quo. Were you happy for these messages to be incorporated between the seams?

CL _ You had a free brief and you challenged the status quo. That was what *BLITZ* fashion was all about – experimenting, challenging, artistic differences.

Did it surprise you when I left *BLITZ* to go to Fleet Street to become Fashion Editor of the London *Evening Standard* newspaper?

ST _ We were so sorry to lose you, but it was clearly time for you to move on and up. The only surprise was that you went from the freedom and unlimited artistic license of *BLITZ* to the more conservative demands of a mainstream newspaper.

CL _ We were very proud of your achievements at *BLITZ* and just as proud of you being offered such an important role in the 'grown up' press. It was like losing part of the family, but you deserved the opportunity.

Tell me about Kim Bowen, who took over the role of Fashion Editor at *BLITZ*? She certainly pulled out all the stops with her mega-designer first issue...

ST _ Kim did a superb job over the next couple of years, but the market had changed completely by the time she took over from you in 1987. The UK launch of *Elle* and other fashion-oriented women's magazines, as well as a host of newspaper fashion sections (including your own at the *Standard*) and dedicated men's magazines like *GQ*, made fashion far more mainstream. We couldn't afford to be as radical or as unconventional as we had been in the first half of the decade. So Kim's spreads focused more on big name designers, were cleaner and less quirky, because that's what designers and readers wanted by then. They wanted to be able to see the clothes!

Why did you eventually close the magazine?

ST _ Closure was not our decision; it was forced on us by the brutal recession of 1990–91, which was just as bad as the recent credit crunch. In some ways it was worse, because it happened so fast and we had no experience of how to cope with it. Our advertising just melted away, and by September 1991 we simply couldn't afford to keep going. Our two main competitors had already secured financial backing from larger and wealthier publishing companies who could carry them through the recession. Foolishly, we had spurned similar approaches ourselves in the belief that we could always remain completely independent. Even now, more than twenty years later, closing the magazine we'd built from nothing and run for more than a decade remains the most painful experience either of us has ever been through. It was like losing a child. Not a happy time.

How would you like people to remember the magazine?

ST _ I hope people remember *BLITZ* for its intelligence and its unconventional breadth of content. Not just the fashion you produced, but also for all our other editorial photography, including superb portrait work from photographers such as Nick Knight, Russell Young, Richard Croft, Robin Barton and others. We also set out to give writers like Paul Morley, Ian Parker, Paul Mathur, Jon Wilde and many others the space and the freedom to give full rein to their considerable abilities, and tackle topics or subjects that didn't get covered elsewhere.

CL _ I hope *BLITZ* is also remembered for its entrepreneurial spirit – an example of how two teenagers, with no experience and no funding, built an international magazine publishing business from scratch. Something that probably could not happen today. Back issues and *BLITZ* T-shirts and memorabilia are now collectors' items, and the entire *BLITZ* archive of issues and images is held by the Victoria & Albert Museum.

Why do you think *BLITZ* has been sidelined to *i-D* and *The Face* in the annals of pop culture media?

ST _ Perhaps we didn't try hard enough to be fashionable? I don't know. We simply set out to do our own thing, and much of the time we got it right. Certainly we lacked the age and years of commercial experience and contacts that the publishers of the other two style magazines already had from working within the mainstream publishing industry beforehand. And we certainly lacked their big company funding that allowed them to ride out the recession and enjoy longer prosperity and wider publicity. But then we consciously chose not to 'sell out', rejected big financial offers from major publishing houses, and in hindsight perhaps we should have followed suit. *BLITZ* has gone down in history as an iconic style magazine of the eighties. Regrets? We have a few … but at least – and with apologies to Frank Sinatra and Sid Vicious – "more, much more than this … we did it our way".

When I left the magazine you gave me a book of my pages with a mock-up of a cover. One of the cover lines read: '5 years of the fashion editor's friends and boys with no tops on'. Does this sum up my tenure pretty well?

ST _ No of course not. That was just a parting joke! Certainly your friends featured heavily in your work, because they were all creative influences in their own right. But you played a huge part in building the success and the influence of the magazine. We couldn't have done it without you!

CL _ Absolutely! *BLITZ* wouldn't have been *BLITZ* without the challenging and out-of-the-ordinary fashion content. You did the magazine proud!

This was the first fashion story I styled for *BLITZ* magazine. I was always looking for opportunities to make pictures, so I was thrilled when Mike Owen asked if I would style a story for a new magazine. I pulled clothes from my wardrobe and borrowed some more designed by my flatmate. I did some sketches to show to Mike. The theme was War, but there was also an underlying androgynous mood. Some pictures were taken on location and some in Mike's warehouse studio. Baillie was a square-jawed hunk who looked good in a vest and was always a laugh. I wrote an accompanying text that referred to Westwood and McLaren's Clothes For Heroes, Robert De Niro (a throwback to *The Deer Hunter*) and fashion casualties. I ended the piece: 'The Invasion of the Falklands, or battling to get into the next Worlds End show?'

At War

Photographer: Mike Owen

Models: Michaela at Models 1, Baillie Walsh at Top Models

Make-up: Debbie Bunn

Hair: Ayo at Schumi

Clothes: Amazon, Flip, Laurence Corner, Rider

Mike Owen, photographer:
I had already shot a couple of stories for *The Face* magazine when I got a call from Simon and Carey asking if I'd like to work on their new project, *BLITZ* magazine. I really liked them and what they were trying to do. It was the start of a great working relationship.

I had a top floor studio in Clink Street near Borough Market, a warehouse on the site of the old prison. It was far less gentrified back then and difficult to get a taxi to take you there. It was a great time to be living and working in London. I was shooting with recording artists such as Duran Duran, Fine Young Cannibals and Terry Hall, and magazines including *19*, *Sky*, *The Face* and *i-D*. The industry was far more intimate then, everyone knew each other and new contacts were found via word of mouth.

It was very early days for Carey and Simon, who were not from a fashion background, so I had almost free rein to choose collaborators. I was very impressed with your enthusiasm and personal style when we met at a photo shoot for *Creamy Editions* magazine and subsequently used you on a hair shoot for a Japanese client, which went well. It was the *BLITZ* ethos to use new, young, raw talent so you were an obvious choice. Further to our discussions and following on from your degree show, which had a war theme, we came up with the military story. I had always liked androgynous looking models, which is why I chose Michaela. By then I had already worked with Baillie several times. I really liked working with him.

Baillie Walsh, model:
This was the first shoot we did together. I think I'd only been modelling a while. They are a great set of pictures and they were in my book throughout my career. I loved the way I looked in them, although my legs look skinny. I grew into those later. It was always exciting working with Mike. The joy of working with you and *BLITZ* was that I'd get to work with really creative people. It was much more interesting than being photographed standing in a pair of underpants for a catalogue, which was really dull. I was usually being used in a very straight way.

Debbie Bunn, make-up artist:
I started working with Mike and Jamie Long at the very beginning when *BLITZ* was still in black and white. I was actually on the cover of the first colour issue. You and I met through Mike or Peter Brown. We might have done work before the war story. It was good the way the shoots evolved. Everyone turned up and did their bit. Did you bring the playing cards? They were very Mike as well. He loved all that nostalgia stuff.

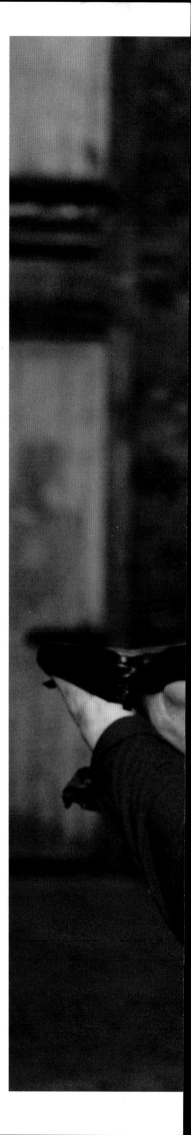

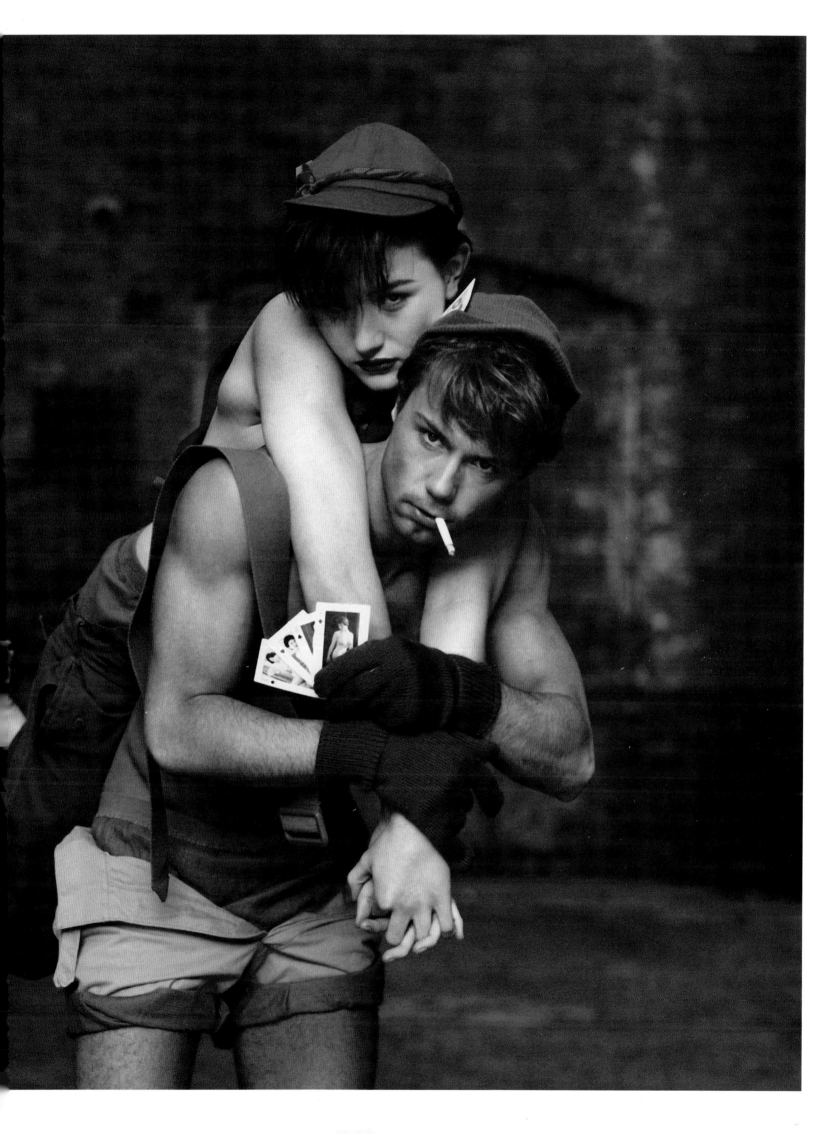

I have always loved Brassaï's evocative photographs of the Parisian *demi-monde* in the 1920s. I saw a lot of parallels among London's bright young things, who were indulging in a nostalgia fest for all things decadent – heavily painted faces, cross-dressing, a little opium and a lot of heroin.

Déjà vu

Photographer: Sally Boon

Models: Hilde Smith, Caroline Houghton, Fiona Nardello

Make-up: Gregory Davis

Hair: Paul Whittaker at Alan International

Clothes: Bernstock Speirs, Adrien Mann, Amazon, Zelona Zaba, Crolla, Lisa Vandy, Donna Weight

Sally Boon, photographer:
I was adrift after finishing college and I believe I met you through Gordon Currie, even though I had been going to the Blitz club and we probably rubbed shoulders there. It was a period of breathless excitement and painful confusion in my life, a little like living in a pinball machine. To get my work published in a cutting-edge magazine like *BLITZ* was an honour. I was thrilled as I felt I was working in a commercial capacity but without compromise. It was the only time that really happened, and I later abandoned commercial photography and focused only on art making.

I loved the 'Déjà vu' story where everything came together so beautifully. The styling was amazing, with many layers, and all the models got into character so realistically.

**Gregory Davis,
make-up artist/designer:**
I remember the girls sitting in a booth when I was doing their make-up, as there wasn't anywhere to do it properly. You just got on and did it wherever. Hilde, Caroline and Fiona each had a strong look and great style. The girls we knew were wearing full-on make-up at that time; that was the look in the clubs but not in *Vogue*. Fiona modelled for me when I did my first collection; it was only about eight pieces.

You and I shared a flat on the Pembury Estate in Hackney. I worked in the rag trade in North London, designing for a company called Oui Madame. I had just launched my own line. It was the first time I had my name on the label. I had a studio behind the BBC that I shared with a bespoke tailor. I remember Ossie Clark came in one day. I dabbled in lots of different things and got involved with a project to promote Jim Henson's *Dark Crystal* film.

You featured my first collection in a shoot based around the film *Blade Runner*. I used heavy, furnishing-type fabrics: silk linens in blood orange, russet red, purple and black. I loved what the Japanese designers were doing; Kansai Yamamoto, Issey Miyake and, of course, Comme des Garçons.

I showed that collection during London Fashion Week at Olympia. I was part of the Individual Clothes Show collective, along with Betty Jackson, Zwei, English Eccentrics and Donna Weight, among others.

I always did freelance projects so I could work with you when I wasn't designing. I've always loved make-up. As a teenager, David Bowie, Lindsay Kemp and glam rock were a big influence. As soon as I moved to London I got into nightclubbing. I loved Yours Or Mine at Sombrero and the Blitz club. It was always about dressing up, and when we went out I'd do make-up for all my flatmates and their friends. The getting ready was the fun bit.

For this shoot the look was a mix of twenties and thirties. Very decadent, dark heavy-lidded eyes, pale skin and strong lips. Properly finger-waved hair. They were definitely supposed to be night people. This story was totally inspired by the old black and white movies we watched on TV on Saturday afternoons. Louise Brooks and Bette Davis were such major influences.

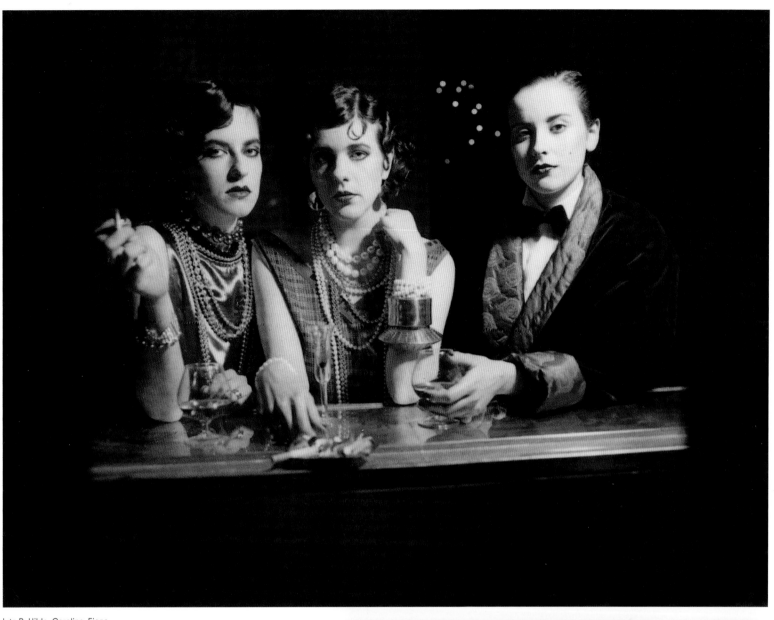

L to R: Hilde, Caroline, Fiona

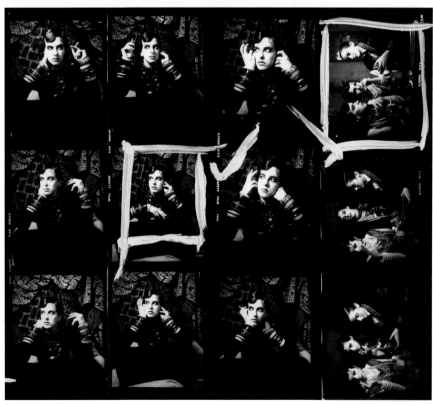

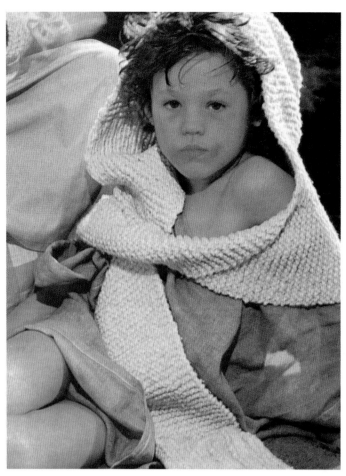

Young designers were taking a new approach to knitting. Eric Holah, Rachel Auburn and the Bodymap duo, Stevie Stewart and David Holah (brother of Eric) produced a selection of basic silhouettes, shaped like things you would make for your teddy, in dishcloth cotton yarns and rag remnants. Walking into Kensington Market and seeing a stallholder knitting new stock, I was reminded of the women who knitted at the foot of the guillotine. There was a revolution happening in fashion, the young taking on the establishment. The imagery seemed appropriate.

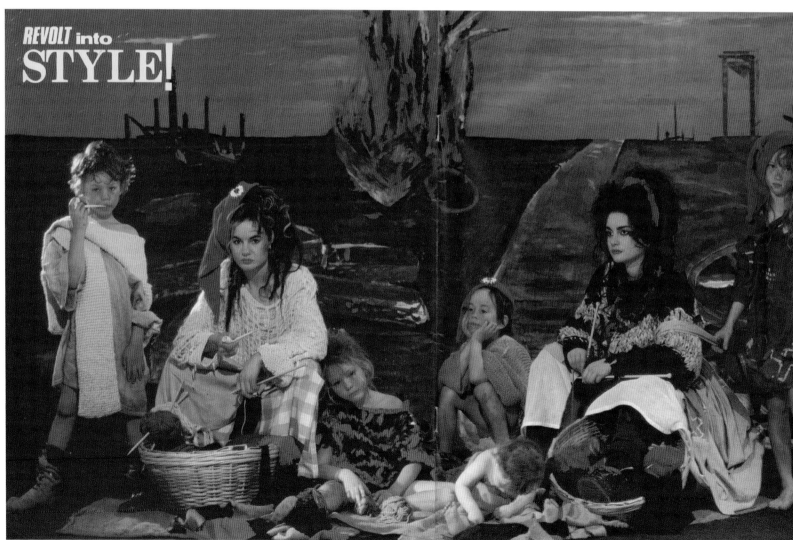

REVOLT into STYLE!

BLITZ #13
July/August 1983

Beat the revolution Revolt into style

Photographer: Jamie Morgan

Models: Princess Julia, Kate Garner. Children provided by Nancy Howard

Make-up: Gregory Davis

Hair: Debbie Dannell and Martin Farino for Antenna

Clothes: Bodymap, State of Undress, Nocturne, Donna Weight, Helen Robinson for PX

Backdrop painted by Kevin Allison

Top: Felix L to R: With children, Kate, Princess Julia

Jamie Morgan, photographer:
This really was one of my first shoots ever. Before Buffalo. The young boy is in fact Felix [Howard], a few years before the 'Killer' cover of *The Face*. This shoot was part of the very beginning for me, before I really defined my Buffalo style. It used the attitude of the New Romantics, a mix between the Dickensian style of Haysi Fantayzee and the pirates of Vivienne Westwood. It was my first look at iconic historical references before I went deep into the icons of men's fashion that became Buffalo. It used sets and backdrops, which I soon abandoned for the clean studio look used in many of the Buffalo images.

Princess Julia, model:
I'd put on a bit of weight due to continual boozing so I did wear quite a lot of layers. I went from the Blitz club look of '79 (structured and tailored) to a more obviously deconstructed feel. The Blitz club look mixed retro and futuristic: thirties, forties, even Victorian – any vague dressing-up things from any era. It was an opportunity to recycle the fancy dress we had got from the sale at Charles Fox, but updated with our take on what the future would be. The early '80s saw a more relaxed approach and quite organic-looking hand knits and hand painting. I hand knitted things for Bodymap. I probably knitted that. I did the patterns, scarf hoodie things, they were all quite blocky. I also did some for Richard Torry and John Flett and I might have done one or two for John Galliano. It was all very craft-orientated. There were knitting machines but they were a big deal and no one had access to them. These things were based on the Seditionaries things.

Scarlett Cannon, model:
Julia looks so young. Julia and I weren't regular models, so we used to say if you're nice, people are more likely to ask you back. Because we didn't get work that often. She was good at knitting in those days. She knitted me a fantastic cardigan with SEX BOMB on the back.

Gregory Davis, make-up artist:
The boys who took the pictures and painted the backdrop were the west London lot. Trendy, handsome and straight. I met Kate Garner when she was doing Haysi Fantayzee. We all knew each other. Julia was a Warren Street girl, always out and about. We were club people and a lot were becoming celebrities within that scene. I can't believe you used Felix before he became a little star and danced with Madonna in that *Open Your Heart* video!

You made hats from my cast-off fabric – 'cabbage', as they call it in the trade. That was from my Cross collection. Ribbed knits in brick red, ginger, milky cream, brown and black. That collection really launched me. I got picked up by magazines like *19* and *Honey* and even on TV. I sold to a lot of stores including Joseph and Harrods.

BLITZ #15
October 1983

I was always interested to go to the end-of-year student fashion shows to see what new talent was emerging. Of course, St Martin's School of Art was always a first port of call. I was really excited by Simon's menswear collection and his presentation, which followed in the footsteps of Stephen Linard's ground-breaking show — both used real-life character models who exuded a sexy, raw manliness that was the antithesis of the well-groomed, almost antiseptic male model look. Foxton took the boxer as his macho muse, adding a punch of Vegas-style glamour to conservative men's tailoring.

Simon Foxton

Photographer: David Hiscock

Models: Mick 'Marciano' Hurd, Baillie 'Sugar Ray' Walsh

Facial Rearrangement: Iain R. Webb

Clothes: Simon Foxton

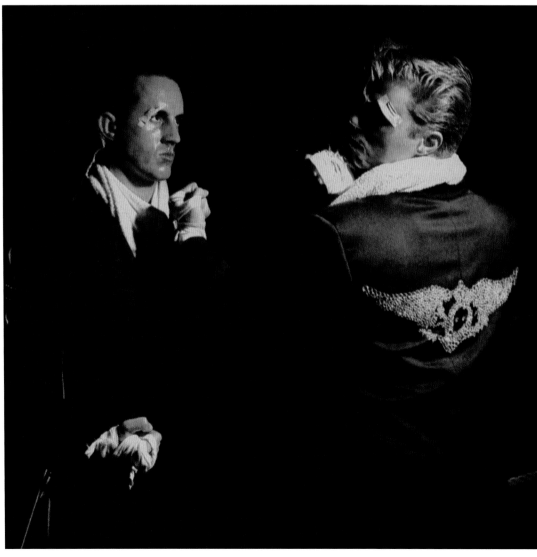

L to R: Mick, Baillie

Simon Foxton, designer:
I have a great deal of affection for this shoot as it was my first exposure in print. *BLITZ* was one of the great triumvirate of style journals of the early '80s (*The Face* and *i-D* being the others) and we used to devour it as soon as it hit the news stands. To have my degree collection featured in it was just amazing. It totally raised my profile, so from day one people had seen my name and consequently doors were open to me that may have otherwise remained closed. Seeing someone else style my clothes was quite an eye-opener. It allowed me to view them in a different way from how I had first envisaged them. I think the styling was spot-on; it still looks good today. I think magazines such as *BLITZ* allowed us to see the possibilities of fashion photography and of styling by reflecting and enhancing the way we all dressed or designed at the time.

Baillie Walsh, model:
I really like all of those pictures that you did. I was always surprised by the end result because I look different in each one. There is a filmic, art school quality that really comes across in all the work, which is why they haven't dated. You could put this in any magazine now. You were using inspiration from varied sources. You were inspired by films and things around you, it wasn't about trends or catwalk. Dave's lighting is great. It's weird, like looking at a completely different person. I've got quite a lot of hair.

I was young and it was fantastically exciting. I didn't know what I wanted to do in life at this point, so working with all those interesting people was informing me about what was possible. I'd been to Art School and I'd been a stripper and now I was modelling. I was the kind of person who took a long time to work out what I wanted to do. I'm so glad that we had that time to play around. That was our way of doing things. Nobody had a career. I was lucky to get a grant to go to Art School. I certainly didn't have a huge debt hanging over me. Now kids need to have an end game, but that's not the reason to go to Art School. You go to find out who you are. What you want to be. We all went to the clubs and we were all doing things, wanting to do things, but there wasn't the pressure. I am really glad that I was a part of that scene.

Gregory Davis, make-up artist/designer:
Mickey looks brilliant, like an East End boxer from a Ray Richardson painting. Maybe he's a bit too pretty though.

Sally Boon, photographer:
I found you to be very kind, quietly supportive and genuinely confident of my abilities to visualise the stories. On the shoots I felt we had an easy dialogue.

Helen Whiting, model/make-up artist:
In 1981 I was working as an air hostess for British Caledonian. They were very strict and I don't think I fitted the company image. I got sacked when I was caught roller-skating in a hotel bar still in uniform. So I thought what would I really like to do?

We met through photographer Chris Garnham. He was taking some pictures of dresses you were making and asked me to model. We did the photographs on the stairs at your flat in Royal Crescent. The dress was really simple and tight around the knees. I remember it gave me a Jayne Mansfield derriere.

This shoot reminds me of *The Last Picture Show*. I have always loved the late fifties and early sixties styling. That was the main reason I got the sack from the airline, everyone else was dressing normal and wearing the fashion of the time. I lived in Holland Park, and Chris and I used to go up to Portobello Market, which was fantastic then, and also Camden Market. I worked in a shop in Portobello called Risk. I used to do alterations on fifites ballgowns and stuff like that, so I also got first dibs on what came in. When I was still an air hostess, whenever I was in the States I used to go to the big warehouses and source stock for the owner.

It seemed to be quite normal to dress the way we did. Perhaps it was the group of people we went around with. Everyone was into dressing up. It was a way of life. It was much more individual than today. Everything now seems much more homogenous. What's happened?

Photographer: Sally Boon

Models: Helen Whiting, Gary

Clothes: Stephen King, Richard Ostell, The Sale, Jenny Barrett (Kitsch-In-Wear), Demob, John Watts

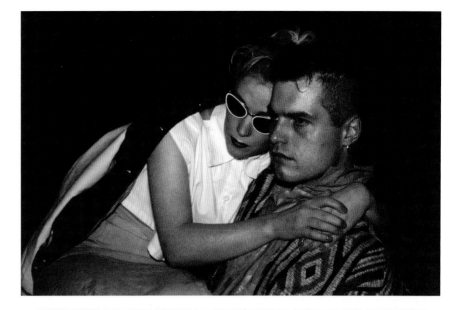

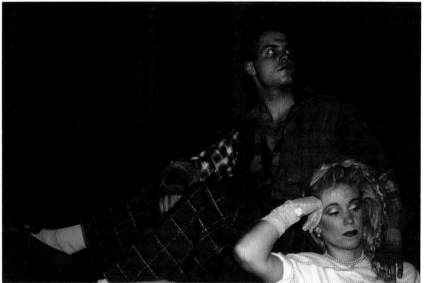

This story (again only two pictures) was part of the 'Style' spreads I produced early on in my tenure before I was officially Fashion Editor. The shoot was inspired by Kerouac's *On The Road*, along with the rockabilly styles that were *au courant* on the King's Road. Helen was a make-up artist I regularly worked with. She had a great fifties look. Gary was the boyfriend of a friend. He looked suitably strung-out in these photos. I don't think modelling came naturally to him although his handsome features often meant he was asked to do just that (he had also appeared in Bodymap's Querelle collection). We shot this in the Gate Cinema in Notting Hill, a venue that became home after dark at the weekends, when they ran all-night showings of cult classic movies. I wrote a mock extract from a possible road-trip novel featuring Dean and Marylou. I did apologise to Kerouac.

Fifties

BLITZ #19
March 1984

Photographer: Sally Boon

Models: Anita Evagora,
Ivan Kushlick

Clothes: Blanche, Laurence
Corner

Barbara Horspool, designer:
Mark and I were studying fashion design at Kingston College of Art, which groomed designers to be commercial and prided itself on placing students at huge fashion brands. Mark was into the London club scene – forever at the Blitz nightclub, he was considered a maverick. In the first year we rarely spoke (I obediently worked long hours designing the Kingston way), but by the second year we became friends because of our obsession with fashion and style. He worked as a Saturday boy for Chloé (Lady Clare Rendlesham ran it then) and I remember having those amazing riding boots from Lagerfeld's cavalier collection.

Our tutor Richard Nott (Workers For Freedom) suggested we start a label together. My mum lent us £500 and off we went with silks and cottons from McCulloch and Wallis, and a trip to Paris where we discovered an attic full of vintage ribbons that became our trademark. Mark had prints by Timney Fowler in his final collection and they also became a signature. Blanche was named after the character in *A Streetcar Named Desire*. We were style magpies. Inspiration came from books, films or characters both fictional and on the London scene. We designed, cut and made all the samples for our first collection, which sold to Joseph and Whistles, whose owner Lucille Lewin called it 'wickedly sensual'.

We lived in bedsits and every penny we made went into Blanche. We lived frugally so we could buy ourselves a few beautiful things. Mark survived on brown rice, bananas, milk and bread so he could buy a Turnbull & Asser white shirt. I freelanced at a dreadful rag trade supplier to Topshop and then started to teach, a route many of us struggling designers took to get some cash. My mum paid for fabric in advance of orders and we had a backer for a short while, but it was really tough to balance the books. Banks didn't like

youngsters starting a new business and shops loved to not pay for six months, or do a runner. There was no business support (and there is little today save for Sir Philip Green) and no advice. I was lucky that my mum was an accountant, but inevitably after six years we could not sustain the label without serious investment or completely selling out our soul and taking the braveness out of Blanche (somewhere in the world we sold three organza and satin tops with monkey skin cuffs!).

For me, the best sellers were usually the things I wore, so I decided to design for mass market at Marks & Spencer and learn how you make money out of selling clothes. But we had brilliant fun from lots of hard work and some amazing parties. I'm not sure if you were at the one we had at our Stockwell house – Fairies, Fantasy and Fashion. Mark was in full eighteenth-century ballgown and corset, and me as Njinsky in *L'après-midi d'un faune*. I remember Stephen Linard, Philip Salon and all, parading down to the Big Apple in Brixton for snacks at 4am in full costume.

These looks were from the 'Querelle of Brest' collection. The nautical element was perfectly illustrated in your pictures. Blanche never did a collection without navy and white. Stripes became another signature, as did pea coats and matelot trousers. Evening looks in black, red and fuchsia represented the whorehouses that the sailors frequented. Historical reference inspired us but the design and styling came from the crowd we went out with. The outfit you shot was inspired by our environment. We had a one-room bedsit in a grotty Stockwell house, and loved the way that certain girls in Brixton wore pencil skirts, bare legs and white stiletto court shoes. I was into the gym so all our looks were underpinned by a Speedo type T-shirt or a ballet rehearsal shrug layered on top. Even the eveningwear mixed a massive dance tutu in black and white silk tulle, a black Speedo swimsuit, a cigarette and a pair of Manolos.

Barbara Horspool and Mark Betty were one of the designer duos that emerged in the 1980s. Their label Blanche had a nostalgic mood, spiced with an underlying sexual tension. Their collections had a filmic narrative so it seemed right to shoot their designs as stills from an imagined movie, probably with subtitles. I chose Anita (one half of hat design label, Fred Bare) to model. She looked like a modern day Anna Magnani. The original shoot appeared on only half a page in the magazine.

Anita Evagora, model:
I loved the Italian 'film noir' feel of the shoot. I am not sure if I even spoke to my co-star, probably a friend-of-a-friend. At the time (pre-celebrity culture) it was all about individual looks and inventiveness and less who you were. The great thing about the post-punk era was that you didn't have to use a model from an agency. It was understood that anybody who was part of the scene focused around the London art schools would get involved in these shoots just for the hell of it. It was just part of the whole creative milieu that everyone was involved with and absolutely thrilling to be part of.

At the time I was at the RCA studying ceramics. Night time was spent creating our personas. Lack of cash made us more inventive. We would make our own clothes – a skirt made from a shower curtain proving lethal near cigarettes – or search charity shops for wacky and odd accessories, and of course plenty of make-up. Only then were we ready to step out to clubs such as the Blitz or Hell. Often we would end up at a one-night-only club, usually in some dark dive, say a basement in Soho, with no ventilation and clouds of cigarette smoke. The only way to find the venue was to be in the right place at the right time. It was amazing how word got round without mobiles. The clothes by Blanche were beautiful, clean-cut and understated, in contrast with the seediness of the shoot. I should have felt quite glamorous but the stilettos were so painful they almost brought tears to my eyes, so I was mainly concentrating on keeping this pain from showing on my face.

Blanche

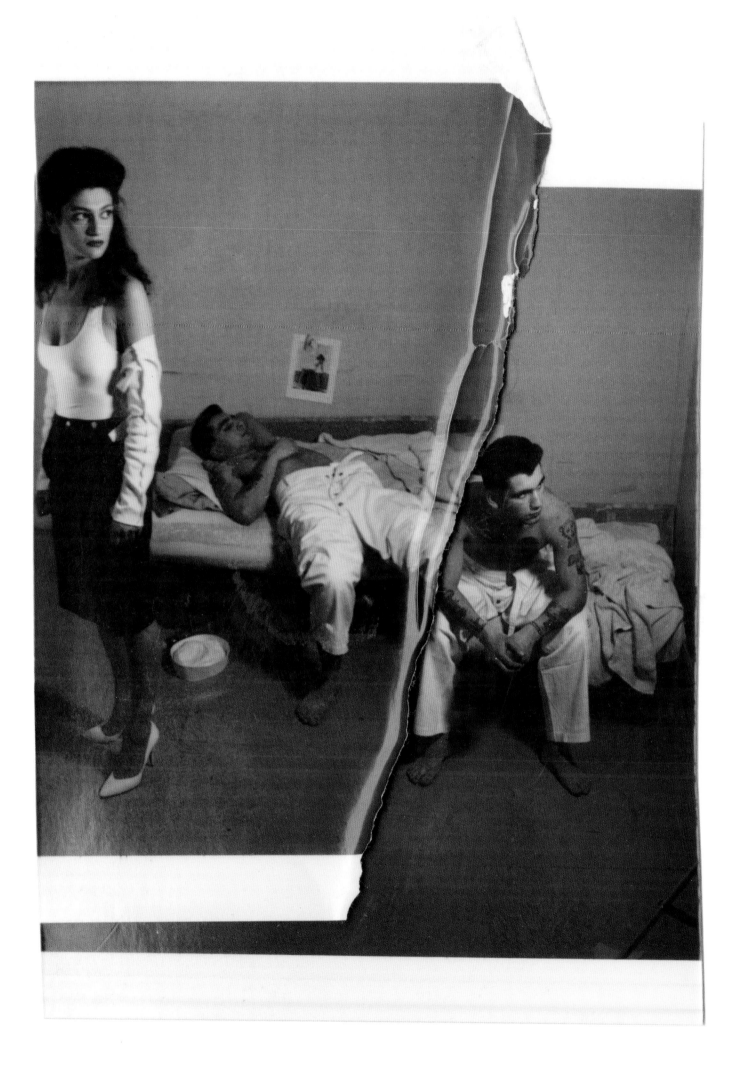

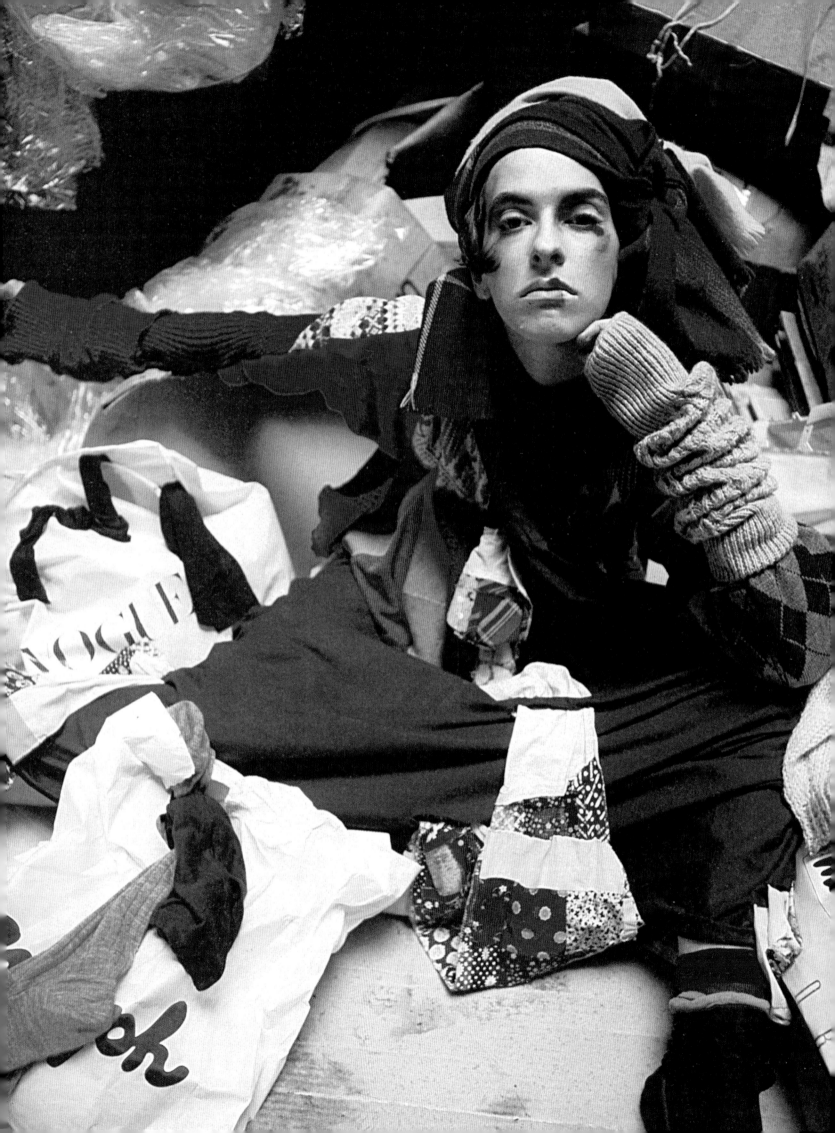

Bag Lady

I was asked to produce a series of images for *The Fashion Year*, an annual publication that packaged all the key looks and trends of the previous year. I put together several looks that represented sportswear, androgyny and Fifties nostalgia along with this one that showcased the vogue for clothes constructed from scraps and cast offs. This unravelling, raggle-taggle look favoured by London's anarchic young designers ran parallel to the deconstructed looks of the Japanese designers. One of the most prolific exponents of this look was Rachel Auburn whose designs sold in New York. Her 'bag lady' styles, as they were described in the press, caused a storm of protest.

Rachel Auburn, designer:
I remember arriving in New York with Leigh Bowery for the first time in 1983 for the New London In New York fashion event launched by Susanne Bartsch. I can remember thinking at the time how different everyone was dressed, running around in trainers and '80s power suits (very *Working Girl*) and how different my things were to what was happening in the Big Apple. My look at the time had a deconstructed feeling. It was about texture and fluidity, the opposite of the hard, sharp and very distinct silhouettes that had gone before. Also, I loved the idea of recycling. I don't think anyone had dared at that time to actually consider selling an item as high fashion in that way. Certainly punk and the vibe of Rei Kawakubo had been a massive influence for me. Anyhow, the fashion show featuring these new London designers was an eye-opener for New Yorkers, and buyers from department stores such as Bloomingdale's and Macy's were immediately 'on it', ordering from the collection, which I had partly made from cutting up old colourful sweaters from Portobello market and joining them together in a new way. All the commotion happened when people found out that customers were buying 'rags' for top dollar money, when people out on the streets were wearing 'rags' because they had to and could not afford to eat.

Photographer: Nick Knight
Models: Hilde Smith
Make up: Helen Whiting/IRW
Clothes: Rachel Auburn

Judy Blame, designer:
Susanne Bartsch was coming to Cha-Cha's and she started promoting a lot of young designers from London. She put on shows in New York and Tokyo that caused lots of interest for all of us. If you look at the list of people involved – Leigh Bowery, Rachel Auburn, Dean Bright, Greg Davis, John Richmond – we were all struggling away in London and no one was taking any notice, but the minute it was taken outside, then everyone took notice. It was funny that it took some Swiss bitch from New York to come to London and stir things up.

I loved going to clubs. Night-clubbing now has become more mainstream. There wasn't anything mainstream about it then, it was about like-minded people wanting to be together and also not being worried, about sharing ideas or supporting each other. Now people are worried about where their next idea is coming from, whereas then we were too busy having them. I mean if you dropped a bomb on Blitz or Taboo or Cha-Cha's in those years you would have wiped out half of creative London. And I loved that there was a massive camaraderie between all the designers. At that time, in the '80s, the designers were fucking each other and now they fuck each other over. Do you know what I mean? There was a lot more communication then and now there's so much more media. It's everywhere. Blah, blah, blah. Fifteen hundred magazines every day. It's been watered down.

Nick Knight, photographer:
What you did was a really important part of the '80s and it was wonderful that it included me and Bodymap, Rachel Auburn and the rest. There wasn't a magazine that reflected that world. *i-D* was busy being reportage and *The Face* was being *The Face*. And *Vogue*? Well, *Vogue* was going its own way and was full of shoulder pads.

Nick Knight, photographer:
In 1981–82 I was at art college in Bournemouth. I came to London and wanted to get my work published straight away. I was at college but doing things for *The Face* and *i-D* at the same time. *i-D* allowed me to shoot people that I liked. I photographed the Rockabilly scene in Bournemouth. For *The Face* I covered the Skinhead scene, but by that time I was coming out the other side of that already. So when I met up with you and *BLITZ*, I had already been doing things for *NME*, *The Face* and *i-D*.

The big moment for me at *i-D* was when I did the 100 Portraits editorial of London's beau monde. You, Leigh [Bowery], Bodymap, Michael Clark and all the others. Doing those portraits galvanised things for me. Previously I really hadn't been out in London and discovering Taboo made me feel like I had a purpose to be there, it felt like it was a place for me.

Anna Paolozzi, model:
At the time, I was working for the fashion designer Bill Gibb and then I went on to design accessories for Whistles, Demob, Liberty, and for bands like Eighth Wonder, ABC and Meat Loaf. My lifestyle was lots of parties, dinner parties and nightclubs and it was really fun.

Nick Knight was really unassuming and nice to us. We did our own hair and make-up and when we finished you said I looked like Arthur Scargill and I had to redo my hair. Gill reckoned that Nick was getting turned on during the shoot. The inspiration behind photographing us as Ron and Reg came from David Bailey's famous black and white photo of Ronnie and Reggie Kray. The belts were originally designed for Richard Ostell's fashion show and they sold out. Everyone bought them including Lynne Franks and Lucille Lewin from Whistles. I used to go to a car dump on the Finchley Road, where the Finchley Road 02 is now, and get the logo badges off old cars. I have still got my belt, and a very old friend told me recently she has still got hers.

This shoot was an extension of the 'People' profile pages. With tongue planted firmly in cheek, Gill and Anna, who were both friends, were keen to present themselves as a modern day approximation of sixties gangsters Ronnie and Reggie Kray. This focus on personal style was a driving force among the new style magazines. There was a lot of laughter on this shoot.

Girls about town

Photographer: Nick Knight

Models: Gill Valenzuela, Anna Paolozzi

Clothes: Anna Paolozzi, M&S, Sex Shop, Dents, Butler & Wilson, Olive

(2) GIRLS ABOUT TOWN..

RON

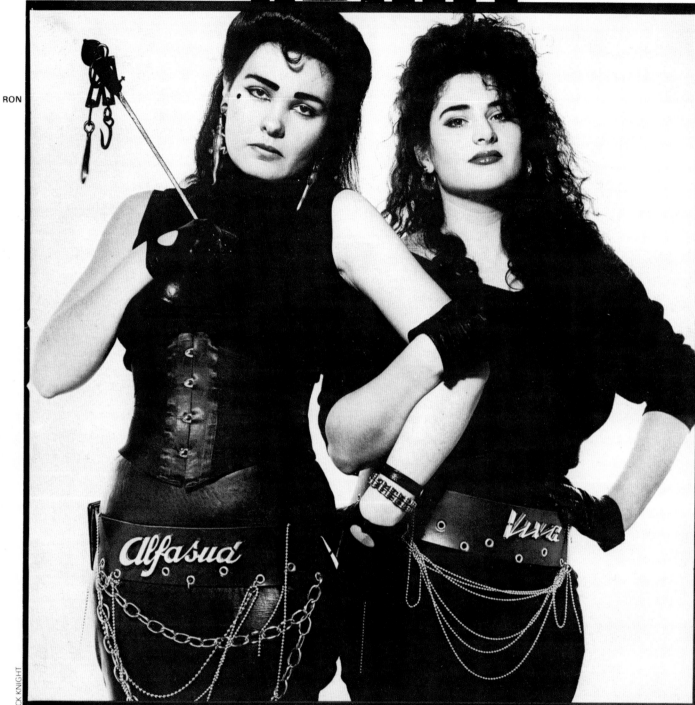

NICK KNIGHT

REG

ABOUT

FIXATION, AGGRESSION, AND THE MURDEROUS GLARE OF THE PATRIARCH... Accessory designer Anna Paolozzi (daughter of sculptor Eduardo) and friend have just finished evening classes in voodoo, and have now taken up G.B.H. full time. Known amongst London's trendier underworld as RON and REGGIE KRAY, their reputation, which began with straightforward threatening behaviour at THE WAG CLUB, has followed them through every shadier nightery they may care to frequent. The belts they are wearing in the picture are created by REG (right) and are a result of the pair's nights Up West smashing and grabbing. Nobody argues with Reg and Ronnie, *alright*?

RON: Top belonged to mother, Olive. Leather skirt, made to measure, £20. Corset, from a sex shop in Soho. Gloves, Dents, £20. Earrings, Scooter (Paris), 300 francs.
REG: Jumper, Marks & Spencer, £7.99. Jersey tube skirt, made by Reg. Gloves, John Lewis, £15. Earrings, Butler & Wilson, £15.

Leather, Chrome and Chain belts by Anna Paolozzi. Available from Pilot, Floral St., WC2, or to order, 01-586 5665.

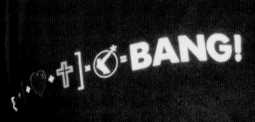

SHOT
6 September 1984

Photographer: Peter Brown

Model: Paul Rutherford

Grooming: Debbie Bunn

Clothes: Frankie Goes To Hollywood merchandise

I made extra cash by styling pop bands like the Pet Shop Boys and Art of Noise, so it wasn't a shock when Peter Brown and I were asked by Paul Morley to shoot images for the Frankie Goes To Hollywood album sleeve. The pictures promoted the band's merchandise, and Paul wanted it done in an alternative way. We had fun with products that included an Edith Sitwell 'Duffle Bag For Life's Little Luxuries' (into which we put Claudia Brücken), the Hugo Ball T-shirt (pictured) and enamel badges, which I pinned through Paul Rutherford's nipple in place of his ring. There was also a Kurt Weill sweatshirt and Jean Genet boxer shorts, and I drew a fake tattoo on Paul's inner thigh. To this day, the closest I have come to a No. 1 pop star.

Paul Rutherford, musician:
I had a wonderful time doing those photographs and to this day the only thing I wear in my nipple is that badge – but it catches on my cashmere these days. I remember my underpants had to show above my waistband (something I still do). Oh yeah and standing in a bin is still very fashionable round these parts. If you ever need a fifty-plus-year-old model, you know where to find me.

Peter Brown, photographer:
We also did a shoot with the Frankies in Heaven nightclub. Do you remember we all walked off in a huge huff? I was like, "I can't work under these conditions. I've never been so insulted!" We were doing a version of the Last Supper with the whole band, and they thought it was blasphemous and horrifying. Can you imagine that a band like that would be so offended by our beautiful Last Supper thing in a gay club? It was fantastic.

How strange that a shot from this session ended up being the cover of *The Face*, a rival magazine. This was an all-nighter shoot in the basement at Holborn Studios. I think we finished about five in the morning. Do you remember we had Claudia in a duffle bag?

Frankie Goes To Hollywood

Paul Morley, writer, critic, co-founder of ZTT Records
People either talk about these pictures very fondly or with disgust. I just thought if we are being forced by the record company to sell stuff then to do it in a poetic way. So selling the merchandise became another collaborative process where the banal and grubby was turned into something delightful and poetic.

That Heaven shoot? Back then the band were often uncomfortable with a lot of the things that actually made them an interesting group. They were most upset doing things like that.

BLITZ #24
September 1984

This image was part of a quartet of photographs themed by colour. This required four different sessions. The other pictures featured Black (a photo of Dencil Williams in leather bike jacket shot by Nick Knight), Yellow (model Amanda Masters drenched in water wearing WilliWear raincoats in Ron Arad's Covent Garden store) and White (Antonia Leslie posing over a mirror dusted with white powder). The Orange image featured Amanda again (I loved her classical beauty and she was game for anything) and John Moore, footwear designer and one of the founder members of The House of Beauty and Culture design collective. This look was based on the Buddhist 'Orange People' I saw daily as they paraded through Soho. Amanda wore a draped ensemble by Comme des Garçons while John was wrapped in a nylon bed sheet that I found in an Oxfam shop. I copied the white and gold make-up of the Buddhist devotees. I have always been fascinated by the symbolism associated with religion, like the Ash Wednesday tradition of the blackened sign-of-the-cross smudges on the foreheads of besuited businessmen I saw in New York.

Gill Campbell, photographer:
I came to work for the magazine through a boyfriend, later to be known as The Compulsive Liar. His flat mate, Mick Hurd, needed some portfolio photographs and said that if I took some pictures for him, he had a mate who would style it. That was the first shoot we did together. Most of the time you would explain your vision for stories and I would interpret your ideas by means of lighting and background.

When we met I had already been working as a photographer for a couple of years. After finishing college I was determined not to take the route of assistant, so I started off as a photo-illustrator, shooting book jackets and magazine articles. I was starting to get into fashion photography, which had always been my ultimate aim, by getting commissions for crappy teen magazines. We all have to start somewhere.

A friend and I had leased a big studio space in Clerkenwell, in a street full of photographers and studios, which we refurbished to live in and work from – illegally of course, but that added to the thrill. It was a brilliant time.

It was great to work for *BLITZ*. I think you were either a *BLITZ* or a *Face* person. Indeed I don't think you were allowed to work for both. It was a fantastic opportunity to get some tear sheets for the portfolio, and I much preferred the layout of *BLITZ*.

Orange

Photographer: Gill Campbell

Models: John Moore, Amanda Masters at Laraine Ashton

Make-up, hair: Harry Kitchener

Clothes: Comme des Garçons, Wendy Dagworthy, Freemans mail order

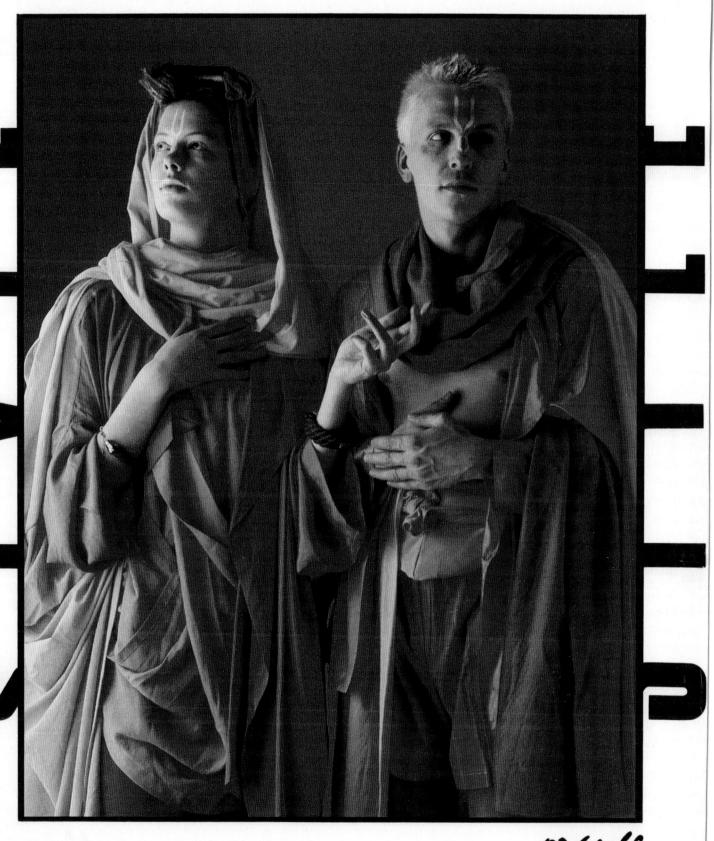

orange

● Photograph by Gill Campbell. Modelled by John Moore, Amanda Masters at Laraine Ashton. Hair and make-up by Harry Kitchener.

him: orange silk jacket by Wendy Dagworthy; orange checkerboard shorts by Williwear; orange footless tights (as cummerbund) by Stirling Cooper; pink woollen scarf by Comme des Garcons; orange sheet from Freemans mail order.

her: orange criss-cross front top, pink rayon satin jacket, red rayon satin pants all from Comme des Garcons; orange suede turban, orange and gilt bangles from Bernstock-Speirs; saffron orange silk robe from Contemporary Wardrobe.

Bodymap were making childrenswear and their PR Lynne Franks had another client, Raleigh, so I wanted to do a sporty story, but one which featured a realistic, possible scenario; hence the locks and the yamaka (by Stephen Jones, of course). Jewish kids ride bikes too. Red-headed Aaron was the nephew of hairdresser Debbie.

Barmitzvah boy

Photographer: Adrian Peacock

Model: Aaron Dryland

Hair: Debbie Dannel-Davis for Antenna

Clothes: Bodymap, Stephen Jones, Lonsdale

Adrian Peacock, photographer:
I can't really remember how we met. I think it was something to do with degree show parties and nightclubs. I went to live in America when I graduated but came back a year later, having got into photography there. I started assisting Mark Lebon at Bow Street Studios. He was doing 'fashion and pop' so I sort of fell into it. I remember doing our first pictures for BLITZ, of film maker Isaac Julien.

I was not a very good assistant and wanted to take pictures too early. I started getting work from Jane Gould at the Mail on Sunday. We did a set of pictures together in Covent Garden. James Lebon did the hair and scratched 'Cuts' (the name of his brand) on the wall, which could be seen in the pictures.

Marcelo Anciano and I took on a floor in a warehouse next to a derelict Hawksmoor church in EC1 and laid it out as a studio, but lived there as well. I had a darkroom in the shower and spent many hours printing and inhaling fixative. I earned my living doing stills on pop videos. Marcelo was a director. I worked on a lot of his shoots and became a regular for Picture Music International. I didn't have much of a portfolio. I think I met a lot of my clients in the Zanzibar.

Paolo Roversi was taking rather beautiful photographs using a 10 x 8 Polaroid camera. I wanted the effect but couldn't afford the film so I bought an old fashioned Polaroid Land camera. It was fiddly to use, but if you shot black and white you could wash the negative it created and then print from that. The negs were very delicate and scratched easily. It was a creative time for me as a photographer and I was experimenting all the time. Luckily you put the weird and wonderful in front of me, and I kept pressing the shutter.

At the time I didn't think it was that odd to do those 'Barmitzvah Boy' pictures as I used to go through Stamford Hill to go to college. However, of course, they were quite provocative.

BLITZ was a magazine of the time. It was competing with The Face and i-D but definitely had its own identity. I think the competition spurred contributors to be more creative. For me working for BLITZ was primarily a relationship with you. We were friends and collaborators. I still work with Louise Constad (make-up artist), who is a close friend, and I always had time for James. He was special.

Debbie Dannell, hairdresser:
We did a lot of shoots with kids. Would it be allowed today? I don't think so. We had them smoking and God knows what. The ginger Jewish locks? I don't know how we got away with that. Everything now is so PC.

Aaron did the Style Council video. Him and Lee, his best mate from school, wearing Crombies and Levi's, pissing up against the wall. The locks were made from the Monofibre we used for the dreadlocks at Antenna. I curled it and stuck them inside the skullcap. Aaron whinged a bit, but I remember us telling him he looked gorgeous. My sister still has that picture up on her wall. It's brilliant but Aaron still cringes.

Lynne Franks, PR:
I'm so grateful to have been part of it all. I guess part of my job was bringing together a melting pot of people. I encouraged and supported the young up-coming designers and then also had big clients like Raleigh and Swatch watches. Cycling clothes were soon being worn to clubs and became part of the club culture look.

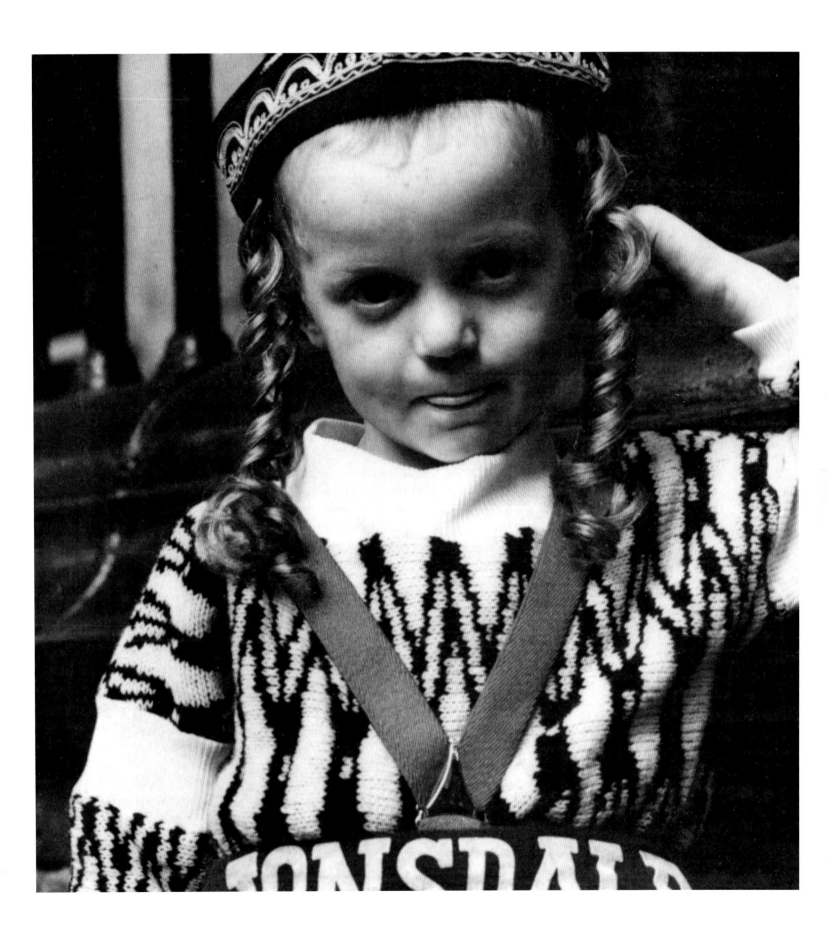

BLITZ #25
October 1984

Man

Photographer: Holly Warburton

Model: Nick Alexander at Models 1

Clothes: Dean Bright, Stephen King, Crolla, Andrew Logan, Mikel Rosen, Adrien Mann

Dean Bright, fashion designer: I was so, so happy with the image you created using my clothes. You got it so right. I was obsessed with the opium smokers of the early twentieth century, the Surrealists, and Cartier-Bresson's photographs of the Paris underworld, so your picture was a perfect expression of my motives to create the Opium Collection, which was the label for those clothes. I still love that picture. I was young and vain and being in the magazine really did go to my head. I was over the moon but at the same time I was troubled by the intense interest in my designs and me. Frankly I was unprepared for the attention that came my way post-St Martin's, but I can honestly say that being in *BLITZ* was a dance-round-the-room-screaming moment.

I couldn't have been happier with your article because it made me appear to be an established label and someone to watch, whilst in reality I was working alone with no backing and struggling to meet the orders that were coming in. I was selling to three of the best shops in the world but they all demanded exclusivity and didn't order that many pieces, so it was hard to make money. But I did glow in the glory of being fashionable. I had just left college and found myself flung into the deep end. I lived with the fascinating Rebecca Du Pont de Bie, and we spent our time hosting surrealist dinner parties and generally dressing up on a daily basis, regardless of the situation or event. During the early '80s there was a hardcore party scene, which I ostentatiously attended with a passion. My diary was packed. I worked at the Royal Opera House as a dresser, behind the bar at the Zanzibar membership club, and did work experience with Bruce Oldfield, as well as going to every party or club on the hit list. I'm exhausted just thinking about it.

Dean Bright was one of a new breed of young British designers creating peacock-style flamboyant menswear. His graduation collection was snapped up by Pete Burns and Dead or Alive and can be seen in their video for *You Spin Me Round (Like A Record, Baby)*. I wanted to create an equally decadent image and asked photographer Holly Warburton to take the pictures. I had originally met Holly on a foundation course at Salisbury College of Art and we had both got places at St Martin's School of Art, where Holly studied fine art and film. Her work was rich and exotic, romantic and fantastical. She created wildly theatrical sets. We did the shoot in her front room, which she turned into a lavish, Bedouin-meets-boudoir environment with lots of drapes (her own furnishings). The look was louche and seductive, so much so that Holly's exquisite silver grey Siamese cat decided to snuggle up next to model Nick. It added perfectly to the hedonistic mood.

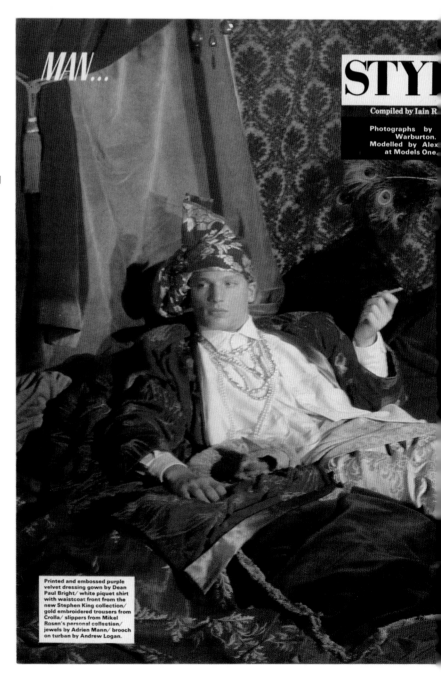

MAN...

STYl

Compiled by Iain R.

Photographs by Warburton. Modelled by Alex at Models One.

Printed and embossed purple velvet dressing gown by Dean Paul Bright/ white piquet shirt with waistcoat front from the new Stephen King collection/ gold embroidered trousers from Crolla/ slippers from Mikel Rosen's personal collection/ jewels by Adrien Mann/ brooch on turban by Andrew Logan.

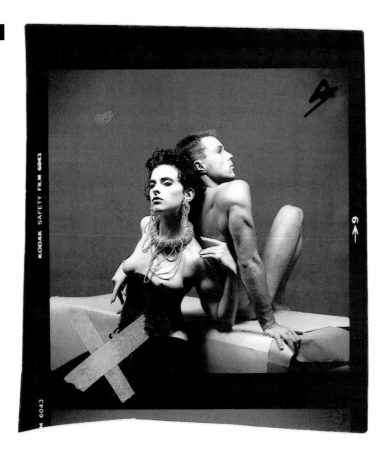

This was another opportunistic shoot. Judy had loaned me some jewellery, so I cajoled Hilde and Baillie into doing a shoot. Hilde had no problem with baring her bosoms and Baillie had the kind of body that seemed to demand him getting naked (in issue 62 Fashion Editor Kim Bowen would cast him in the same role). The poses were supposed to emulate classical Greek statues, something that was enhanced when David did his magic, scratching away at the print in the darkroom. The mood was also heavily inspired by the films of Jean Cocteau.

Judy Blame

Photographer: David Hiscock

Models: Hilde Smith, Baillie Walsh

Make-up: Gregory Davis

Hair: Not listed

Clothes: Judy Blame

David Hiscock, photographer:
During the time we worked together I was an assistant in a studio in Shorts Gardens in Covent Garden, and we could only use that one in the evenings or weekends. Then I went to the Royal College of Art, where the photography department was opposite the Natural History Museum (what is now, I think, the French Embassy) and they had fantastic studios. My work changed between Shorts Gardens and the RCA because the equipment at both was completely different. These were lit with really, really old lights, these beautiful dish lamps. That was the first time I'd come across them so I sort of lived for those beauty lights. Lovely. I love that these contacts still have the dots and the little taped cross because that's how we used to go through them to edit them, didn't we? One person would use a gold dot or a biro star or some masking tape. I can remember sitting with you and saying "Well, I like that one" and you'd like another and say "Well, we'll come back to that one". We never shot much film, because basically we were paying for it ourselves. At Shorts Gardens we might be able to put through an odd roll here and there on a job.

Judy Blame, designer:
Inspired by punk, I ran away from home in Devon at seventeen. I came to London and just thought I'd get off the train and bump into loads of people but it didn't really work out. London was a bit snobby so I got a train to Manchester. During 1977–79 I met lots of brilliant people like Malcolm Garrett, Peter Saville, Howard Devoto, the Buzzcocks, The Fall. Manchester had the biggest scene outside of London but was much more relaxed; it wasn't so fashion-orientated or cliquey. We didn't have to go to SEX every week for a new T-shirt; we made our own stuff. Rather than going to a boutique, we went to a jumble sale and would buy a shirt, then wreck it, stencil it with words and join it back together with safety pins. I was playing around a lot with my own appearance, we all were.

Baillie Walsh, model:
The reason that I got any kind of work as a model really was because in those days, apart from the Americans and Bruce Weber boys, most models didn't have great bodies. So people would use me because I had a decent body, so I was like, fine... It was like being a hand model really. I was a body model. It was no problem at all. In this photo it's treated like a piece of sculpture. And Hilde got her tits out, which was great. She's just got great attitude. Classic. I'd worked with her a few times, she was so great and again she was really creative. I think Judy was there that day and brought his jewellery along in a plastic carrier bag, because he was always late with things. He's still churning it out now. These pictures are very Horst, but David's made it more modern. Horst would have had a piece of sculpture in the background and instead you've got me. Horst would have had a horse's head. I love this picture and David made a poster of it for Athena but scratched my face out. My face was gone. That's what I mean. I wasn't booked for my beauty.

Take the blame

Monica Curtin, photographer:
I was Jamie Morgan's assistant. This was shot in his studio, probably in the evening. We were always working late at night. Somehow we fastened the fabric to the rafters and then you or Jalle wrapped it around her head. Scarlett couldn't move or it all went a bit wonky. I remember the palaver of gaffer-taping it up to the ceiling and trying to get the billowy silk to stop moving with the heat of the lights. It wasn't an easy shoot, but then it never was.

Scarlett and Judy were big mates. It was lovely that the models were more odd-looking. That was definitely exciting for a photographer.

Photographer: Monica Curtin

Model: Scarlett Cannon

Make-up and Hair: Jalle Bakke

Clothes: Judy Blame, Penny Beard, Sue Clowes, Laurence, Bernstock Speirs

I remember that one with the dead flowers, and Jalle cursing about you putting pennies on her eyes because it covered up his make-up, but then he did that fabulous gold splodge. When I originally met Jalle he was wearing dreadlocks, fake tan and a home-made outfit and I just burst out laughing. I thought, 'God, take a look at that!' We said hello and then later he turned up at the studio with hairdresser James Lebon, and we became friends right away and moved in together in Notting Hill Gate, which was difficult because he didn't speak great English. We did tests together and took them to magazines if we got the chance.

I got to know Judy Blame on London's club scene. He was an original thinker and, like many British design iconoclasts, his work was an extension of his personal style. He fronted the nightclub Cha-Cha (a backroom at Heaven gay discotheque) along with Scarlett and Michael Hardy. Judy's accessories were made from discarded detritus he found around the East End wasteland. The shoot was a nightmare for Scarlett, who was pinned into everything and had pennies stuck onto her eyes with masking tape. Judy had made a crown that Irish Tinker royalty might wear, so this was a tribute to the burial tradition for the dead to pay the ferryman to Heaven. Just like Judy, I scavenged my inspiration from wherever – romantic, punk, folkloric, organic, confrontational, historical and urban.

Judy Blame, designer:
I met you at the Blitz club, and I was becoming more knowledgeable about fashion because Stephen Linard was standing over there, and Stephen Jones and Melissa Caplan were starting to make a living out of it. For me that was an exciting period because punk had become so uniform, but the New Romantic thing was very much about the individual, about everyone wanting to be different.

Then Michael, Scarlett and I were asked to run a club at Heaven called Cha-Cha's. I was on the dole so I made up the name Judy Blame just so I could still sign on. We couldn't afford a new outfit every week, so I had my David Holah chemise (a long shroud-like dress made from cheap muslin) and just used to make a new piece of jewellery. I do blame David Holah because you needed something large to go on top of his chemises. I started using materials that weren't normally used with accessories design. That was purely because of finances. England is brilliant at that – when we haven't got the money we have to use our imagination. I used to go and scavenge by the river Thames. Because of punk rock I didn't have any fear about using something that wasn't a classical jewellery material. Me… and the other genius, of course, was Tom Binns.

Scarlett Cannon, model:
The quality of these images is so fantastic because they were shot on film, of course. I remember I had to be very still even when things needed to be fiddled with around me. How fantastic is that other frame with no coat? I have never seen that before. Why didn't we use that?

You and I met in the ladies toilets at Bang gay disco. We knew a lot of the same people. We'd always say, 'Hi, what you doing?' And then suddenly we were in a studio making fantastic images.

I was a Saturday girl at The House of Beauty and Culture. Judy was doing jewellery as if it was clothing, almost, and you were the person who picked that up.

Very early on at Cha-Cha we were wearing shrouds – a bit of old fabric wrapped around, with a fabulous bit of big old Judy Blame jewellery that was almost a piece of sculpture made of rubber, fabric or whatever. This was real salvage, sprayed gold. How fabulous.

I really liked this shoot because it looked almost sepia, even though it's a colour photograph. They have that old Hollywood look. I wasn't lying down but it looked like I was. I was champion at standing still in those days.

The clothes were just fab and the make-up was fantastic. Jalle did the best make-up for me ever. He did the best eyebrows for me. And that gold glob down my face.

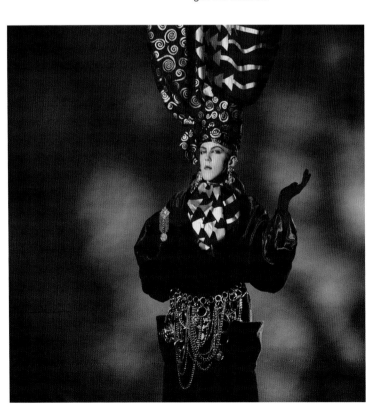

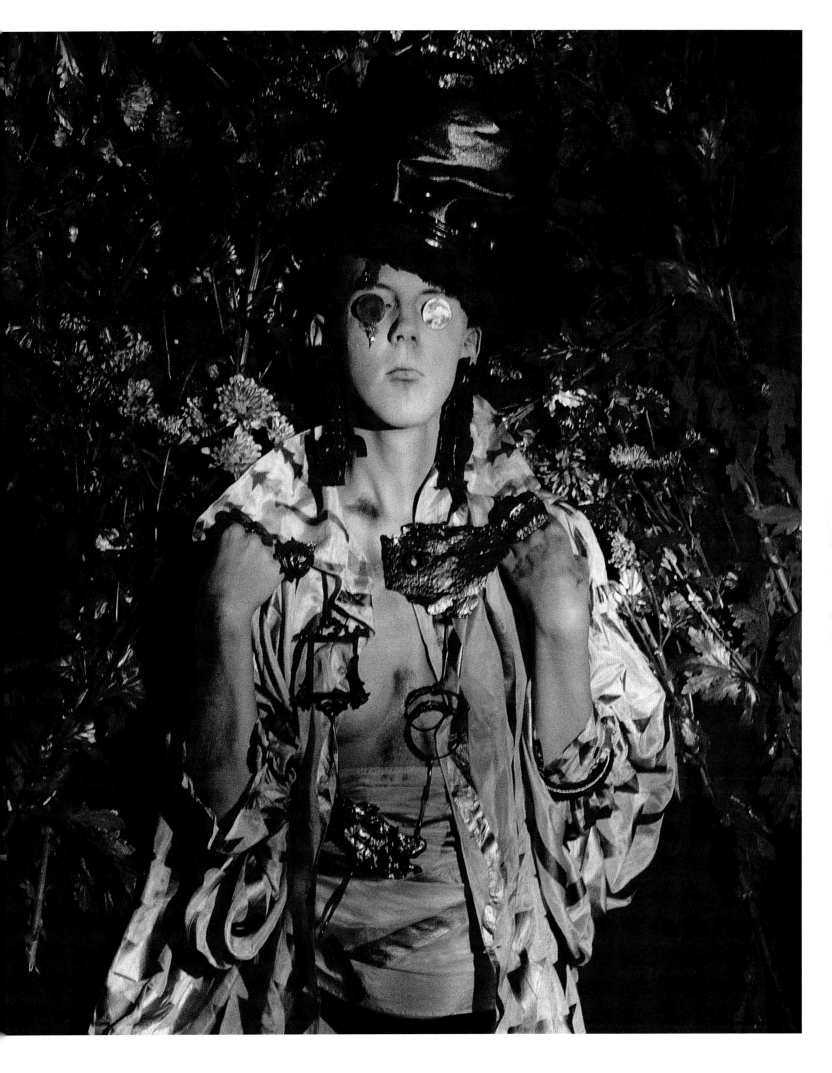

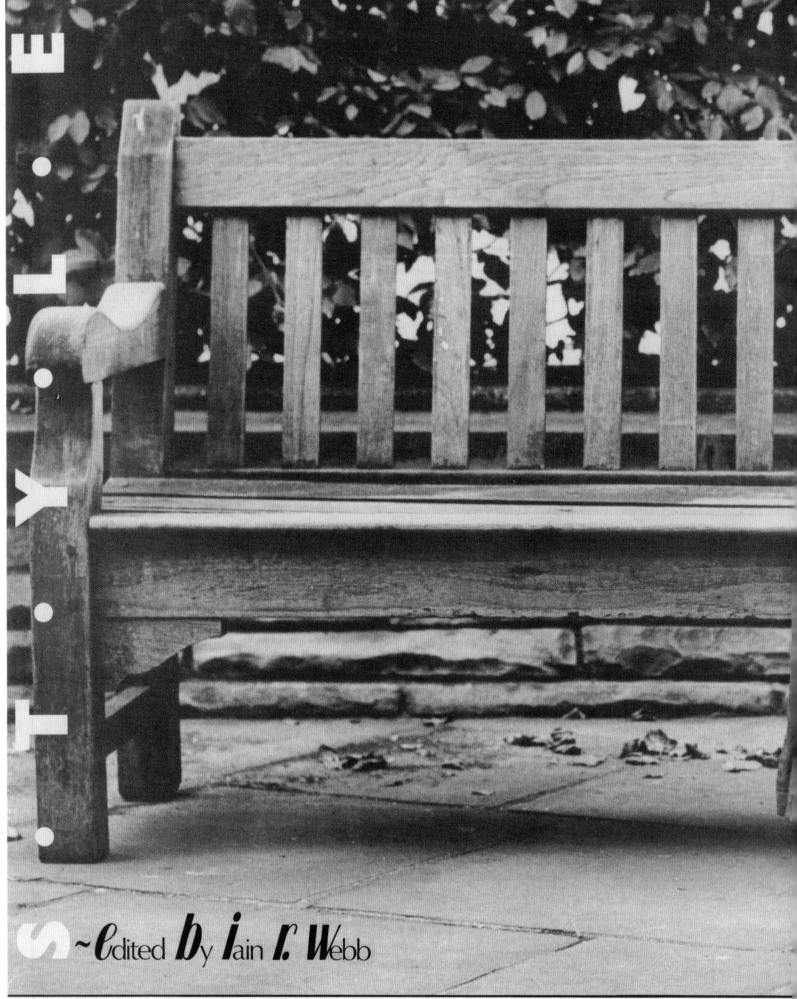

S ~*e*dited *b*y *i*ain *r.* *W*ebb

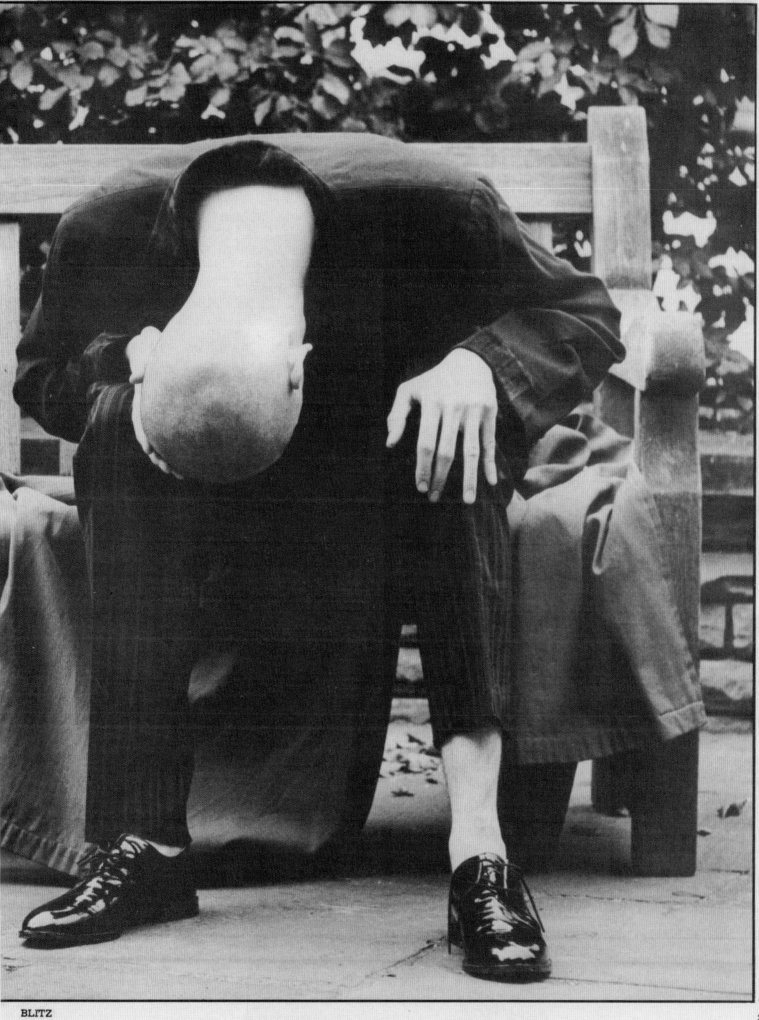

*

Photographer: Peter Brown

Models: Paul Morley, Claudia Brücken

Make-up: Debbie Bunn

Hair: Debbie Bunn

Clothes: Katharine Hamnett, Coup de Coeur, Chelsea Girl, HN's

Peter Brown, photographer:
Can you imagine we made people do things like this? But it was kind of fun. We did get people to do the most extraordinary things. And everybody was willing to do it.

Paul Morley, writer, critic, co-founder of ZTT Records:
After the *NME* I had actually written for the first few issues of *The Face*, in the days when nobody paid, so you were supposed to be doing it for the honour of working for them. *BLITZ* was perceived to some extent as second tier, but there was something about it that I liked. Maybe I preferred to work for the underdog, but I was excited by the energy that it had and, of course, there was Tim Hulse, who was a really good editor. I found a home for my writing, which is really difficult. *BLITZ* was sort of under-the-radar, and I liked that. As great as *The Face* was, I think *BLITZ* was more maverick and it gave me more freedom to experiment with my work. I remember I wrote a very conceptual piece about Cabaret Voltaire for *The Face* and when I handed it in it got short shrift. While *BLITZ* was seen as something of a pretender, it very quickly developed its own identity that lifted it up, and that was a big feat because *The Face* had quickly achieved a kind of iconic status.

BLITZ was started out of a fanzine mentality and it gave me access to a lot of different people. I profiled Martin Amis and Rowan Atkinson and Steve Martin. I invented a TV column that was way ahead of its time. It was called 'Telecide', from a quote by Bruce Willis on *Moonlighting*. I had great fun writing about TV in an almost academic way. I got a chance to play. I was introduced to a whole new world, and I met people like you, the people I needed around me. I had started ZTT, which was the conceptualising of a record label. One of the most wonderful experiences was when we put Art of Noise on *Top of the Pops*, and we worked together to present them almost like an installation. It was very much the presentation of the band as an object. I liked the idea of doing something disruptive, of putting that into the mainstream, doing something to stir things up. I learnt a lot during that time about surrounding a piece of music with context. We instinctively knew about the look, the photos, the clothing. I could make the record, make the photograph, write about the record. The concept of the multiple CV started back then. Nobody had a fixed role. We were earning and learning at the same time.

The thing I remember most about this shoot was thinking that I was going to die. When you wrapped my face with the ties, a total feeling of claustrophobia set in. It was horrendous. I thought it was going to be a real problem but I stuck

with it and it was worth it. This shoot got me into trouble with the group and the record company as, although I was the writer, I was also supposed to be running the record company; so appearing like that caused a lot of tension, but I don't regret it at all, as they are a really great series of images. They have a real energy that is very rare. Your fashion pages were challenging. A lot of the magazines that I look at wouldn't run them now. But I'm always happy to fly the flag for the radical. And they were timeless. The things we did were not about the moment, they were about an idea in the moment.

Debbie Bunn, make-up artist:
I liked Claudia's face. I loved it. I actually liked doing real people rather than models with perfect features. Mimi Potworowska also had a wonderful profile. She had a strong look as well. You have to use their features. It was more about their features than the make-up.

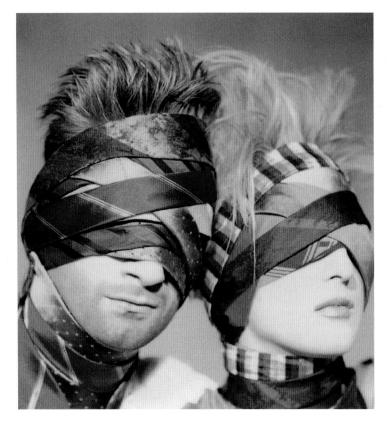

Beauty and the Beast
(or just more ZTT propaganda?)

Paul Morley was a contributor to *BLITZ*. His writing in the *NME* had been a massive influence for me so it was a real treat to meet him. We got along well and after a while he asked me to style some of the bands on his ZTT record label: Frankie Goes To Hollywood, Propaganda and Art Of Noise. I adored his then girlfriend Claudia Brücken, who was one of the singers in Propaganda. They made a cute couple, so it wasn't long before we did a fashion shoot together. I dressed them in identical outfits and I was surprised how they were totally cool with the looks. Except one: for a portrait, I wrapped their faces with a selection of patterned silk ties. Unable to see, Paul began to freak out. But we got the shot, and I was thrilled when a very similar image appeared on the cover of Italian *L'Uomo Vogue* a month after the story was published.

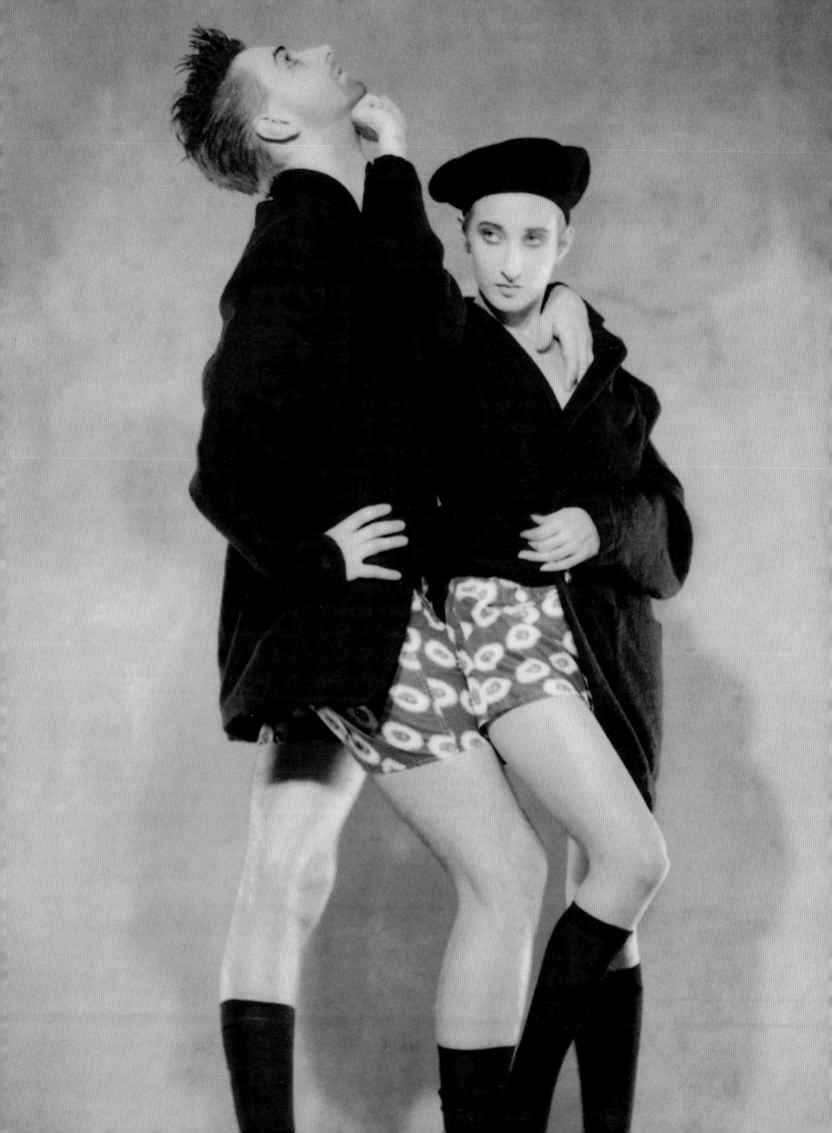

Propaganda

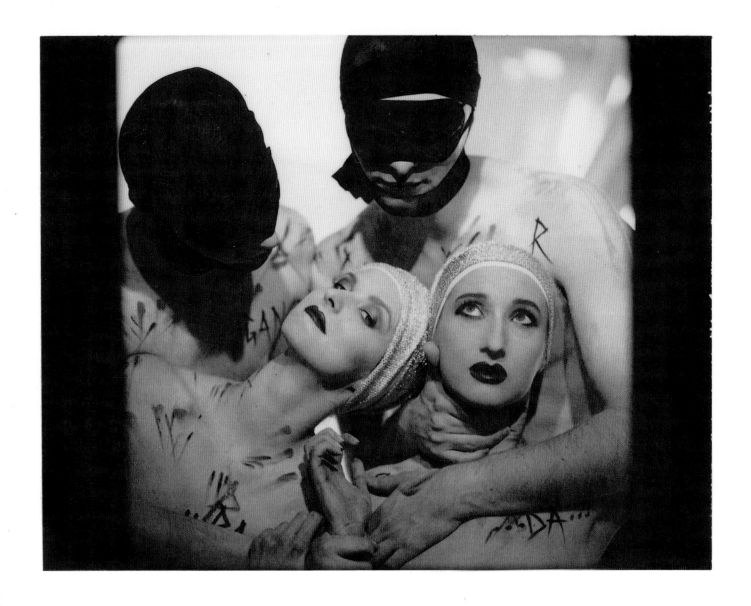

Propaganda featured Claudia Brücken along with Susanne Freytag and two blokes. We wanted to make a picture that was filmic and disturbing. We drew on movies such as *Psycho* and *Metropolis* for inspiration. The girls were made up perfectly to resemble 1930s starlets. I wrapped their heads with Lurex tights, which looked both clinical and robotic at the same time. I added sleep-masks for the boys. We shot several versions of this picture, starting with a relatively straight portrait. We then added the band's name as though carved into their necks and chests, along with a frenzy of blood-red slashes. It looked like they had been attacked by a crazed fan. Various images from this shoot were used for the album, single and in the music press.

Photographer: Peter Brown

Models: Propaganda

Make-up: Not listed

Hair: Not listed

L to R (front): Susanne, Claudia

Peter Brown, photographer:
We made people look fantastic. Pure Marlene Dietrich and Greta Garbo, but also very fetish. We did love the weird mix of inspirations. It's a fantastic image. Damn, we were good. Wouldn't it have been great if they had used these for the cover instead of the safer options?

Paul Morley, writer, critic, co-founder of ZTT Records:
It's all curating really, which I know is a very fashionable word at the moment, but it is about putting things together. It's about making events, producing occasions. And this was pre-internet. Today images are devoured every single day. It was great to work with photographers and stylists like yourself. I didn't really know what a stylist was then, and they weren't all good. On one shoot a girl turned up with a rack of clothes and it just depressed me. It was like she was a retailer. But I loved working with someone like you, when there was the conceptualisation of an idea. These are great images and still look very contemporary. The record company really didn't understand at all. They kept asking, 'Why are you making the girls look ugly? Why aren't they smiling?' This image also flirted with something kind of gothic, and I loved all that. I needed people like you and Peter. I could write it but I couldn't actualise it. The process worked really well and it was a pleasure when we were all thinking the same thing. This really does not look dated. You worry when you look back at things that they will look quaint and silly, but we took things out of their time. It all comes down to having a good idea, whether it's making a record, or making a poem, or making clothing. At the heart of it is the idea, and that can be a comment about yourself, about other people, the place you're at, or somewhere you'd like to be. And that will work if the person is comfortable in the area – be it music, fashion, whatever. Basically, those strange collaborations were really successful because we all worked to bring together the ideas we wanted to express.

The 1980s was the video age, and colour media was brand new. It was really a big deal. It wasn't that long after colour TV and suddenly you had all these colourful glossy magazines, so it's not surprising that the groups exploited the opportunity to appear in them. Suddenly you had all these colourful groups who were all about image. Now, the most important thing is the image and the music is the soundtrack to it.

Debbie Bunn, make-up artist:
I have in my diary: 'Propaganda. Video shoot. Midnight. Farm Lane, Fulham. £200 cheque.' I worked with Propaganda a lot. I did the videos and I did the pictures with Claudia and Paul Rutherford for the Frankie's album.

Claudia had an amazing look. She had such a strong look, whereas the other girl was much more classical. The big magazines like *Vogue* were very anti-make-up at the time. They were into natural make-up and we were piling it on. I always enjoyed doing strange stuff. Did you do the writing on them? I don't remember doing that. It was all about expressing yourself.

It's very Hollywood. I'll be really upset if I didn't do it. The make-up looks fabulous. I'm frantically scouring my diaries to see if I did it. I'm hoping I did. It must have been me as I was doing all their videos. I remember one time, Paul Morley saying that he wanted it 'really Joel Gray' and I said, 'Is that a colour?'

Claudia liked to have the same person doing her make-up. It's funny because bands were even more insecure about their image, they don't have the confidence that models have. In this business you are meeting someone new all the time. Part of being a really good make-up artist is to make the person feel good about themselves. Actually I don't think most models feel that good either but they are more used to putting on a look.

BLITZ #27
Dec/Jan 1984/1985

Le matin après le night before

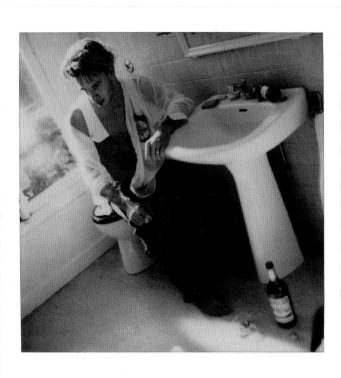

Ben Shaul, model:
Can I make some shit up? I'm not sure I can remember much. And did we consume all the liquor? That might be why?

Paul Bernstock and Thelma Speirs, designers, Bernstock Speirs:
We [Paul and Thelma] met at Middlesex Polytechnic in 1979 on the Fashion and Textiles BA course. We soon became friends, and part of a gang that would dress up and go out to the nightclubs that were a vital part of the alternative fashion and music scene bursting through. There was a sense of freedom and excitement that we could create something new and relevant to our generation.

We decided that we wanted to work together, and in 1982 established Bernstock Speirs. Having limited funds we decided to focus on accessories and began making and selling them. Fiona Dealey introduced us to Susanne Bartsch, who was planning a huge show of young London designers' work in New York. Our first designs were bought by Joseph Ettedgui, whose Joseph shops sold the best of exciting international fashion. We found a studio with Gregory Davis in Dalston and began working there.

You were one of our earliest supporters and soon became an important contributor to our work, doing illustrations, and styling photos and videos for us, as well as championing our designs in your editorial pages in *BLITZ*.

Gill Campbell, photographer:
Because there was never much of a budget, we shared a hotel room. How romantic! We even shot Ben in the bathroom. It was really small so I think I balanced on the bidet at a very jaunty angle. The thing I most remember about that trip was that you got the hump because the Gaultier tickets didn't turn up and so you took to bed in a sulk. I got fed up and despite a torrential storm, I went to the location to try and blag my way in, which, of course, you said I would never be able to do. Security was massive, aware that sophisticated Parisian ladies, dripping in jewels and fur, were clambering through tiny toilet windows to get into shows. But the weather was in my favour as everyone was soaked through waiting to get in. I was wearing a huge leather biker jacket with layers of jumpers and scarves and stuff underneath, but came out in a cold sweat when the crowd surged forward as the doors opened, all waving their invites and press badges. I was determined to get in just to prove you wrong. When security stopped me, I made a huge song and dance of trying to pull out my non-existent press pass, which I assured them I had under all the layers of clothes. Due to the masses of people pushing and shoving and the general chaos, security gave up and let me through! I even had the audacity to turn round and grab hold of a boy, who earlier had told me he was an aspiring photographer and also didn't have a pass, and tell security he was my assistant. The madness of it all! When I got back to the hotel you were still in bed. I will always remember your wry smile when I told you I had just shot the Jean Paul Gaultier show. My fashion photography style verged on still life. I loved to light. Even if the subject was chaotic, there was a calmness and clarity to my work. I think that was why we worked so well together. I especially loved to work in black and white.

Photographer Gill Campbell and I went to Paris for the Spring/Summer '85 collections. Outside one of the shows we bumped into Brit model Ben Shaul and got chatting. Before we knew it we were organising a shoot. We didn't have many invitations for the shows so we wanted to make the most of our trip. Ben came to the hotel the next day and I dressed him in the latest collection by Bernstock Speirs that I had borrowed to wear at the shows. I remember we stalked the hallway of the hotel taking empty bottles of Ricard and beer from room service trays left outside other rooms. I even wrote the caption in very bad Franglais.

Photographer: Gill Campbell

Model: Ben Shaul at K-Z

Clothes: Bernstock Speirs

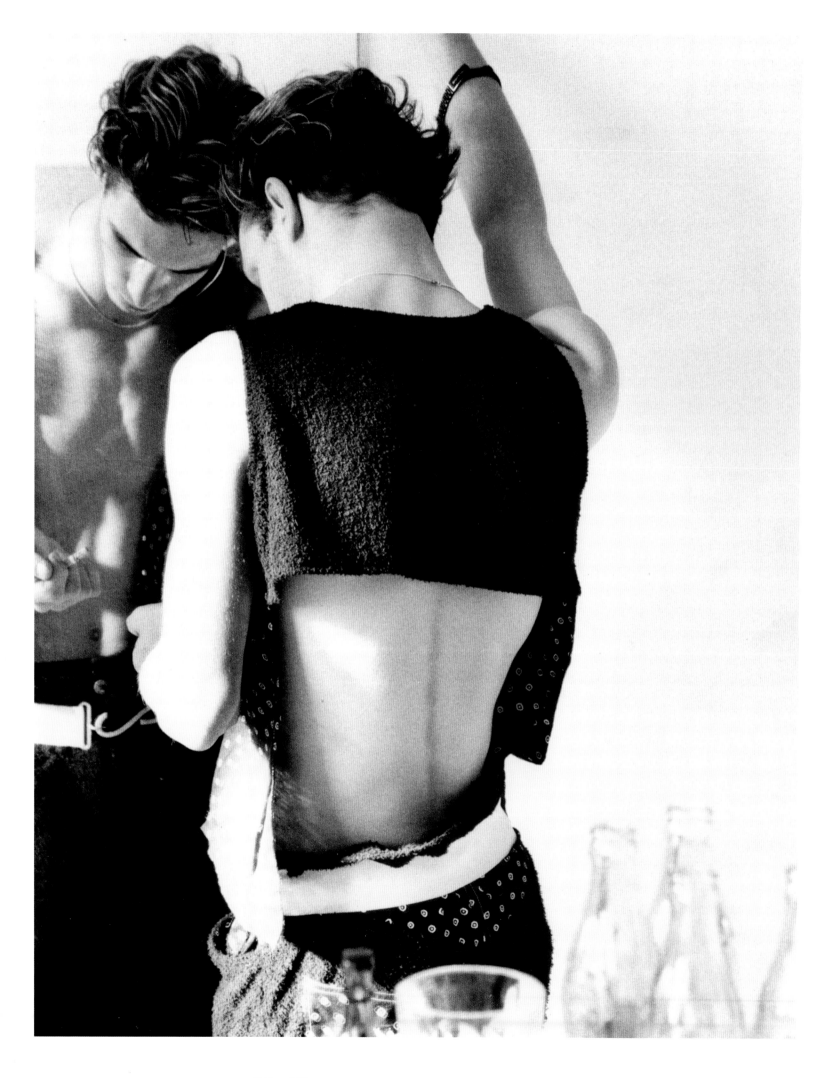

I first wrote about Stevie Stewart and David Holah in issue 14 (Sept '83) as part of my 'People' column. They were part of the New Romantic club scene, and I met them through mutual friends at nightclubs like Billy's, Blitz and St Moritz. Their label, Bodymap, became one of the beacon brands of the early 1980s, inspiring a new way, not only to design and make clothes, but how to present them on the catwalk and in photographs. In the spirit of collaboration, they asked if I would like to illustrate several of their collections. The artwork was done at a photo session. Amid the craziness I sat on the floor with my layout pad, sketching. Their cartoon-cut designs were easy to capture and I wanted the illustrations to resemble a child's colouring-in book. I featured the drawings in the magazine, to accompany news stories about the duo.

Stevie Stewart and David Holah, designers, Bodymap:

SS _ David and I graduated in 1982 from Middlesex Polytechnic. We met on the BA Fashion course. We had a mutual friend, Melissa Caplan.

DH _ I was living in the Warren Street squat with Melissa. She was doing her Pallium Products fashion label. She was in the year above us at college and said we had to look out for each other. And we hit it off.

SS _ We worked together on projects. At that time there was intense competition between Middlesex and St Martin's and we were always pushed forward because we made good PR. We were pack leaders. While we were at college, we were already working on freelance jobs, selling things.

DH _ My chemise things.

SS _ I had a market stall and David helped me. We sold prison flanelette pyjamas that we dyed in five different colours and styled like Jap, with diagonal slung jewels. When we left college, the lecturers wanted David to go to work for Lagerfeld and me to go to Armani. So, we went to Milan and went to see Anna Piaggi at Italian *Vogue*. We had older friends in the industry but we thought it was all too old and cliquey. We were young and vibrant London designers. We didn't want to be an assistant for somebody. We wanted to do it ourselves. We were already selling things. We were making quite an eclectic look, with tweedy things and dishcloth knits, tartan wool skirts. For the knits we had to make a jersey toile, a test garment cut in jersey, and all of a sudden the jersey pieces became interesting.

DH _ We wouldn't have been able to work for anyone else. We wouldn't have been able to do the things we did, cutting things up, doing things the way we wanted to do them. I went to work for Hardy Amies. I thought, I'm never going to do things like that. I was never very good at sewing so I had to invent ways of doing things. Instead of putting in a zip, we invented our pull-on skirt.

SS _ In 1983 we showed at the Individual Clothes Show and we won the Most Innovative Designer award. We've still got the cup. It was all quite scary.

DH _ It was great.

SS _ You loved being on the catwalk.

DH _ Being in *BLITZ* meant that we could go to stores. We could show buyers that we had great publicity. It was important on the right level. And when we were in Italy designing for Goldie, when they saw our stuff in these magazines they couldn't get enough of it. That's exactly where they wanted to be. *i-D*, *Face* and *BLITZ* were much more important than *Vogue* to them. *BLITZ* was majorly important. You had different ways of shooting things. The way the things were shot, the androgyny thing, Martine Houghton. We loved that.

SS _ Then we did the 'Barbee Takes a Trip...' photo shoot with Mario [Testino] and you just came along to draw it. Layla [d'Angelo] was doing the hair, Lesley [Chilkes] was doing the make-up and you were doing the illustration. You were all part of the Bodymap family.

Barbee takes a trip around nature's cosmic curves Lovely Simple Designs

Illustration: Iain R. Webb

Clothes: Bodymap

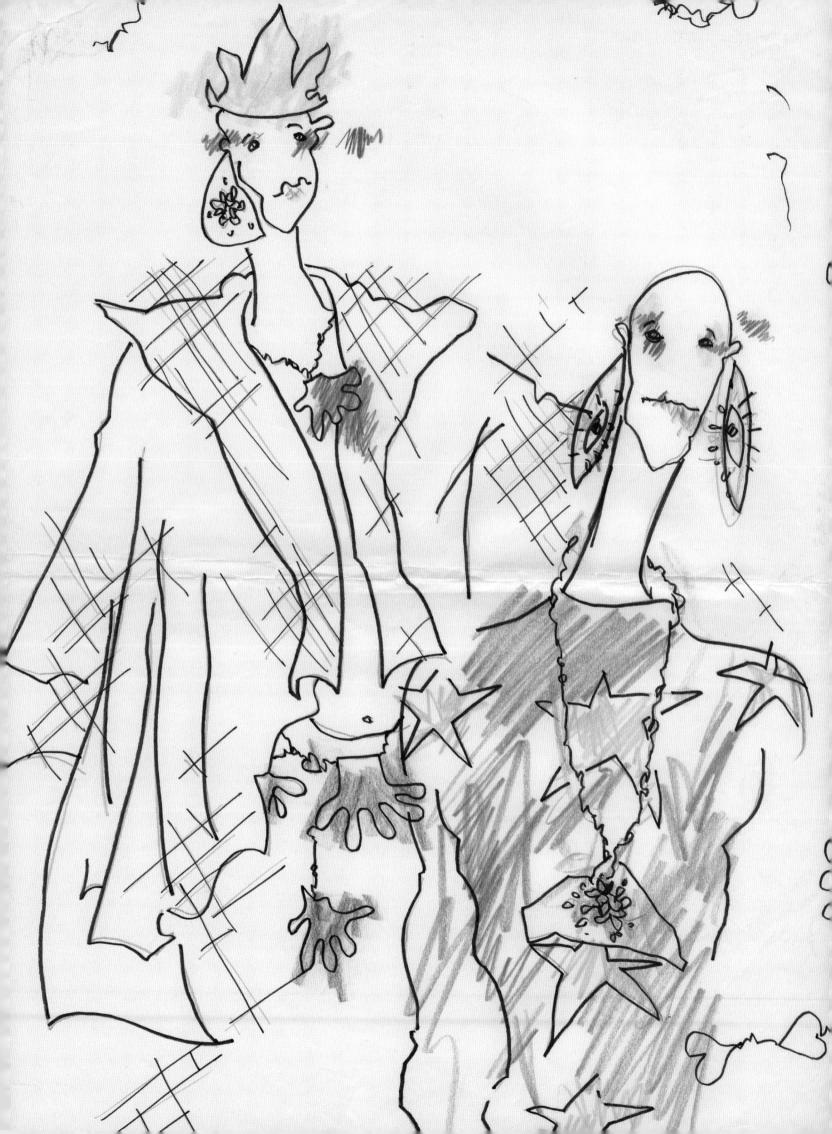

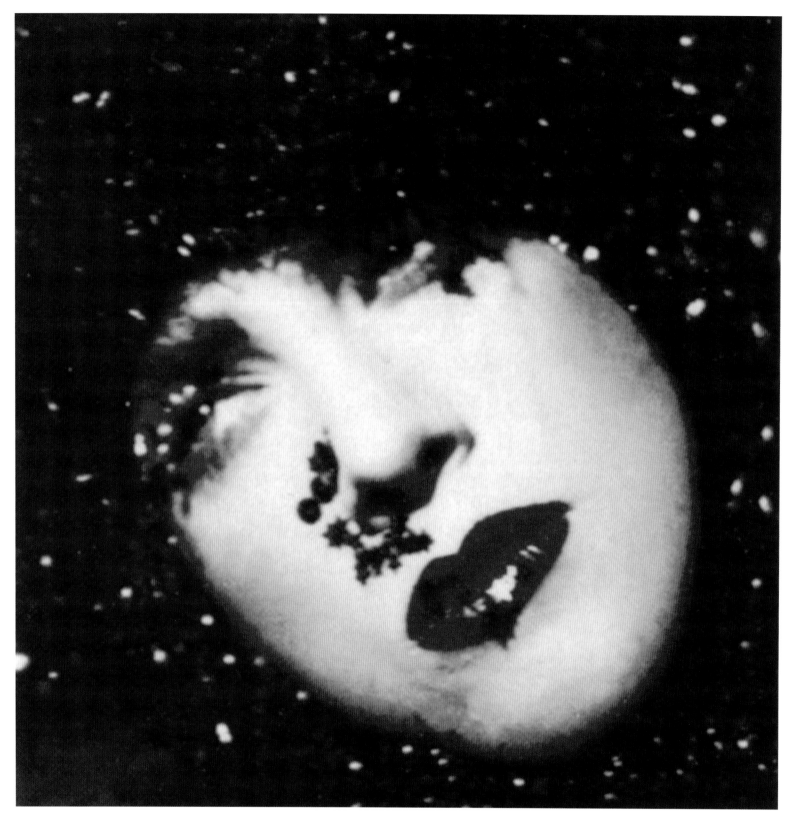

For this series, I put together looks with a vague winter
wardrobe theme but couldn't resist throwing in some
particularly curve-ball styling. There were odd Glam Rock
references, perhaps to add a Christmas feel: a hat decorated
with 7-inch singles including Gary Glitter (whose gleam has
since tarnished), half-mast Lurex tights, and another sheer
pair stretched bank robber-style over the model's face.
There was also a peculiar price point element to this story,
so washers (*very cheap* from a local hardware store) were
worn as rings and accessorised an *expensive* Nordic-look
sweater from Browns. The clothes were listed in order
of price from 'Buy It' to 'Beg, Borrow or Steal'.

I never went to school, so during my photography career I always felt very insecure about that. I always felt I was a B-list photographer instead of an A-lister, so I worked really hard. I studied artists' work and lighting, and I was very influenced by people like George Hurrell, so I bought old movie lights which I've still got. So I really know about lighting.

I love the photo of just the chin, and the washers as rings are so good. Why not? It was so creative, a genius time. But I love the labels now. You know why? The quality. The fabrics are more durable!

Johnny Rozsa, photographer:
I used to work for *BLITZ* , *i-D* and *RITZ*. David Litchfield, the co-owner of *RITZ* was really helpful, because not only did I shoot pictures but I was also featured in their gossip columns at parties. I think that's how I got in with Simon and Carey, who were really fabulous to me. I was also doing lots of things for *19* and *Honey*, and I did lots of things for *The Sunday Times* for Meriel McCooey and Michael Roberts. That's how I earned money, how I lived. It was not very much, but it paid so I could do things like *BLITZ*.

This shoot is brilliant. Did we do it in my studio in Holland Park? It was like a flat. She's lying on a duvet. It was in a mews, a carriage house, where they used to keep horses, and I converted it into a studio. I had my Buddhist chanting space and then the front room was used as a studio.

These Polaroids are divine. Terry Jones [editor/founder of *i-D*] gave me a Polaroid camera to take to clubs to shoot people and I was convinced that it was the way of the future, so I think I came to you and said 'let's use Polaroid!' I have thousands of these Polaroids. I used to just hand them in as a page layout. I remember saying "I'm going to do heads and middle bits and bottoms, shoes and feet". I think I did it on a commercial camera that just popped the Polaroid out, not even a pull-one like professional photographers used, but so what? They had the white strip at the bottom.

Paul Coster, model:
At the start of my career, my agency sent me to see Johnny Rozsa. He helped me out a lot and took some great arty pictures of me. He was a good man. Very cool. He gave me quite a few tips, like always be presentable when you turn up for a job, put on a bit of aftershave. That stuff really matters.

Photographer: Johnny Rozsa

Model: Nicole Bordeaux
at Premier

Make-up: Louise Constad

Clothes: Mark & Syrie, Cathy Renshaw, Sue Clowes, Krizia, Katharine Hamnett, Stephen Sprouse, Adrien Mann, Johnsons, Modzart, Goldie, Jay Musson, hardware store

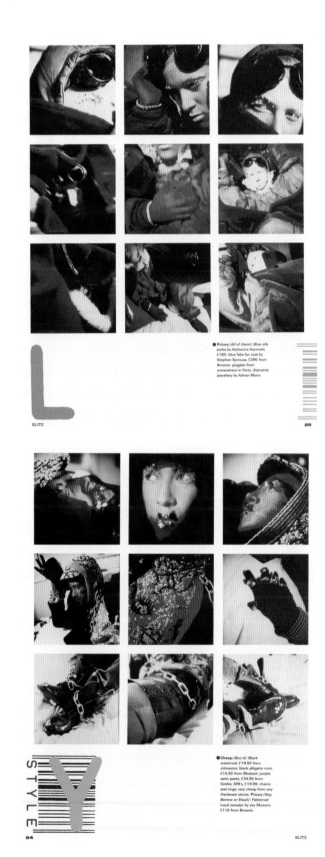

Style

Photographer: Nick Knight

Model: Nathalie

Clothes: Katharine Hamnett

Nick Knight, photographer:
BLITZ provided a beautiful flamboyance in the '80s and you brought that to *BLITZ*. You had an artistic fashion vision, which is why I worked with you. It was a lovely and important part of my life. *The Face* and *i-D* never really represented fashion. They never captured that love of fashion and the understanding of the power of fashion as you did. You crystallised that vision. *i-D* was focused on what was happening on the streets and *The Face* was very cliquey and was more interested in the experience of fashion, and that came from Nick Logan who had been a Mod.

When you and I met up it was an eye-opening moment for me. You showed me a life that was different to how I had perceived it. I met you and everybody in London that centred around Taboo nightclub, and there is nothing more exciting that discovering a world that you don't know about. The experience was extremely exciting. So much of it was about breaking down barriers. Discovering that world was a springboard for me onto Yohji Yamamoto. Art director Marc Ascoli saw the '100 Portraits' I did in *i-D*. To go from Taboo to Paris was a really head-swirling moment.

What was lovely then was that there was lots of experimentation and enthusiasm. You lose that open-mindedness. Those tender years were amazing. You just can't stop doing it, even if it is three o'clock in the morning. It was very much the same in Paris as the way we worked together. It could be two, three, four in the morning. We were always wanting to push it. It wasn't until the mid-nineties that I suddenly came across people in studios saying, 'it's six o'clock, why aren't we going home?' That was when the fashion thing became driven by very powerful forces like LVMH and US *Vogue*. Suddenly money shaped everything.

In *BLITZ*, your bits were the best. There should have been much more of what you did and less of the music and the acting.

Katharine Hamnett, fashion designer:
It was an amazing time. Everything seemed so easy. It was so much fun and we thought we could change the world. *BLITZ* was great, considered really cutting-edge, and you had to be in it. You were a laugh. Why don't people have parties like that anymore? I remember the interview. You were sweet, so young, and if I remember rightly, your tape recorder was not working.

Katharine Hamnett was big news. She cleverly introduced a very utilitarian look that featured the kind of clothes you might find in flea markets in Paris or Laurence Corner in London. But the people who desired (and could afford) Hamnett's designs weren't the type to ferret through stall after stall of second-hand clothes in the hope of finding the perfect raincoat or jacket, so instead the designer offered a wardrobe full of desirable classic pieces. These were cut from equally utilitarian fabrics like gabardine and glazed cotton. Her catwalk shows were wild affairs with the sexiest girls and boys running riot on the runway. Hamnett cleverly sexed up politics while Tony Blair was still at prep school. Some of her basic designs made from brightly coloured parachute silk resembled religious robes, so we wanted to create an image to accompany the interview that was quasi-ceremonial. Almost sacrificial. The ultimate fashion victim?

Hamnett

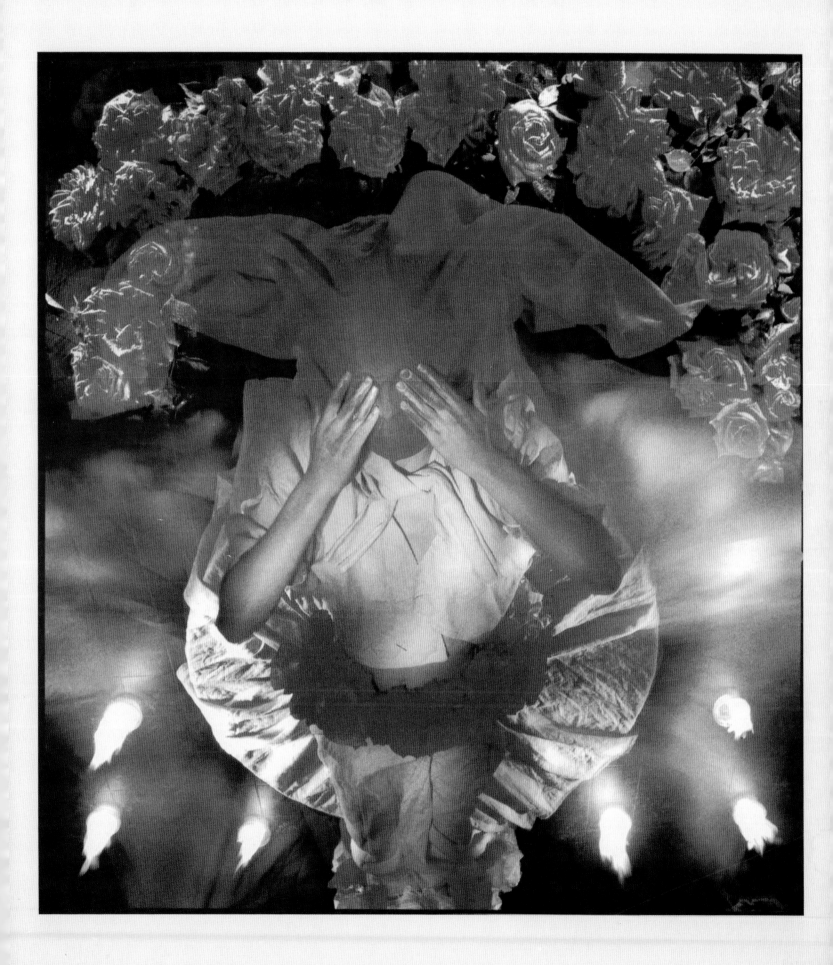

Photographer: Peter Brown

Model: Astrid at Premier

Make-up: Debbie Bunn

Hair: James Lebon

Stylist stand-in:
Bertie 'Berlin' Marshall

The Fashion Year

In 1984 I contributed a chapter to *The Fashion Year*, an annual publication that charted that particular year in fashion. The theme was street style, so I enlisted Nick Knight to shoot some images that represented the various looks that had been popular. Simon and Carey also produced a chapter about *BLITZ*. The following year, I was asked to co-edit the book with Lorraine Dicky. She was a joy to work with, pretty much giving me an open brief. We compiled a hit list of topics and collaborators. It was a fantastic Who's Who of 1980s fashion freaks: Michael Roberts, Amanda Grieve, Stevie Stewart of Bodymap, and Lynne Franks. It featured rock writers Paul Morley and Julie Burchill, who both succeeded in writing totally enigmatic entries. Burchill penned one of the best sentences ever written about fashion: 'The only reason to put clothes on is to get someone else to take them off.' There were interviews with the style queen Diana Vreeland and transgender model Teri Toye. Models of the year were painted by Trojan, Leigh Bowery's self-styled side-kick. The cover was another *BLITZ* crew production: Astrid was the perfect cover girl, wrapped and pinned into a silky evening gown. At one point during the evening shoot, she fainted with such precision into hairdresser James Lebon's arms that I still am not sure how real the vapours were. I don't know many who would not have done the same, given half the chance.

Peter Brown, photographer:
Astrid was our model *du jour*. She and James got very friendly on the Luisa shoot, didn't they? Standing her on blocks made her look about eight feet tall. And Bertie was hanging around as usual. And everyone in black. That was the styling. Everyone had jet black hair, except you.

Debbie Bunn, make-up artist:
My diary says: 'Thursday 13 March 1985, Fashion Year Book. 7pm.' Another evening shoot. In the day I did a job with Mike Owen for *Hair and Good Looks* magazine. I got sponsored for *The Fashion Year* shoot by Cosmetics à la Carte. £100. I used to love them. They were one of the first companies to mix foundations to match your skin colour. They had a little shop in Motcombe Street and a factory in Battersea. It doesn't say if they actually paid me or not! I always used to try and actually use their make-up for the job. A lot of the big magazines used to just sell the credit later and it was most likely not the actual make-up used. But I had a good relationship with them and so if I could sell them a credit I would. It was good for them I guess.

That shoot was done at the London Bridge studio. What does my hair look like? James always looked gorgeous, didn't he, and he was charming to everyone and just so cool. Astrid's hair is really theatrical. Maybe he was using his Cuts hair gel. Maybe he gelled my hair. Or maybe that's how I looked every day. Atrocious!

I remember you told us all to wear black. I had my new cowboy boots on. They had gold bits on them so I think they distracted in the picture so you told me to take them off, and I remember thinking how short I must look. That's why Bertie stood in for you. We all had black hair. Mine was dyed at the time. I was really surprised when I saw it on the cover. I didn't expect it to go on a book.

Katharine Hamnett, designer:
We used James a lot. He was cool, beautiful, fun and sweet. He was in endless catwalk shows, starred in our short-lived magazine *Tomorrow* and an Ellen Von Unwerth advertising campaign. We did a catwalk show in Paris once, at Circe d'Hiver, where he got so drunk backstage before the show that he could only crawl down the catwalk. He was still great. The girls all loved him.

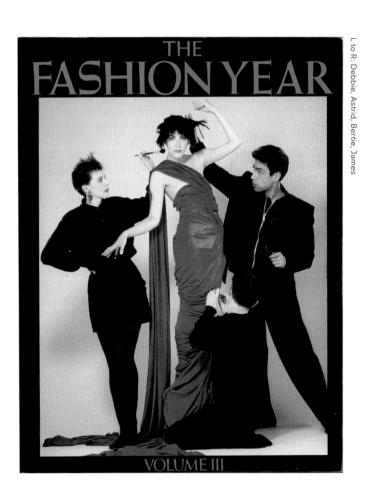

L to R: Debbie, Astrid, Bertie, James

BLITZ #29
March 1985

Photographer: Gill Campbell

Model: Ken Flanagan at
Marco Rasala

Make-up and Hair: Debbie Bunn
represented by Lynne Franks

Clothes: Laurence Corner,
Demob, Wendy Dagworthy

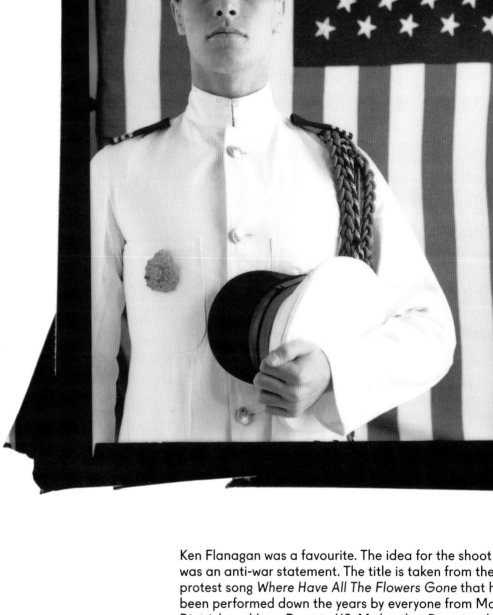

Gill Campbell, photographer:
Ken Flanagan was a favourite, of
course! A few years ago Pete made
a giant lith positive of this picture
and fixed it in a big light box. It's
in our living room. A lovely way
to light a room.

Ken Flanagan, model:
I remember Gill being very serious
and you being super-friendly and
reassuring. Hair and make-up were,
as always, an odd one. I had no
idea how the spread was going to
look but trusted you completely.
At the time I thought I was an odd
choice for the story, but once I saw
it I could see that it worked in a less
obvious way. I was as naïve as the
kind of boys that would typically go
off to war, and to that extent there
was a certain strange truth to it.

Barry Kamen, model:
The braiding on that jacket is
beautiful. The smashed picture.
Sometimes one double-page image
was all you needed. Everyone now
is, 'Oh, if I haven't got 16 pages
I'm not gonna do it'. Blimey, we just
used to do the back page of *The
Face*. That was a big deal.

Where have all the young men gone?

Ken Flanagan was a favourite. The idea for the shoot
was an anti-war statement. The title is taken from the 1961
protest song *Where Have All The Flowers Gone* that has
been performed down the years by everyone from Marlene
Dietrich and Joan Baez to U2. My brother Dave used to
sing it during his Bob Dylan phase. We did the shoot over
two sessions. The first time, we photographed Ken in a
white officer uniform from Laurence Corner Army and
Navy surplus store, and also in kagool coats from Demob.
Gill made the prints and then we re-shot them in a still life
scenario. The shattered glass was meant to evoke the sense
of destruction. The Stars and Stripes flag is draped over a
box, possibly a coffin. I guess the image was intended to be
part tribute, part warning. I had used images of the Vietnam
war (photographs by Don McCullin) in my final year at St
Martin's School of Art. In February 1985, Paul Hardcastle
was in the pop charts with *19*, dedicated to the young
American soldiers who served in Vietnam.

WHERE HAVE ALL THE YOUNG MEN GONE?

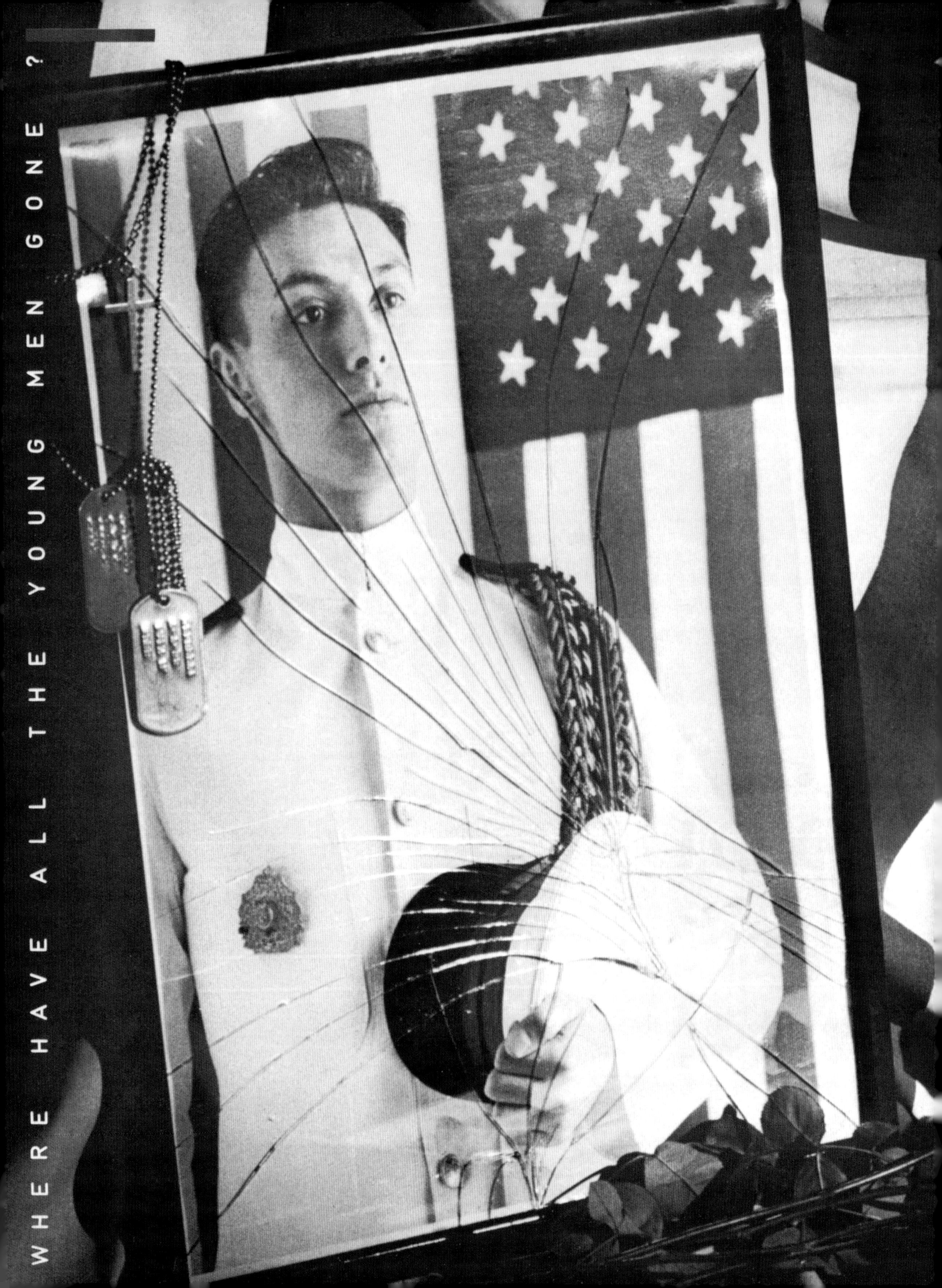

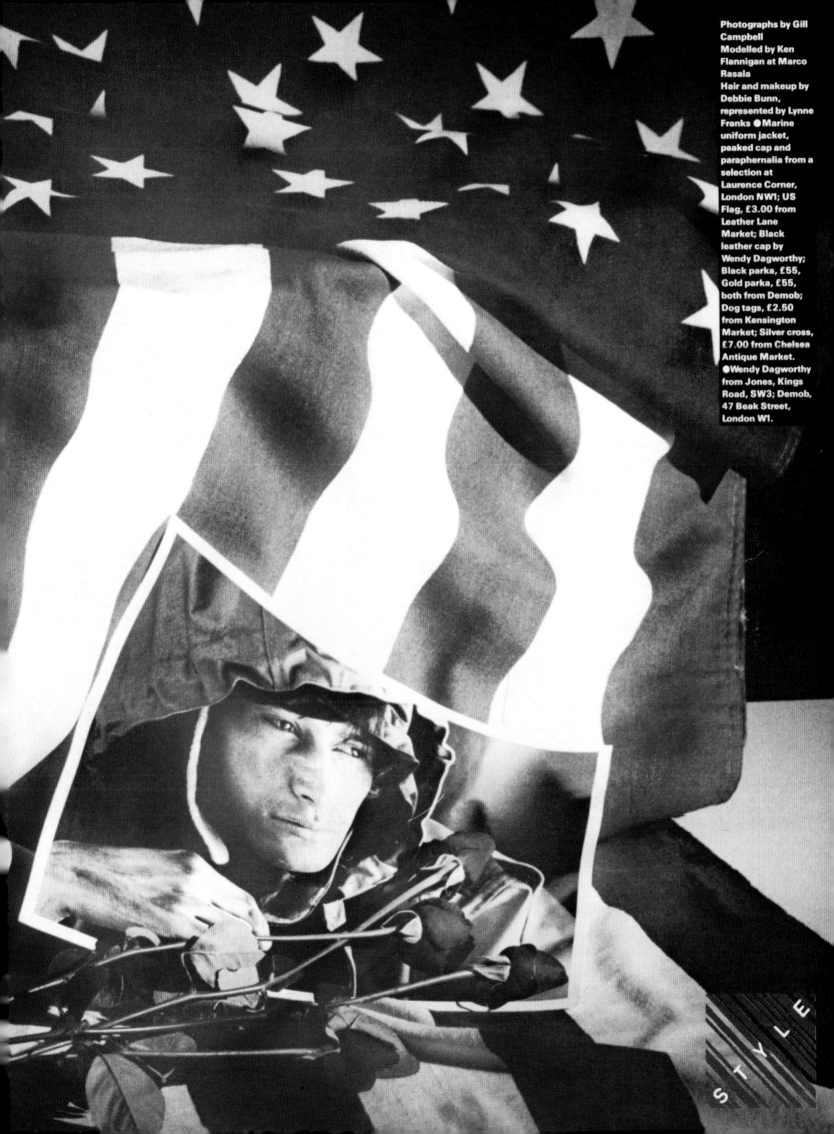

Photographs by Gill
Campbell
Modelled by Ken
Flannigan at Marco
Rasala
Hair and makeup by
Debbie Bunn,
represented by Lynne
Franks ●Marine
uniform jacket,
peaked cap and
paraphernalia from a
selection at
Laurence Corner,
London NW1; US
Flag, £3.00 from
Leather Lane
Market; Black
leather cap by
Wendy Dagworthy;
Black parka, £55,
Gold parka, £55,
both from Demob;
Dog tags, £2.50
from Kensington
Market; Silver cross,
£7.00 from Chelsea
Antique Market.
●Wendy Dagworthy
from Jones, Kings
Road, SW3; Demob,
47 Beak Street,
London W1.

STYLE

Where there's smoke

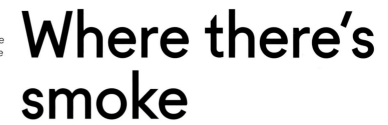

Peter Brown, photographer:
I was obsessed with all that old Hollywood imagery, but this image could also be from a French movie starring Simone Signoret. And androgynous too. Girls like boys, boys like girls. I think it was a test. Missy wanted a beauty shot and you came along and styled it. If the model got a picture for their book and we got to use it for the magazine, they were like, 'Yeah, you can use it for that'. It was not like, 'we have to be paid this'. It was shared. We might have got advertising on the back of this picture or the model might get work. We were all young and we were all coming up together and helping each other out.

Missy was a big runway girl, she did all the shows. We used a lot of runway girls in print, which in those days was unusual. Michele Paradise, girls like that, there was a different aesthetic for the runway and for print. Nowadays it's absolutely the reverse, the print girls are the runway girls. And no retouching! Everything was just how it was. Certainly no one had any money to do hand retouching.

Photographer: Peter Brown

Model: Missy at Z

Clothes: Not Listed

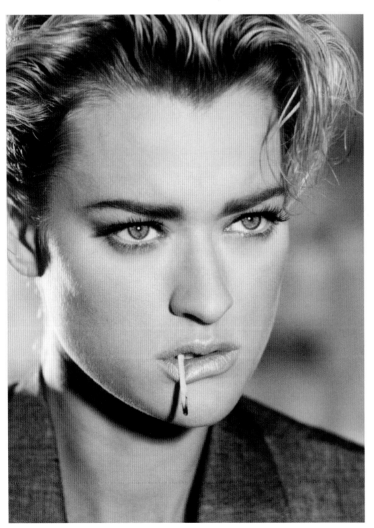

Missy, model:
These photographs, well, there's so much to say. I remember the shoot but never realised how much it would propel and launch my fantastic career into the great future I had. These photographs became the favourites for many people: designers, clients, photographers, editors and magazines worldwide! Of all my pictures, these are still my favourite and captured the real Missy that I was, and still am in my soul. This photograph became Jean Paul Gaultier's favourite. It launched me on to opening his fashion show and I worked for him for ten years. I was one of his favourites. This picture became an inspiration for designers' collections. The image is androgynous and evoked old black and white movies as well as classic French elegance. Yohji Yamamoto, Claude Montana and Ray Petri loved them. Marc Ascoli loved them too. City Models loved them. It goes on. These photographs got me my first shoot at French *Marie Claire* and major advertising campaigns for Ferragamo, Missoni, Trusardi and Krizia. They got me on every catwalk in London, Milan, Paris and New York. Whenever I went backstage at the fashion shows, this image was the one used for the line-ups. They got me on every airplane, to every imaginable destination all over the world and more.

Ziggi Golding, model agent, founder of Z:
There were so many rules. You were either a show girl or an editorial girl. We tried to do everything. Missy could have just been a show girl but look how much editorial she did. Another agent might not have taken her on but I thought she photographed like an exquisite statue.

Missy was another favourite. I cannot remember if this photograph was taken to illustrate a story I had written on images of smoking in fashion magazines, or if I wrote the piece inspired by the picture (I re-wrote this story several times over the years for a variety of publications). Again, a wonderfully lit portrait that harks back to the classy Hollywood portraits of George Hurrell, the plume of smoke evoking sophisticated sirens. This is probably one of the most timeless images I produced. The black and white image was used in the magazine, and it was not until I met with Missy again for the purpose of this book that I was shown the beautiful colour image. I am now torn between them.

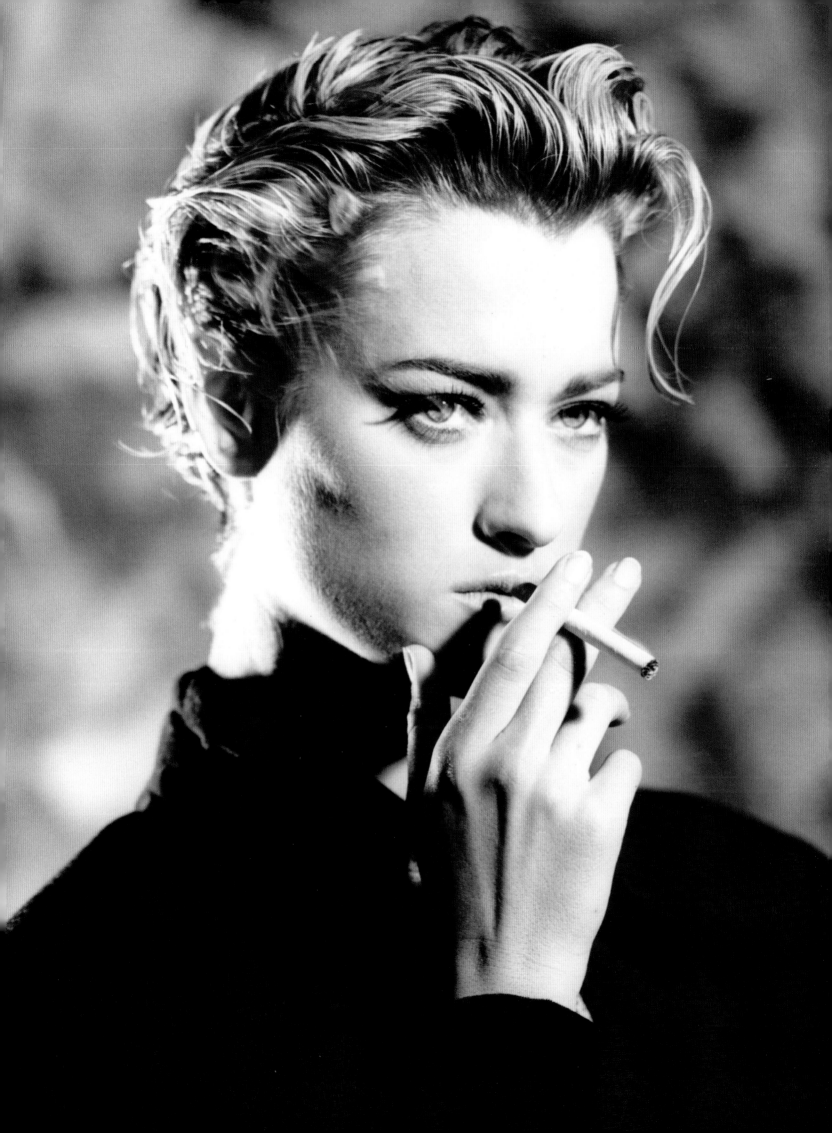

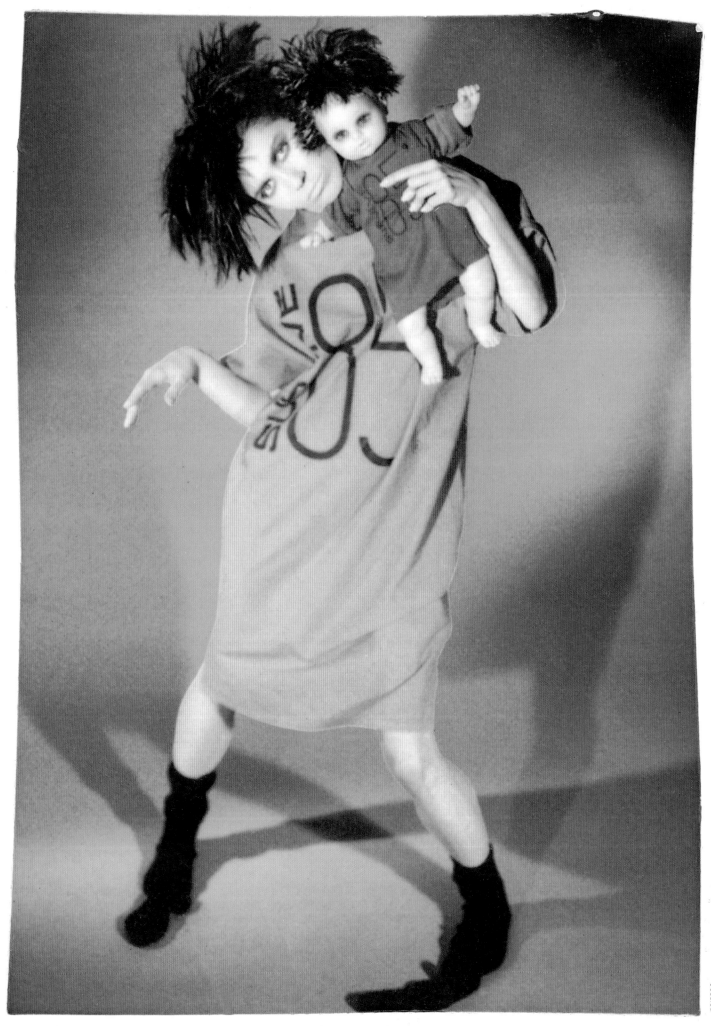

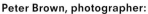

SHOT
21–22 March 1985

RESHOOT
4 April 1985

Photographer: Peter Brown

Art Director: Dick Tyson

Model: Sherry at Premier, Jessica at Z

Make-up: Debbie Bunn

Hair: Not listed

Clothes: C&A

C&A

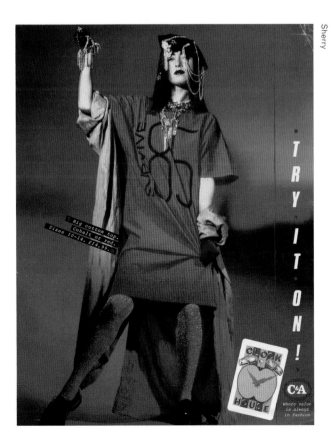

Sherry

Peter Brown, photographer:
Oh my Lord! Can you believe what we did? The 1985 T-shirt was a re-shoot because the original shot pushed the boat out a little too far. It was so kind of *Carrie* goes crazy, with a voodoo edge. I love it – but for a commercial high street store, what on earth were we thinking? One time, as inspiration for a shoot, I made the entire corporate staff of C&A sit down to watch Derek Jarman's *Angelic Conversation*. I said, this is how I want it to look. Poor old Dick Tyson, although funnily enough the account went on to win him two or three awards.

You were certainly gilding the lily. Do you remember the belt you made of little dolls but it was rejected, so we toned it down to this much more conservative image. Too funny. I remember we were howling with laughter when we shot it.

Dick Tyson, art director:
I was an advertising agency art director working on the younger Clock House and Avanti sections of C&A. At first I had to work with an in-house stylist, who not only organised all the accessories but also chose the photographers. Being conscious of how awful the clothes and styling looked, and how much harm was being done to the brand, I talked my creative director and the client into letting me loose to try and improve the look. They gave me a budget of £2000 and a free hand. I came up with the 'Try It On' strap-line for Clock House and decided to do just that.

At that time *Face, i-D* and *BLITZ* were the cutting-edge fashion magazines, so it seemed obvious to me that the talent I needed would probably be involved with their brilliant fashion editorial work. I approached a couple of the photographers that impressed me most, Peter Brown at *BLITZ* and Martin Brading, who was working with *i-D*, and offered them each £1000 to do test shoots for me.

I had no idea whether or not they'd want to work on C&A (it could have wrecked their careers had it become widely known), but I persuaded them by giving them a free hand with their choice of stylists, hair and make-up artists.

Of course, I loved the results. And, for the most part, so did my Creative Director and the buyers at C&A (who were the real gods!). So suddenly I was in charge of advertising the two brands. At last kids would see that some C&A clothes, if styled with flair and imagination, should be on their shopping lists.

We had tremendous fun doing the shoots. Advertising was much more liberal then than it later became. What was the point of doing all that work if you couldn't enjoy yourself doing it?

Pushing the boundaries was an essential part of trying to keep the lines up-to-date and relevant. It did occasionally go tits-up (the 'Survive 85' re-shoot springs to mind), but that was okay. It had to be edgy or it wouldn't have worked so well. I never went back to working in the old way.

Working with Peter, I met Maxine Siwan and you and many others, and Martin introduced me to Kim Hunt and a load more brilliant visionary stylists. With all of you on board I couldn't really fail. In my opinion, out of the three biggies, *BLITZ* was the most cutting-edge, gritty magazine, not only in fashion (that would have been down to you, of course), but also in graphics and editorial. Mind you, I didn't know of any fellow art directors that didn't buy all three.

Peter and I worked on several extra-curricular jobs. These usually paid well, which funded our editorial efforts. One of the most enjoyable collaborations was with C&A, the high street store. Although decidedly middle-of-the-road, the brand was eager for an update. Peter and I were employed to give the clothes the *BLITZ* edge, although this sometimes went a bit too far for the client. I am still surprised at how certain key people embraced our off-the-wall approach, specifically art director Dick Tyson, who masterminded the C&A advertising campaign, and Diane Grant Davidson, whom I worked with on the store's catwalk shows. They were both truly generous in their encouragement and open-mindedness.

Debbie Bunn, make-up artist:
Working for C&A was probably the only time we ever made money. £100 for half a day seemed a lot at the time. I got more detailed with my notes in my diaries over the years: £20 oooh, £10 oooh... of course, zero cash on the *BLITZ* jobs. Nobody got paid for *The Face* or *i-D* either. Make-up artists got paid by make-up companies.

The best thing about C&A was that we could do what we wanted. We used to make the clothes look mad. They were such normal clothes. And Dick loved what we were doing, that was what was so exciting. Perhaps C&A closed down because they stopped taking risks.

You really needed to have editorial tear sheets but they were never very commercial so I'm not sure how much they helped me get jobs. I loved working with you at *BLITZ*. I really loved Simon and Carey too. I did Carey's make-up at their wedding.

BLITZ #30
April 1985

Knits

New photographers often turned up at the office in Soho, but I first encountered photographer David LaChapelle when he was dancing on a podium in White Trash nightclub in Piccadilly wearing tiny satin shorts. He had arrived fresh from America, and via the Bodymappers, we became friends. Simon and Sherry were two of my favourite models. I liked their similar androgynous features and long, poker-straight hair. There was lots of giant-sized knitwear around, including cardigans big enough for two, so it seemed logical to photograph them sharing one. I love functional jersey pieces like long-johns and granddad vests. With David I was always encouraged to push the styling to the limits. I think he enjoyed the opportunity to make fashion pictures that were not cataloguing product. He was handsome too, and tremendous fun to be around. His enthusiasm and playfulness was incredibly infectious.

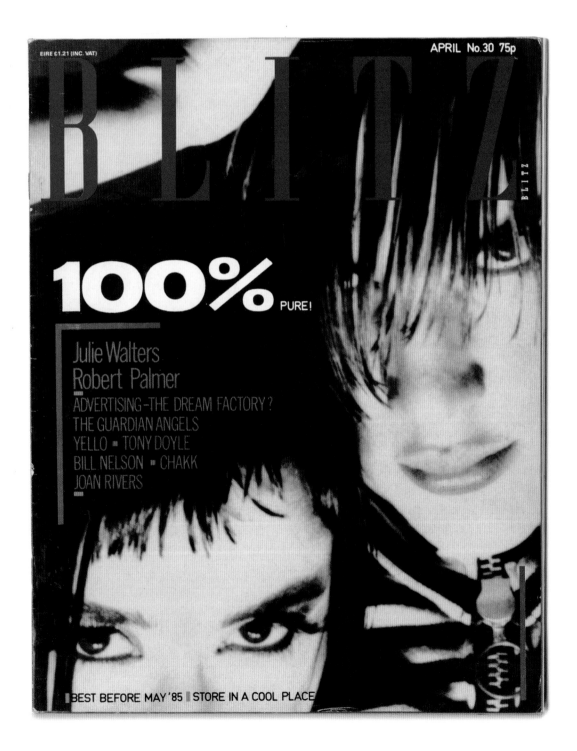

Photographer: David LaChapelle

Models: Simon Ringrose at Z, Sherry at Premier

Make-up and Hair:
William Faulkner

Clothes: Martin Kidman,
Ten Big Boys, Bazooka

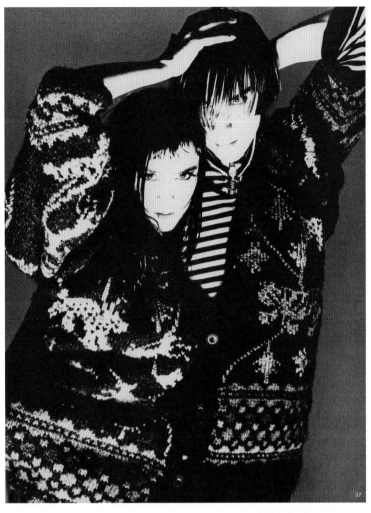

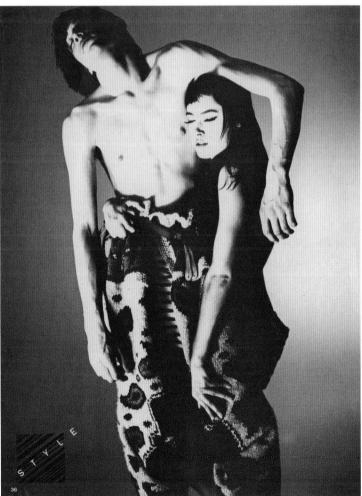

I had a good friend, Gareth, who was also at Z agency, and he was staying with you. Gareth had invited me over for a cup of tea and some porridge (as we didn't have any money this was our staple diet), prior to going out to a party or club. You had styled him, dressed him up in a tablecloth wrapped around like a kilt, and he looked great. I think you asked me to do some pictures the following Saturday. The shoot felt like I was having an 'out of body experience'. To be on the cover was pretty cool. Wow, what an honour.

Ziggi Golding, model agent, founder of Z:

How amazing that you worked with David LaChapelle right when he was starting out and he shot these beautiful, simple black and white pictures. You can't think of him now without imagining a wild and colourful fantasy scenario. He had come over from New York and was just this really young club kid. If he hadn't done anything in London, where would he be now? You were the first to do pictures with him and encourage him. Imagine if he hadn't have done that. Everyone on the scene was young and starting out. I remember we used to do castings for Marc Ascoli and the Japanese designers, and Mario [Testino] used to come to our offices in Gee Street, which was in real east London, especially back then when it wasn't trendy at all. But Mario loved to do castings there. All the other agents were really pissed off.

Sherry Lamden, model:

My friend Claire [Ringrose] said that I would be working with her little brother Simon, and that it would be his first shoot and that he was very shy and therefore pretty nervous. So, of course, on the day you told us to strip off and get into jumpers together! It might as well have been getting into a bed. We were neither of us professional models, so we did not just drop our kit off easily. However, David was great and, as I recall, you and he were really funny and happy with the way the shoot was going, and because of that the atmosphere was really good. Simon was made to feel like the Adonis that he was, which did wonders for his shyness.

The cover was brilliant, as it wasn't a supermodel but us. The beautiful black and white close up of Simon's equine face and my eyes was not like anything else on the news stands. It was very uncommercial and didn't feature a big advertiser's collection piece. I think that it was David's first cover too. When I saw him at a party soon after it came out, and although it was only my eyes that featured, he kept calling out during the evening, 'Hey that's my cover girl!' He was so happy with it.

Simon Ringrose, model:

My sister Claire was based in London and had been modelling for eighteen months or so, working in Tokyo and Australia and doing really well. I was working as a trainee forester, which I enjoyed as I loved climbing trees and hanging out in the countryside having bonfires – a real country boy at heart (I still am). I always knew my future lay in the natural world but I was curious to see the other side of the coin – city life, the bright lights, great night clubs, the glamour and art – so I immersed myself in '80s London and loved it.

Pam Hogg

We introduced this feature to package and promote emerging designer talent. As people were interested in the person behind the clothes, we also included a short Q&A interview to provide a little background. Pam was as colourful as her pattern and print (she had studied textiles in Glasgow and at the RCA) and her bright orange hair (now yellow) made her a wonderful portrait. Oddly, Peter and I decided to print the pictures in black and white. During my research I found a colour Polaroid, so we must have shot some colour film.

Photographer: Peter Brown

Models: Astrid at Premier, Pam Hogg

Make-up: Debbie Bunn represented by Lynne Franks

Clothes: Pam Hogg

Peter Brown, photographer:
We used to love the shapes. So we made Astrid do shapes. She was so androgynous. It could be a guy, couldn't it, really? There is a certain sort of drag aspect too. This was pure Hollywood lighting. I blinded many a model. I don't know how many models' retinas I ruined? 'Stare into the light!' It made you look flawless, which was the aim. Pam does look amazing. She almost eclipses Astrid in that picture, doesn't she?

I was always so critical of myself, I still am, but in those days it was never good enough. Now I realise it actually wasn't too bad. If you are never satisfied, you always strive to do better. We set ourselves such high standards. We were very driven and nothing was ever good enough, and I think all of us were a bit like that in a way. Everyone had to do better, do better, do better. There was that pursuit of perfection.

Pam Hogg, designer:
I'd been living in a squat just off Queensway in west London for a while, and then discovered a community housing flat in King's Cross one night when I went to record with my band. It was an amazing place called Stanley Buildings, right beside the station. I ended up living there for nineteen years. I'd also just started making mini fashion collections and had a stall in Hyper Hyper in Kensington High Street.

I used to see you at Blitz club every week, you were so beautiful and excitingly aloof, we never spoke but you'd often shoot me a good look. I was quite shy and never spoke to anyone. You all seemed to be in an exclusive bubble that I never dreamed of popping, I just hung on the outskirts and enjoyed the scenery. But we actually met much later.

I was devastated when I was turned down by the management of Hyper Hyper for a place in their fashion show. They announced in the same breath that a team was being brought in to produce the show and would be checking all the stands of the chosen designers. By some miracle, it turned out to be you heading the team, and when you passed my stall you stopped to have a look, wondering why I wasn't on the list. When I explained I'd been rejected, you went straight to the office and demanded that not only should I be in the show, but I should have the finale. So that's how we eventually met, and you got me that finale.

I knew how great *BLITZ* magazine was. You were excited to turn each page, to see who had made it into the magazine that month, and see who and what was new. I think they stand up well to the best of the magazines out there now. They are still inspirational. Of course, I was really excited when I was asked to do the shoot. I remember anxiously arriving at the green door of the studio like it was yesterday. It was my first ever portrait for a magazine and I was so nervous I blinked constantly as soon as I was placed in front of the camera. Peter was laughing when he showed me the twelve shots he'd taken. My eyes were shut in every single one except the last, but luckily it was the best and everyone loved it. It was so gorgeous I couldn't believe it was me.

It was awesome when the feature was published. I felt I'd finally arrived and was part of something. The collection was actually called Psychedelic Jungle, after the Cramps album. It had that tripped-out hippy feel to it, stretch velvets with silver prints. Maybe that's why you referred to it as 'The Great Big Hippy Trip'.

Debbie Bunn, make-up artist:
Astrid looks amazing but so does Pam. She still looks the same. I did her make-up that day and she didn't normally let anyone else do it. She had her own look and used to do her own make-up. But she liked it, which was nice. Peter liked a strong face light. Black lipstick. 'Less is more' did not apply here.

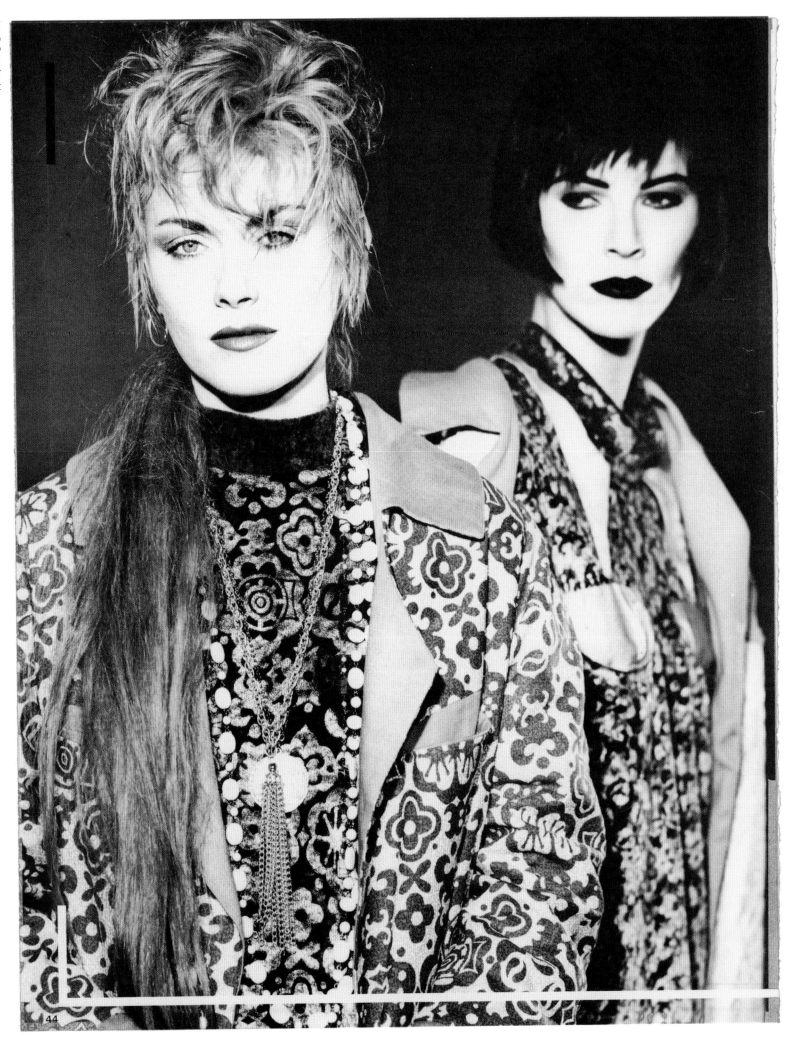

Peter Brown, photographer:
You didn't really know what the actual outcome on film was going to be; it was a whole different thing. The Polaroid was just an indication. Remember we used to take them and cluster around like the three witches in *Macbeth*. But you never knew exactly what you were going to get until you got down to the lab. You could do things with the film and change it, pull it and push it and process it differently and stuff. It made it all rather exciting. There were tragic mistakes, but sometimes the tragic mistake would be good. It happened to me a few times on jobs where I'd have to push the film fifteen stops or so and you'd think 'It's going to be a disaster', but actually it ended up being kind of interesting and everyone loved it. The happy accident doesn't really occur anymore with the digital age because you always know exactly what is going to happen and it's all so controlled.

Barry Kamen, model:
That was early on. It was a Swanky Modes dress. What I like about this shot is that it's completely clean. There's nothing else. That's the styling. That is editing. I remember Rei [Kawakubo] asked Ray [Petri] to help her on one of the Comme des Garçons shows, so he looked at all the outfits and said, 'Everything you are doing is right but get rid of all the shirts. No shirts.' It was a continuous look that went right through the show. It was just one comment.

I never, ever, ever had a problem with being asked to wear weird stuff. I just loved it. I enjoyed the communication that went on. Meeting you, hanging out with you, talking, getting vibed up – it was very relaxed, whether on the pavement, eating a peach wearing found dungarees, a Kenzo boilersuit and a rubber shirt from Stephen Linard or a Swanky Modes dress. It was when I would get a job with Next and I had to put on a nice sweater and shirt and a nice pair of trousers, then I didn't want to be party to it. I had no problem wearing stockings and suspenders or skateboarding down the catwalks for Bodymap. It was being a groom in *Brides* magazine that I found a problem.

Robert Ogilvie, photographer:
He was an amazing model. A Swanky Modes dress? Amazing that he had the confidence to let you do that.

Photographer: Peter Brown

Model: Barry Kamen at Laraine Ashton

Make-up and Hair: William Faulkner

Clothes: Swanky Modes

Tall, dark and handsome

Barry Kamen was the nearest thing *BLITZ* had to a poster boy. I liked his androgynous features, his long/short hairstyle with tumbling curls juxtaposed with a shaven undercut. I wanted the photographs to focus directly on Barry's beauty, an odd new way to look at men, but one with a tradition of adoration that harked back to Michelangelo and David. Peter Brown lit and composed the photographs so that Barry was central to the image. The choice of clothes – long, black and fairly anonymous – did not distract. It was only if you read the credits that you realised that Barry was wearing a dress. This further enhanced the androgynous imagery that was being played with by young London style-setters.

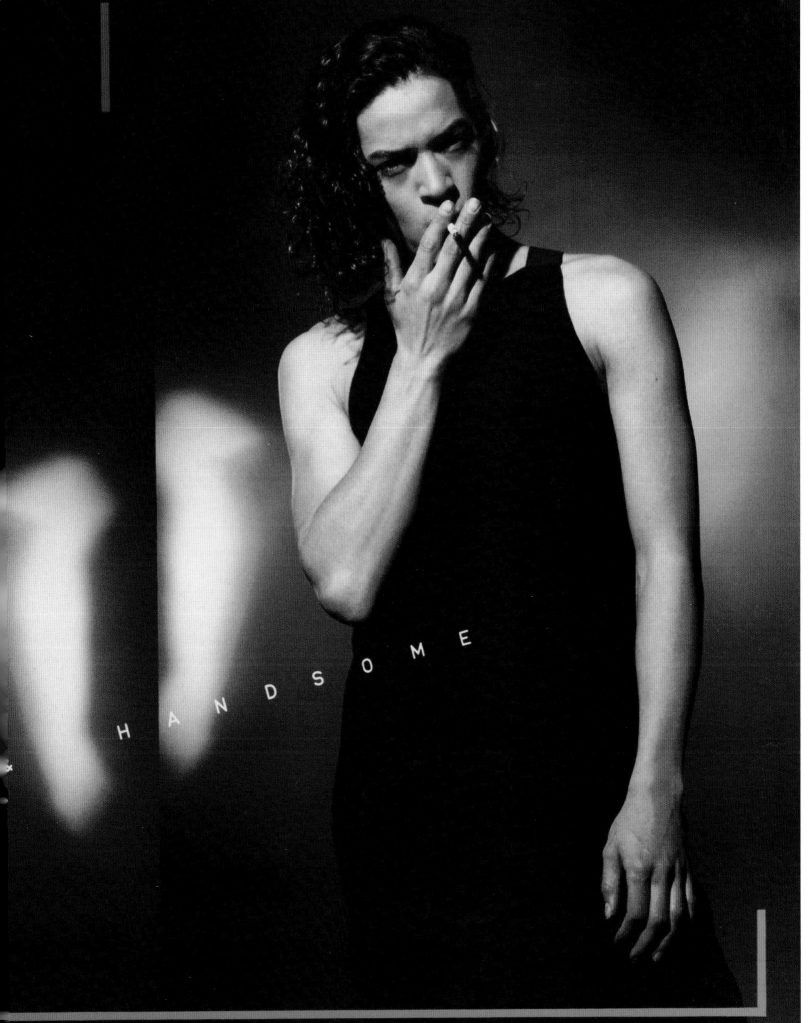

HANDSOME

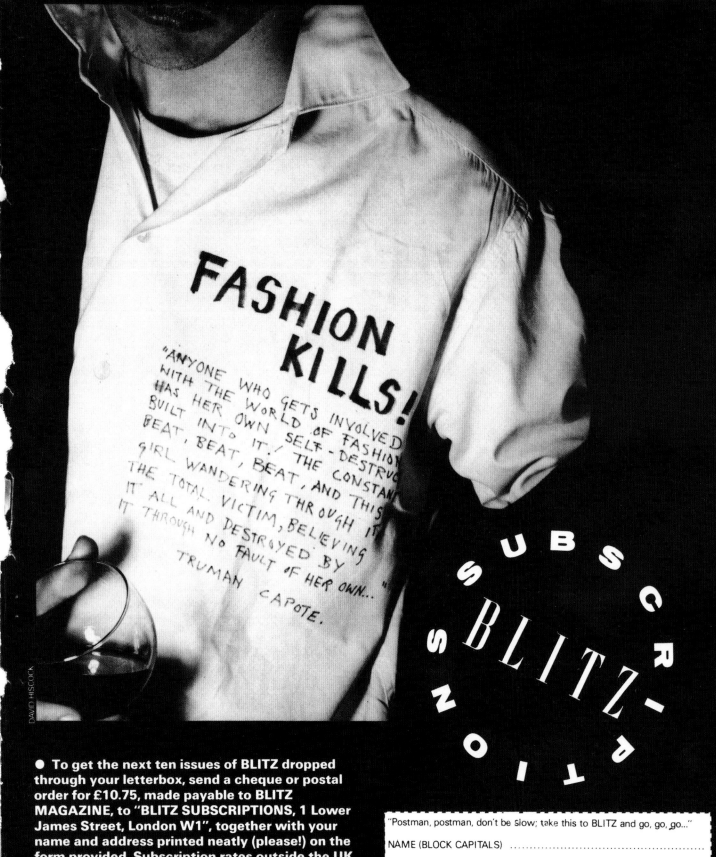

FASHION KILLS!

"ANYONE WHO GETS INVOLVED WITH THE WORLD OF FASHION HAS HER OWN SELF-DESTRUCT BUILT INTO IT./ THE CONSTANT BEAT, BEAT, BEAT, AND THIS GIRL WANDERING THROUGH IT THE TOTAL VICTIM, BELIEVING IT ALL AND DESTROYED BY IT THROUGH NO FAULT OF HER OWN..."

TRUMAN CAPOTE.

DAVID HISCOCK

SUBSCRIPTIONS BLITZ

● **To get the next ten issues of BLITZ dropped through your letterbox, send a cheque or postal order for £10.75, made payable to BLITZ MAGAZINE, to "BLITZ SUBSCRIPTIONS, 1 Lower James Street, London W1", together with your name and address printed neatly (please!) on the form provided. Subscription rates outside the UK are as follows: Europe (surface mail) – £13.50; Outside Europe (airmail only) – £28.00. ALL payments MUST be made in pounds sterling. We recommend international money orders as the simplest method.**

"Postman, postman, don't be slow; take this to BLITZ and go, go, go..."

NAME (BLOCK CAPITALS) ....

ADDRESS ....

.... COUNTRY ....

(If you don't want to cut up the page, apply by letter instead)

BLITZ #31
May 1985

Fashion Kills

I enjoyed writing on my clothes. This was undoubtedly a throwback to punk when, inspired by Westwood and McLaren, The Clash and the like, I merrily stencilled and felt-tipped provocative messages over anything at hand. I have enjoyed an odd relationship with fashion; it has been my undying driving force, yet often I have wished not to be in its grasp. I adore it, and it has afforded me a rich, wonderful life; yet its shallow and cynical constituent appalls me. Fashion is a creative industry peopled by flocks of sheep. I think I was having a bad day when I scrawled this quote onto my white shirt (an Oxfam shop classic). Truman Capote's words refer specifically to Edie Sedgwick but they are relevant to every last woman or man involved in the industry. Don't be fooled by the glitter, don't be this year's thing! I wore the shirt to the launch party for London Fashion Week. This image was recreated in the studio. About a month after the image appeared, I attended the Pitti Trend fair in Florence and was surprised to find a designer sporting a white shirt bearing the same printed message. I was even more shocked to discover a rip-off T-shirt emblazoned with the words in the window of a Carnaby Street tourist emporium. Fashion, huh?

Photographer: David Hiscock

Model: Iain R. Webb

Stefano Tonchi, journalist:
In the 1980s, London was the point of reference for anyone working in music, design and fashion. London had a creative energy that you wanted to be a part of. Fashion was no longer fashionable. A new kind of fashion was christened Style, and this was a new category used to describe many areas of the creative arts that came together. Music dictated a lot of the emerging trends, and there was a lot of experimentation in both photography and graphic design. But fashion was the area where these exciting changes were most evident. Think of the Bodymap shows – they weren't just about the clothes, but involved music, graphic design and theatre.

And that's what brought you and me together. We were both operating in the same world, in this new area that offered a multi-sensorial kind of experience. This was not like the fashion experience we had known before. It was a new way of thinking about fashion.

When I came to London, I gravitated to the world you inhabited, and I wanted to share those ideas and bring them back to Italy, which was yet to experience these kinds of adventures. We had a lot of friends in common so there was immediately an interesting connection.

In Florence there was Pitti, which was a trade fair organisation that offered a platform to promote Italian fashion. They had a lot of money and set up a fair that featured classic and contemporary menswear. We were given money to finance a new project, Pitti Trend, a young fair for young designers showcasing this new energy. They let us spend the money how we liked, so we invited people like you to see what was happening in Florence. It was an interesting way to reinvest in the talent. I think this new, open-minded approach brought you closer to Florence. I don't think you would have developed the same personal relationships in Milan.

David Holah and Stevie Stewart, designers, Bodymap:

DH _ The style mavericks that people hark back to – Leigh, Trojan, Mark Vaultier – wore outrageous looks. I used to wear skin-tight leggings, a skirt over the top and then something else I found somewhere over that. We weren't putting a fashion look together; we were putting a *look* together. That definitely came from punk. The idea that you can create your own look.

SS _ When we showed our first collection in the Individual Clothes Show, we were proud to be English and individuals. *BLITZ*, *i-D* and *The Face* promoted young people to be individuals.

DH _ Now it's about having sex. In those days you didn't think, 'I need to look sexy'. Back then it was a freak show, totally. It wasn't following fashion; it was about style. You'd put your look on and go anywhere.

SS _ People would stare at us whatever.

Princess Julia, model:
We were aiming to make something lasting. We were all living in a precarious way, weren't we? So it felt like, well, it's not strictly fashion, but it is. We didn't want to be the mainstream and we're still like that, aren't we? The things we were doing were bound up with the people that we were. I was super-snobbish. I still am a bit, but not in a negative way. I was very definite about what I liked and what I didn't like or what worked and what didn't work, but also being able to stand outside and say well, 'I didn't think that would work but it did', or vice versa. We had the privilege of being able to experiment and put slogans, ideas, images out there, and that's why these magazines were so important and pivotal in creating a platform for this prevailing attitude.

BLITZ #34
September 1985

Amanda Cazalet, model:
I was quite new to London. I had moved into Phoenix House, behind Euston, a massive squat inhabited by all sorts of creative people: musicians, photographers, Tom Dixon was there, stylist Mitzi Lorenz and make-up artist Kay Montana. Mitzi was going out with Jamie Morgan, and his assistant was Monica Curtin. Mitzi suggested I did a test shot with Monica, and we might be able to get it in *BLITZ*. It was a magazine that perfectly captured where we were at; it was different and had a new voice. It presented fashion and ideas in a new way. I was seventeen. It was a perfect medium for me and my mates. It was exciting to be part of it. When I came into modelling I didn't look like most of the models. There was this alternative culture blossoming that was challenging accepted ideas of beauty. The fashion was outspoken. It made a point about awareness, choice and possibilities. It was all very left-of-centre, which is very me, so I loved it. I had a very radical hairstyle. I was happy to be accepted looking like that. I found the styling and the clothes very enticing and very exciting. I enjoyed the sense of experimentation that the *BLITZ* team engendered, using fashion to get a message across, like Katharine Hamnett and her T-shirts. It was vanguard imagery that highlighted issues such as the superficiality of fashion and conscious consumerism. There was humour too. I am proud to have been involved in the pushing of ideas, boundaries and attitudes, and challenging accepted concepts.

Photographer: David Hiscock

Model: Amanda Cazalet at Marco Rasala

Fashion Kills

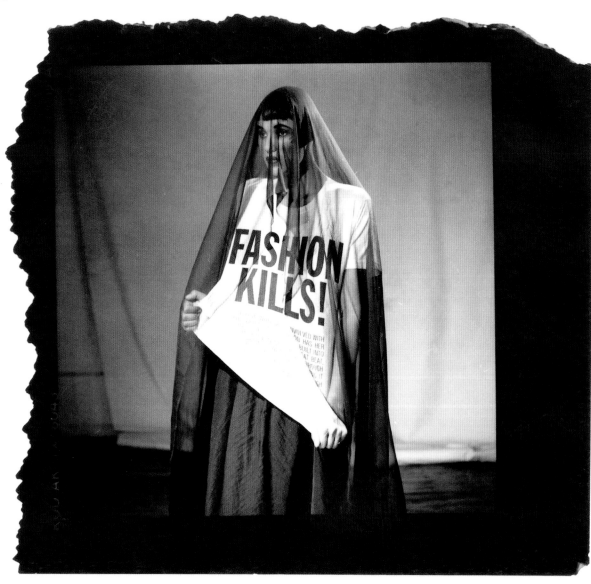

**Paul Bernstock and
Thelma Speirs, designers,
Bernstock Speirs:**
Your work was particularly
interesting because of your breadth
of knowledge and interest in fashion,
from the most rarefied to the street.
Your pages mixed and celebrated
both, in a way that was fresh and
provocative. One of our favourite
images was when you showed our
red silk slip dress with huge crushed
Coke can earrings. We loved the
mix of pop, trash and glamour.

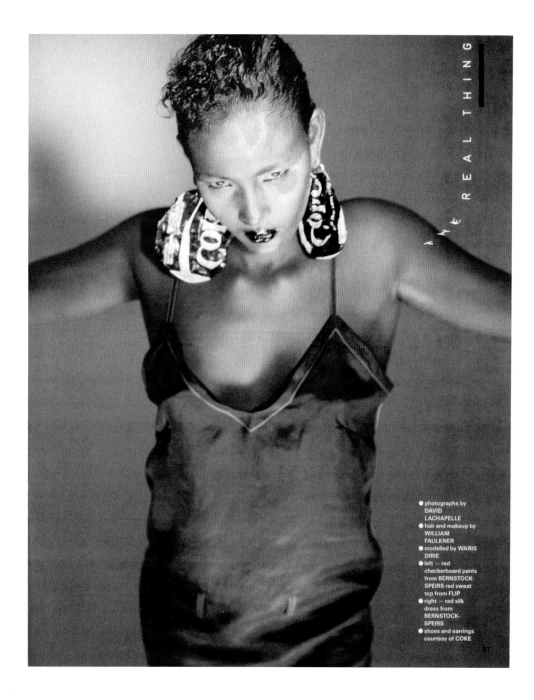

THE REAL THING

● photographs by
DAVID
LACHAPELLE
● hair and makeup by
WILLIAM
FAULKNER
● modelled by WARIS
DIRIE
● left — red
checkerboard pants
from BERNSTOCK-
SPEIRS red sweat
top from FLIP
● right — red silk
dress from
BERNSTOCK-
SPEIRS
● shoes and earrings
courtesy of COKE

The Real Thing

Another recurring theme that interested me was the way
in which big companies were making a march across the
world. I guess these were the first inklings of global branding.
African toys made from discarded tin cans also intrigued
me. I loved the inherent resourcefulness and creativity
expressed by the makers who, without very much, could
fashion something so precious. I liked how they would often
pose proudly with their logo-covered belongings. So, why
not jewellery or shoes? Waris had just arrived in the UK. She
reminded me of Iman. She went on to become a Bond girl
and a human rights campaigner. The clothes were all red,
emphasising the Coke brand. I crushed a can and attached
an earring fitting. For another picture, I made shoes using
strips of jersey cut from a T-shirt tied around her feet.
Waris balanced on the cans so they looked like eccentric
platforms. David decided to use that picture upside down.

Photographer: David LaChapelle

Model: Waris Dirie

Make-up and Hair:
William Faulkner

Clothes: Bernstock Speirs, Coke

Luisa Via Roma

Because the imagery we created in *BLITZ* was causing something of a stir, there were often industry clients that wanted to get the *BLITZ* look for their catwalk or advertising campaign. Luisa was a store in Italy that was heavily buying into the exciting new London labels. This shoot, for a promotional brochure, was organised by fashion consultant and stylish muse, Victoria Fernandez. The team consisted of A-list *BLITZ* regulars: Peter, Martine, Astrid, Carol and James (who, as usual, managed to muscle in to several shots thanks to his devilishly handsome looks). We shot over a weekend, and the results were stylishly provocative: I veiled Martine and Astrid in wafting black chiffon that was part ethereal, part Arab. The shoot threatened to spiral into mayhem when several of the team decided to trip out on hallucinogenic drugs. But we got fab pictures, and the production of the brochure was of the highest quality.

Photographer: Peter Brown

Model: Martine Houghton
at Marco Rasala

Make-up: Carol Langbridge
(now Carol Brown)

Hair: James Lebon

Clothes: Tom Binns

Peter Brown, photographer:
This shoot was a celebration of London style, so we shot it on the bridges down the Thames. Martine summed up the mid-1980s like Twiggy had summed up the sixties. She is pure androgyny and walked the runways as a girl and a boy. Now that Polish boy, Andrej Pejic, is bringing it all back, walking the runway as a boy and a girl. We were strung out on MDMA for the entire shoot.

Carol Brown, make-up artist:
Perceptions of beauty were being challenged, boundaries pushed. Sometimes the models were extraordinary and fabulous and a pleasure to work with, sometimes just strange. There were so many times I turned up for the shoot and asked, 'What do you do?', thinking that they might be the stylist's assistant, to find out that they were the model for the day. It was a very transient time for most, but the opportunity was available to the strong and the wrong; anything but bland. I loved that Martine had quite masculine, almost straight, eyebrows. I would exaggerate them into solid black rectangles and they just got bigger and bigger.

Martine Houghton, model:
When I was about fourteen, my sister Caroline was already living in London with her friend Hilde Smith, who did textile prints for Bodymap. I was still at school and was very bookish but they said I could be a model so I thought, 'Oh, alright!' I was living in Royston and Caroline and Hilde were living a certain way, dressing a certain way, that seemed very exciting. So I assisted Hilde, which was really just a way to get to London. Through Hilde I met David Holah (one half of Bodymap) and he said, "Yeah, be a model". They took me to the Marco Rasala agency. I guess I thought, 'If I don't do it I'll regret it.'

I didn't really like modelling. It was often painful. The 'Luisa Via Roma' shoot was extremely bonkers. Everyone was acting mental. I was like, 'What am I doing here?' Following the shoot, I was inter-railing around Italy and showed up in Florence and … 'Ooh, that's me!' I was in my tracksuit and there were these glam pictures of me everywhere. Very odd. Very funny. I got a bit scared. It was relentless.

Sam Brown, photographer:
While I was digging around in the loft, the best pictures I found, and the best memories for me of back then, were definitely of Martine and Amanda [Cazalet]. Their old agency, Marco Rasala, was tremendously influential. Visiting their office was like a trip into ancient Greece. People mocked them, but they discovered a lot of good models.

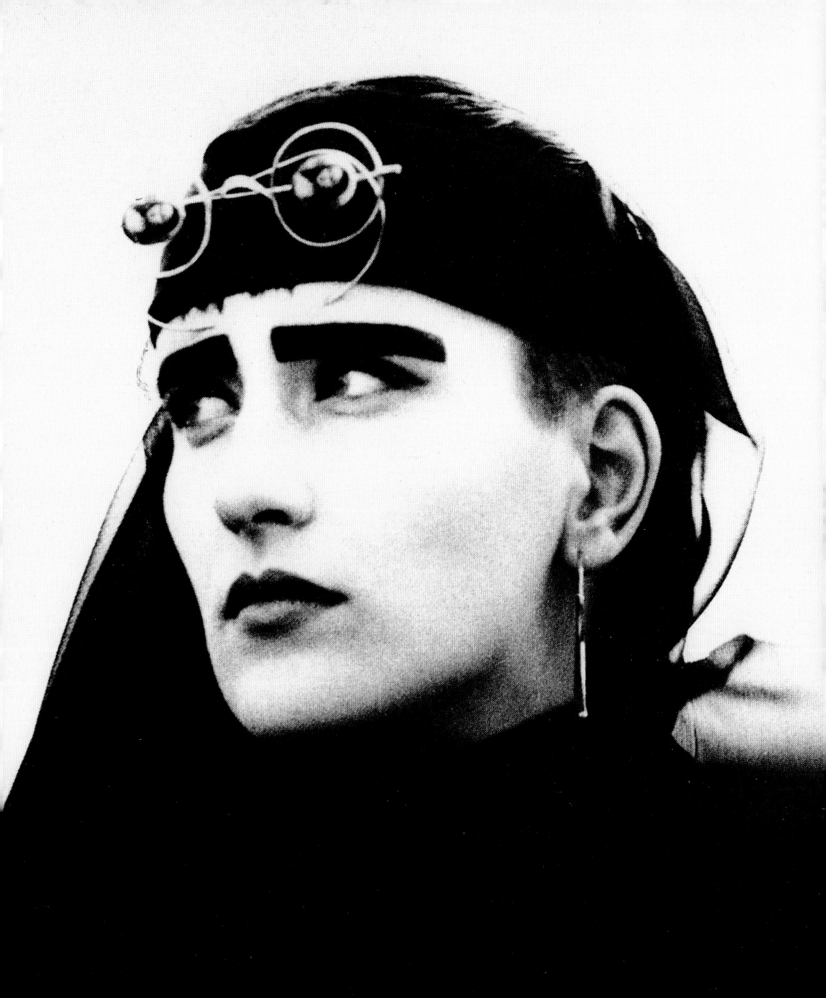

The personal style of textile designer Hilde and Caroline (designer, fledgling DJ and sister of Martine) was a combination of tradition, exoticism and urban references. It was so outside the mainstream that they even got taunted in gay clubs. At one point they both cut their hair into radical identikit Henry V bobs. I wanted to style and photograph them to emphasise this double vision. I put them in almost identical outfits: checkered jackets (one by the classic house, David Hicks, that Caroline designed for, and the other a bondage jacket from BOY) and George Michael T-shirts. In the magazine, the images were used much smaller than I would have liked and overprinted with graphics, but this portrait has had a life beyond the shoot, becoming the cover of the *BLITZ Exposure!* book and a poster. In January 2011, I was tipped off that a story in Italian *Vogue* by Steven Meisel shared a striking resemblance to this look.

Body double

Photographer: Pete Moss

Models: Hilde Smith, Caroline Houghton

Make-up and Hair:
William Faulkner

Clothes: David Hicks, BOY

Pete Moss, photographer:
I was sharing a house in Richmond with two other photographers [Nick Knight and Richard Croft] after leaving Bournemouth College of Art in 1985. One of them was going out with Hellen Campbell, who was your assistant, and she was looking for photographers to work with, so I did a shoot with her. It wasn't great but somehow it got printed. I came into the tiny offices in Golden Square to drop the prints off, and had my portfolio with me. You looked at it and then somehow we started working.

I was trying to work out how to become a photographer without having to assist some awful advertising photographer full time. I was saying yes to every job, from photographing staircases for an engineering company, to weddings for friends of friends. I was hanging out with musicians and had started to get a few record company press office commissions from labels like Stiff Records, Rough Trade and Mike Alway's El Records. I was getting a few extras parts in pop videos, signing on and existing on air. I was certainly very thin and had a fair old hair gel habit as well.

This was shot at Marden Hill, the house in north London where my friends Mark Daniels and Matt Lipsey were brought up, and close to where I used to live, so it was a familiar location. It was a warm evening and we had as much time as we wanted, which was lucky, as the 'identical twin' make-up that looked totally amazing seemed to take forever. I was using a long exposure technique so Caroline and Hilde had to stand very still for a minute or longer. On one of the shots, I placed a hand flash right above the lens on the camera, as the light was too low to see anything, and over-exposed to really burn all the information onto the film. It was a bit of an accident really, and pulled right out of the air, but it worked perfectly and created one of the best shots I think we ever did. The use of the George Michael T-shirts was quite inspired. It's my favourite shoot without a doubt. It was the start of a whole new direction for me.

Martine Houghton, model:
We all lived together at Anson House in Islington – Caroline, Hilde, Thelma [Speirs, of Bernstock Speirs] and me. It was very creative environment. The Anson Girls were a hub of creativity. Being that much younger, I was very much inspired by all the people around me. I think for the most part we were oblivious to the real world. I can't remember what the real world was like; there were a lot of us and that was our world. Thank God there were these magazines to justify our choices.

Jeremy Leslie, *BLITZ* art director:
On the whole, I think we ran our own little departments and had a slightly begrudging respect for each other's work. I wanted to decorate the fashion pages, you wanted to keep them simple – the usual art/editorial wrangle. You were right, of course. You had a strong grasp of magazine fashion history.

L to R: Hilde, Caroline

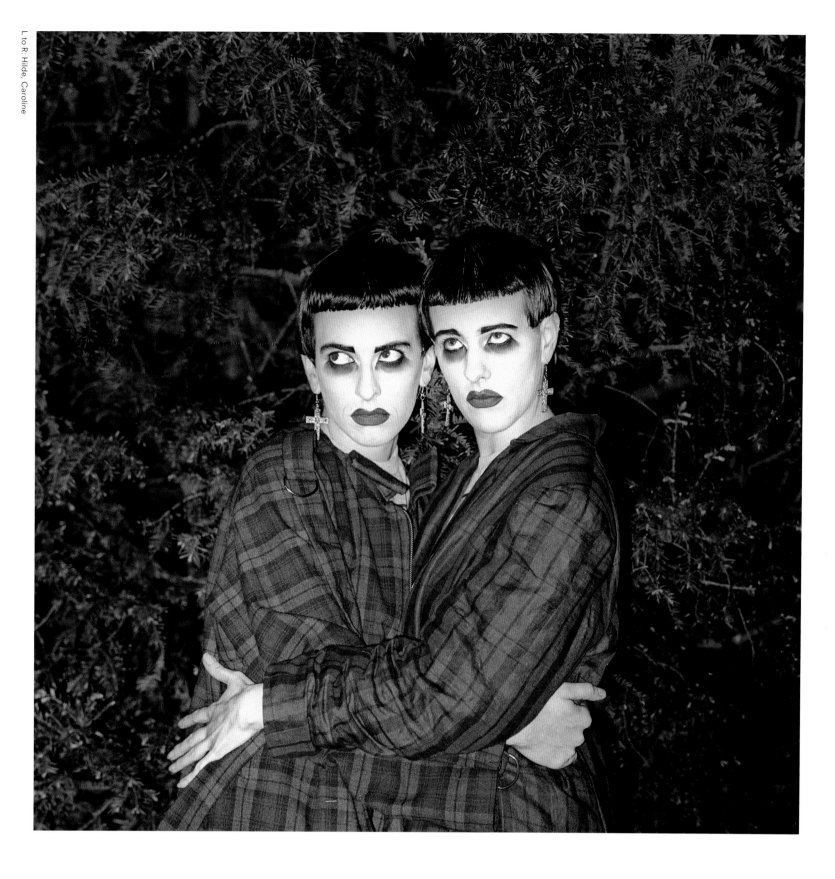

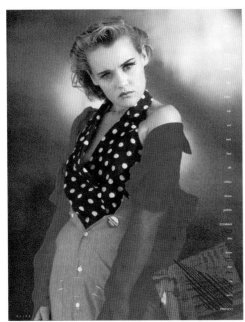

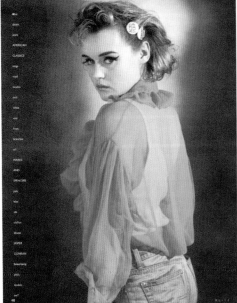

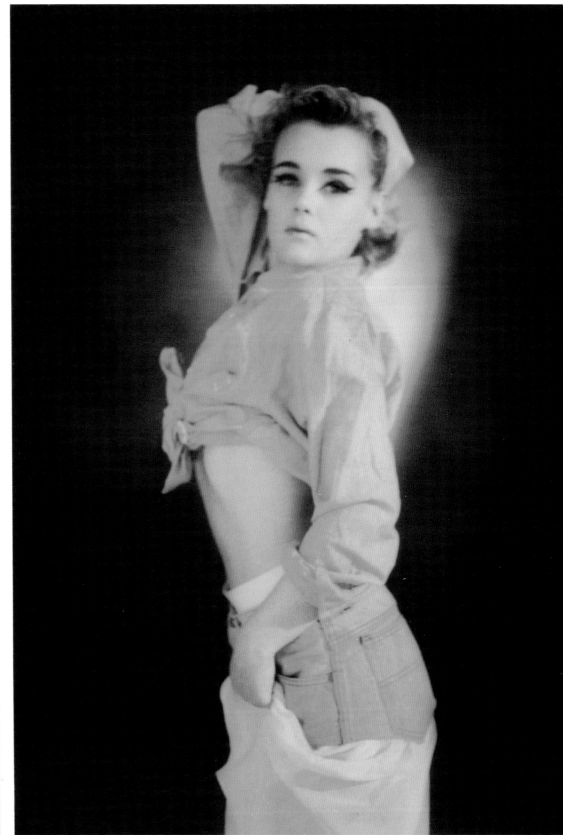

BLITZ #33
July/August 1985

This was an attempt at a more mainstream fashion story. Something like what the trendy girls at *Honey* magazine were doing. Denim was always a favourite. I love how clothes made from it look better the more they are worn and washed. I pulled together some pieces including a battered old jean jacket, and a pair of jeans on their last legs that I cut into a mini-skirt. There was also a much-loved chambray shirt. A lot of the clothes were from my wardrobe or borrowed from friends, along with a couple of sexy sheer shirts by Jasper Conran. I mixed them with pieces of leather. I guess it was a kind of homage to the uniform of the rebel — the styling included badges, one picturing Marlon Brando and another saying ACID PUNK. I knew Sibylle from working with Stephen Jones and John Galliano. I loved her pouty, Monroe/Bardot persona. This was emphasised by Carol's fabulous cat's-eye make-up. Sam was a new young photographer. This was the only shoot we did together for *BLITZ*, but we worked together again when I was fashion editor at *The Times*.

Blue

Photographer: Sam Brown

Model: Sibylle de Saint Phalle

Make-up: Carol Langbridge (now Carol Brown)

Hair: Thomas McKiver

Clothes: Jasper Conran, Fiorucci, American Classics, M&S

Sam Brown, photographer:
At the time I think my best pages were probably from *Honey* magazine, and other things I did with Judith Eagle and Kim Hunt after *Honey* folded. I guess I was doing what every young photographer did at the time – trying to seem busy – although I think I was more 'glass half empty' than some, which really wasn't a good thing. I was testing as often as I could with Carol and Thomas. Getting on in work was a big part of my life. It was the '80s, so you had to have your Comme outfit, a flat and a GTi. My urge to go clubbing had dried up a bit by the time we worked together.

I enjoyed doing the job. I did want to photograph Sibylle in a warm colour, not blue, but really didn't mind either way because it was always about trying something different, especially in an editorial. I was always too introverted, especially when I cared about the pictures. I remember Thomas sidled up to me and said something about giving you the impression that I was unhappy, while really I was just fretting about the end result as usual. I don't remember if you had worked with Carol and Thomas much before, but I always tried to book them because I liked what they did. I knew they could add something extra and also tell me I was crap if necessary. I really liked the looks you put together, but I look at photographs from then and wish I could go back and do them again.

Carol Brown, make-up artist:
We took the black eyeliner from discreet 1950s elegance and sixties cat eyes, and used it in a raw, tougher, exaggerated way. The studio that we used is now a block of flats. Sam and I had our wedding reception in there and Jane Packer did the flowers *à la* Miss Havisham's room.

Sibylle de Saint Phalle, model:
What I remember most about the *BLITZ* magazine experience was the freedom. It was like another planet, how free we were. There were no boundaries, no obligations. You could do whatever you wanted to do. The image was the most important thing. It was all about the image. It was never about the labels, or who would wear what. Now, even the new young hip magazines are restricted by having to feature a certain number of advertisers. It's no fun anymore, if you have to feature what someone else is telling you to use. There is no point, when you are asked to use clothes that will ruin your story. This shoot was back in the good old days when you could cut up a sample, but more than likely it wasn't even a sample; it was probably something from a flea market or an Oxfam shop. We tend to forget how much we lived in a world with such a rich creative freedom. That will probably never happen again. And we always, always managed to have a laugh as well, whatever the situation. We didn't have money but we managed to carry on living and make amazing images, whether it was for fashion shoots or to go to Taboo.

Jasper Conran, designer:
It was exciting because you were doing the same with Jean [Muir] and Rifat [Ozbek] and me, so it was right across the board. What you did was heaven. Even though it might have looked crazy, you were still very respectful in that you knew what you were doing – and anyway, you knew that whatever you did I would have loved it. Like how you photographed those chiffon blouses. I remember showing them over black bras so it was supposed to be a bit trashy. You got that. Not many people did.

Beholders of Beauty

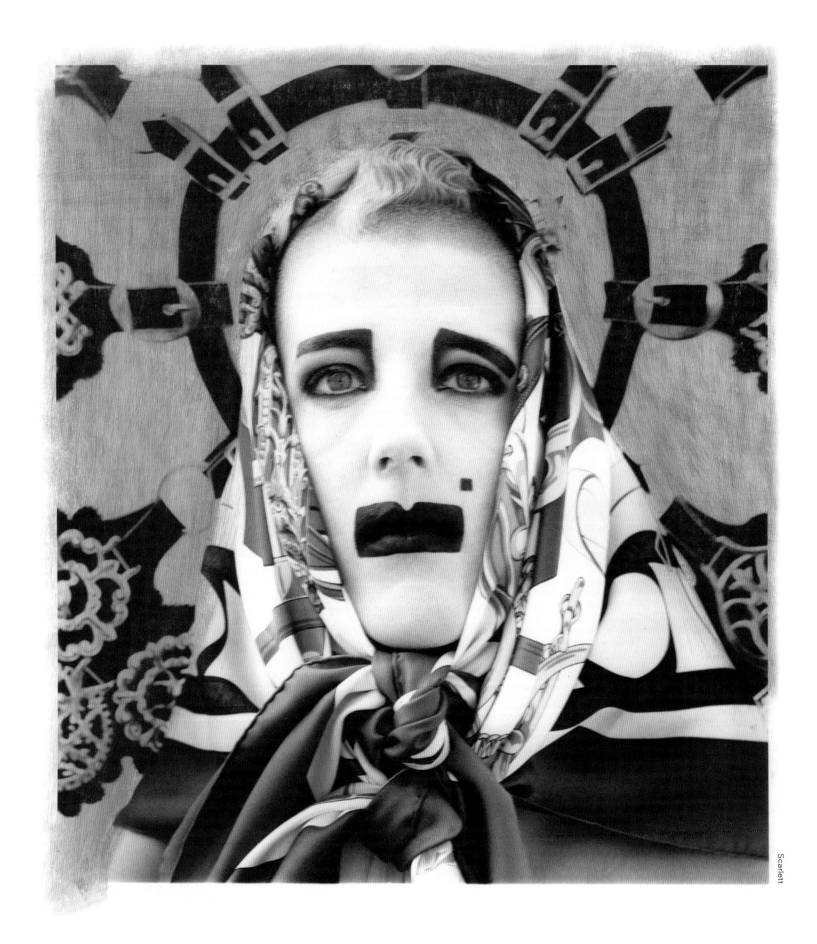

Scarlett

David Hiscock, photographer:
Because I wasn't very good at printing in the dark room and couldn't burn the background, I just used pencil or ink. The process was very uncontrived. The photo of Scarlett was taken outside on the fire escape, with the scarf held up behind her. It would be interesting to see the contact sheet, because there was probably only one picture where it was central. I don't think we were looking for that halo effect, but we had all done our art history, so it was maybe an innate thing to do, not a conscious thing. Maybe that's what makes strong images. I hate images when you are force-fed the idea.

The starting point for this story was a scathing attack in one of the daily newspapers on the new breed of 'ugly' models. This shoot was a celebration of the quirky and individual, the alternative and different. It was a flag-waver for the ethos of the magazine. I picked models who had the kind of looks that had confused the fashion hack and provoked the diatribe. I found their strong features and gender confusion inspirational and to be applauded. The session took place over several days in July, and produced one of the most iconic *BLITZ* images: Scarlett wearing Hermès headscarves. A subversion of the conservative. It could be my calling card.

Photographer: David Hiscock

Models: Amanda Cazalet at Marco Rasala, Chris Hall at 7, Barry Kamen at Laraine Ashton, Scarlett Cannon

Make-up and Hair:
William Faulkner

Clothes: Hermès, Kenzo, Stephen Linard, Jasper Conran, Norma Kamali, Jean Paul Gaultier, Mark & Syrie

Scarlett Cannon, model:
This is my all-time favourite picture. It was the day of Live Aid and it was roasting hot. We were in a warehouse studio and all the windows were open, and I remember us all rushing over to the television when Paul Weller came on.

When the make-up was being done I remember thinking, 'I LOVE THIS!'

The thing I loved most was that it was an Hermès headscarf. This was our take on Thatcher and Sloane Rangers. It's such a classic. An Hermès headscarf was something out of most people's reach. It was quite an old lady look, which I've always been a huge fan of, especially when you're very young. What a glorious thing to be wearing an Hermès headscarf and you're only twenty-two. This was right up my street. I wish I'd known they had that picture of me in the boardroom, I'd have pitched up and been on the blag for sure.

My hair was shaved and Marcel-waved by Ross Cannon, who was an absolute genius. It was permed and then set with fingers, clips, boiled sugar and water. I wanted to look like a black and white photograph, something I strove at for years. There were lots of references here, from Josephine Baker to Jean Harlow to punk Jordan. In 1985 I was still modelling, off to Japan. I wasn't doing clubs, but I did occasional one-off parties. It was quite a good time for modelling because people didn't mind a bit of weird!

Amanda Cazalet, model:
In the early days, I would go to see photographers on castings and people would ask, 'Are you a model?' It was embarrassing. It was very exciting to be around people who weren't into the normal idea of beauty. Your pictures presented a new way of observing this. This new movement generated by people like you became big business and people really bought into it. It changed the world, changed attitudes. It was really important to be involved. From that opportunity, I went on to do very well.

I felt very safe on the shoots. Throughout my life, I'd always felt like an outsider. My family had moved a lot and my childhood was pretty turbulent. Doing this, I felt wanted and embraced. We had loads of fun and were too drunk sometimes, but it was a very nurturing environment. It felt good to be part of something new and different. It was a new way of looking at life, engaging with life. It was like a whole new world. *BLITZ* made me feel like I had come home. It felt like family. The work you were doing was really powerful in giving us misfits and vagabonds a home.

Barry Kamen, model:
I used to work in Stanley Adams in Kingly Street, just off Carnaby Street, and Ray [Petri] came in and asked me if I wanted to do a casting for Levi's. I said I couldn't, but told him about my brother Nick, who was a model at Gavin Robinson. And then I was at college, and Nick phoned me up one day and said, "Ray wants to do a picture of you for a magazine called The Face." It was Kay Montana's very first shoot, Susie Bick's first shoot. It was all sportswear, and that was the first *Face*/Buffalo shoot, although it wasn't called Buffalo at that time. Then I got a phone call from David and Stevie of Bodymap, and another from you, so immediately I started working with you. Then Ray didn't want to use me anymore because I had long hair, so I just kept working with you.

My agent, Sarah Doukas, was totally into what we were doing, as she knew that I'd never make any money. She'd say, 'Brown boys don't make money'. But she loved that I'd work with Gaultier, go to Japan or have pictures in *BLITZ*. I was earning just enough to keep going. Sarah knew that if I kept doing stuff like this, then the agency looked cool. It wasn't about the money. The point was making the pictures. And to be honest, it still is.

Barry

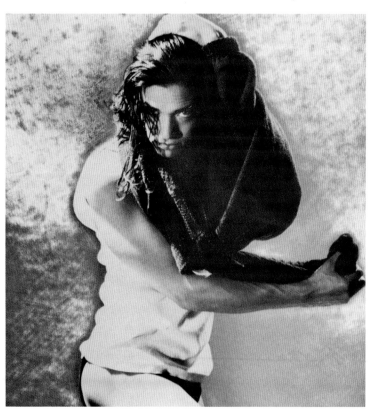

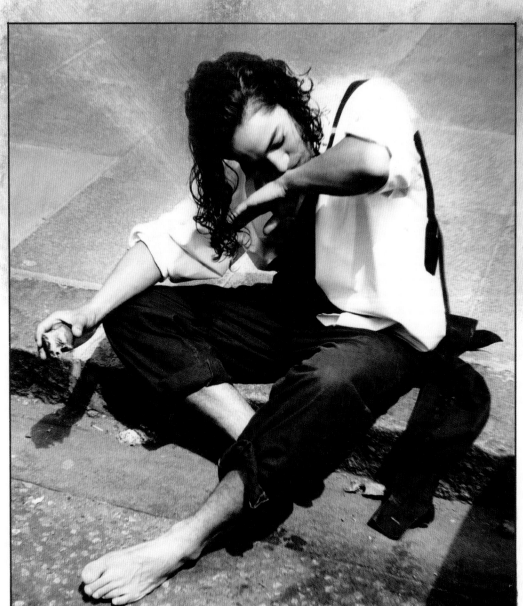

Barry

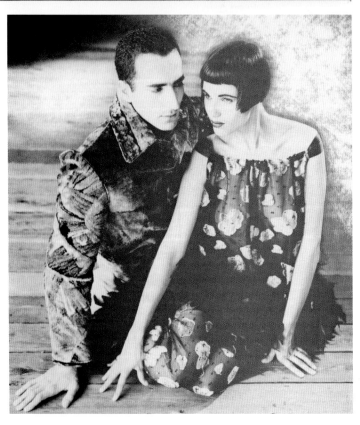

Chris, Amanda

L to R: Simon, Martine

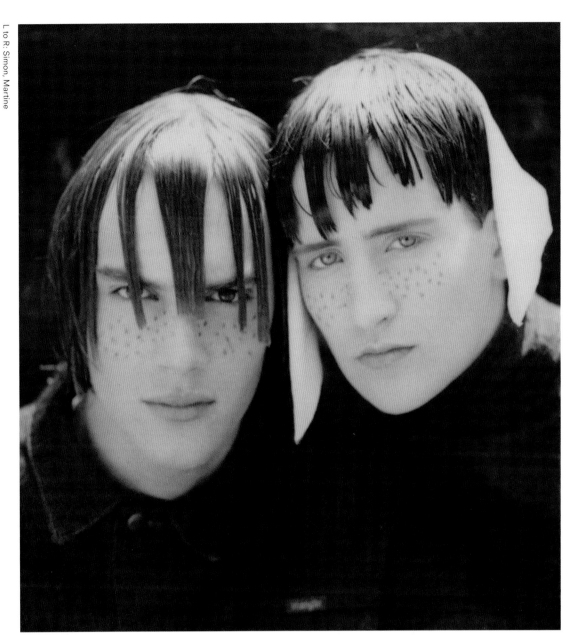

Peter Brown, photographer:
This is such a beautiful image, isn't it? Martine looks at her most beautiful here, as pure as possible. It's one of her best ever pictures. Simon too. They did work so well together. Exquisite beauty. And are they two boys or are they two girls? It is a stunner, and you could put that on the cover of Italian *Vogue* today and it would hold. They were stood on the river wall. I had a thing about shooting by the river. The wide open spaces. The light. But it's pretty far removed from Amish. If you showed it to any Amish person they'd be like, 'What the hell?' But, I know what you were meaning.

Simon Ringrose, model:
Ziggi, my agent, loved them. This picture is my favourite. It's Pete Brown and Martine, and the natural light is fantastic. It was always so much nicer for me to be working outside. Martine looks fab, and the backdrop of the long shot featured one of my favourite trees, the London plane.

Martine Houghton, model:
I didn't feel that what we were doing was cool. It was all a bit more goofy than that.

Photographer: Peter Brown

Models: Simon Ringrose at Z, Martine Houghton at Marco Rasala

Clothes: Wrangler

A quickie

I loved the film *Witness*. I have always admired the purity and unpretentious practicality of the Amish uniform style of dressing. Their favoured fabrics were functional and hard-wearing, so when I decided to do an Amish shoot it wasn't a surprise that I would use denim in some way. Wrangler kindly supplied me some of their classic denim jackets and jeans, which I naturally customised to achieve my version of an Amish wardrobe. For Simon, I unpicked the inner leg seams of a pair of jeans, added a triangular panel and stitched them onto the bottom of a jean jacket to make a full-length coat. For Martine I made a long skirt from another pair of jeans and then unpicked the crutch of another pair so they could be slipped on like a jacket. We shot just one look, with the pair standing on a wall by the river. Peter was obsessed with the clarity of light these open spaces provided. We also did a beauty shot. With the addition of Nivea-ed hair and highly stylised all-American freckles, they look particularly freaky.

Few stories were ever straightforward. A new retail collective, Hyper Hyper, had opened in Kensington High Street (I had styled their much-hyped catwalk show during London Fashion Week), so I borrowed clothes from the designer concessions. However, instead of just photographing them, I asked top-ranking London designers to do whatever they wanted with them. I guess this was continuing our thing for customisation and pursuit of personal style. Leigh Bowery refused to entertain a harlequin jumpsuit: 'I'm sorry, I racked my brains to make these garments look interesting, something I'd be seen in ... NOTHING WORKED!' He dressed Trojan in his own designs and dumped the jumpsuit on the floor. I don't know how we got away with it?

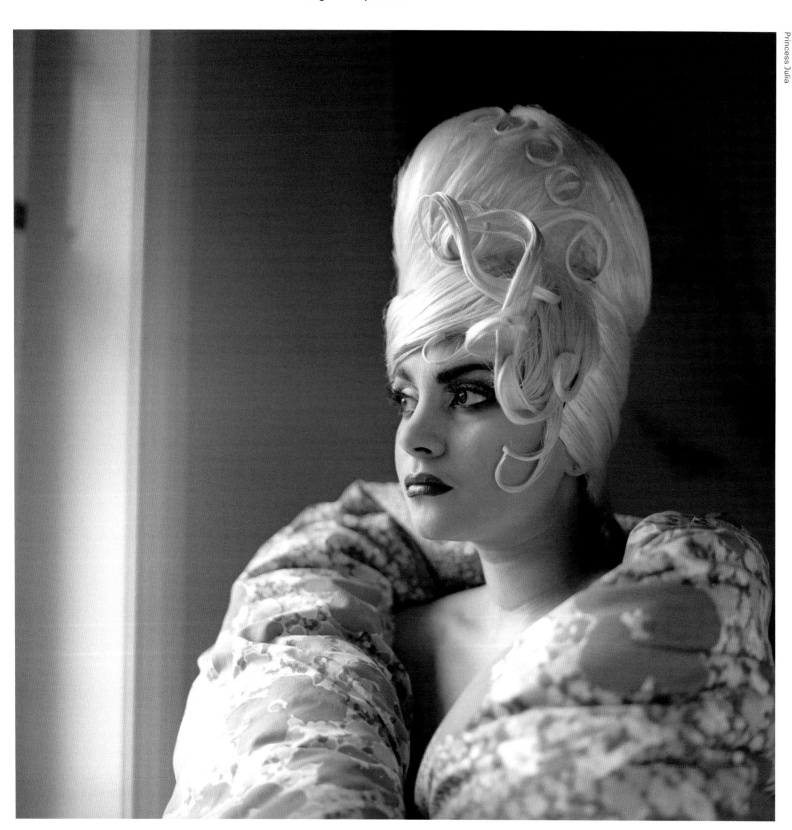

Princess Julia

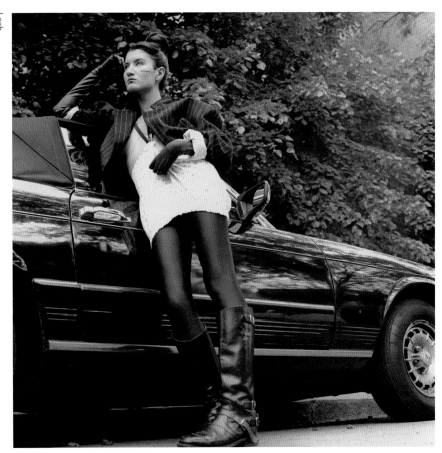

Leah

Maria Cornejo, designer, Richmond Cornejo:
You asked John [Richmond] and I to do a lot of projects. Coming right after punk we thought we could do anything. Now even students have a business plan. Most of the time we were just winging it; everything seemed possible. We were naïve and ignorant, but that was a positive thing. There was no reason not to do things.

We made a pretty cute outfit out of a pair of boxer shorts. It always spurred on new ideas. There was a real playfulness and joy to it. We loved doing things for you. In those days we had time. If you asked me today, I would have a heart attack. We made some special things for Mrs Obama. We made time.

The whole impromptu thing was key to *BLITZ*. It was great being part of something orchestrated by you. The energy was really great and that was you. Your approach was more intellectual. You pulled so many creative people around you. You were surrounded by creativity.

That picture of Leah still looks cool and relevant. When you look back at most fashion magazines, they look like old lady clothes. The pictures you did in *BLITZ* still look edgy. Maybe you were too edgy. Maybe that's why the magazine didn't last. You didn't ever compromise. I'm still a bit too edgy for *Vogue*. It is what we are.

Photographer: Pete Moss

Models: Leah at Z, Princess Julia, Darryl Black, Trojan

Make-up: Audrey Maxwell at Creative Workforce (Leah), Leigh Bowery (Trojan)

Hair: Thomas at Daniel Galvin (Leah/Darryl)

Clothes: Richmond Cornejo, Bernstock Speirs, Leigh Bowery, Stephen Jones, Hyper Hyper, M&S, Lewis Leathers

Pete Moss, photographer:
This was a hilarious shoot. John Galliano got the wrong address and spent an hour sitting in the reception of the old people's home opposite my flat.

Stephen Jones, milliner:
That wig was candyfloss pink. Marie Antoinette meets Wilma Flintstone meets Jayne Mansfield. I remember Julia loving it. I think it's totally bonkers but it was right for the client. Did you credit the duvet? It's so funny, because a year afterwards I did a show in New York at The Palladium, and for the final scene they were all naked with duvets wrapped around them. *BLITZ* was important so that people out in the middle of nowhere might think, 'Yes, I'm a freak but there are other people like me. My God, she's got a pink Marie Antoinette wig on!'

Princess Julia, model:
This wasn't a very structured a day. The duvet wasn't intended to be in the shoot. It was just lying around. It was totally spontaneous but it really works. It was the ultimate DIY. I just turned up, did my own make-up. You had a few key things and no choice. That's why I like working with you because you know what you want to do but you're spontaneous as well. It's that element of experimentation. It could be a still from a Garbo film or a John Waters film. I'd like to get a print please.

Leah Seresin, model:
We did this shoot at the photographer's flat and people were coming and going all day. I was impressed by what Maria and John had done. They were very sweet, but all the designers seemed really nice. There was a huge sense of camaraderie and support, especially with *BLITZ*. I never felt intimidated. I felt totally secure and part of a team. I wasn't just a dumb model. I felt very looked after. When I did tests, often I would find myself stuck in the middle of nowhere and feel vulnerable. I never felt like that with you. Sometimes the shoots were a bit gung-ho and made up as you went along, but you see that in the pictures. It wasn't precious. There was never any sense that there were things we couldn't do.

Uptown goes Downtown

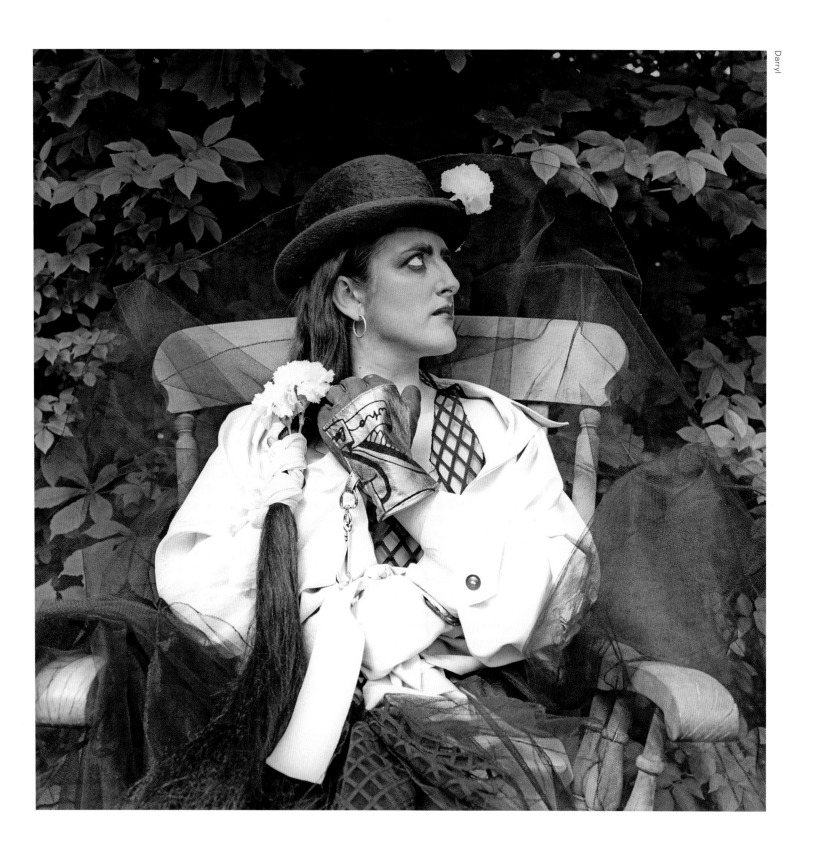

Darryl

Darryl Black, fashion assistant:
That's scary. That was in the garden at Lyndhurst Gardens. I've still got that hat. I left Middlesex Polytechnic in 1984 and then worked for Bodymap, and then with Paul and Thelma [Bernstock Speirs], and that's when I met you. I remember you coming into their studio with your page proofs and you were all excited and I think I just got off on your passion. It was like stars in my eyes. I want to do that. That looks like fun. I didn't know what to expect. And when I got to work for you, it was like getting a little doorway into your crazy mind. There was a crossover when I was working for Paul and Thelma for a pittance, and for you for nothing. But that's what you did.

Paul Bernstock and Thelma Speirs, designers, Bernstock Speirs:
Our first assistant was Darryl Black, who had been in the year below us at Middlesex. Darryl had great style and a similar sense of fun. She became an important collaborator.

Nick Knight, photographer:
You cultivated the world that was inhabited by Bodymap, Michael Clark and David LaChapelle. i-D touched on Leigh Bowery but The Face wouldn't ever go there.

Trojan

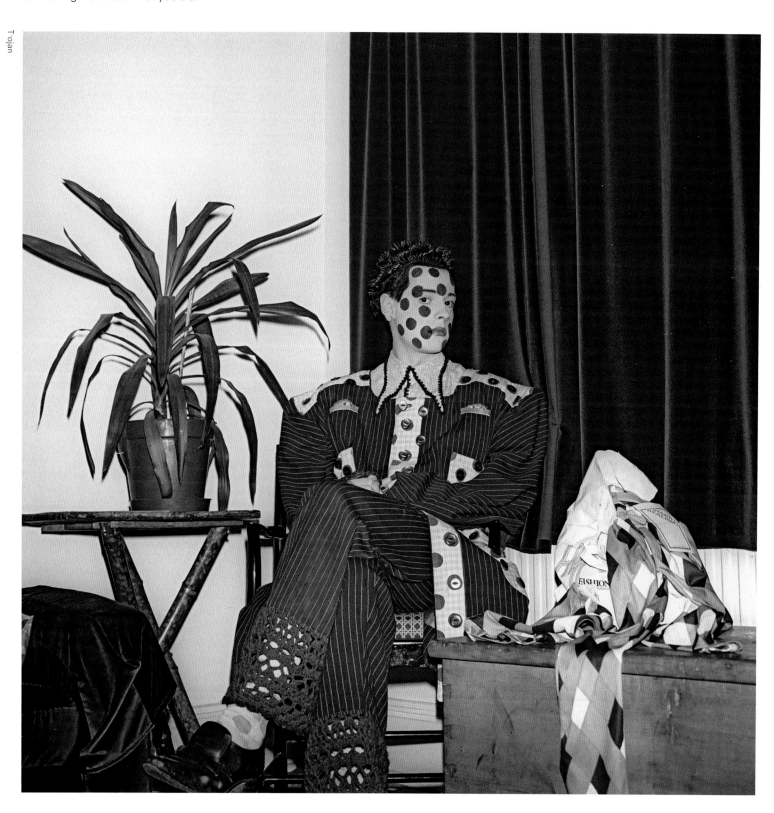

BLITZ #36
November 1985

Photographer: Pete Moss

Model: Michele Paradise
at Models 1

Make-up: Kim Jacob

Hair: Fraser Francis for Phountzi

Clothes: John Rocha, John
McIntyre, Bernstock Speirs

Pete Moss, photographer:
It wasn't difficult to get good
pictures at all as Michele Paradise
was (and still is) so elegant and
the horses were so photogenic.
It was a very classic English look,
but stretched a bit, which is what
you were very good at – subverting
establishment dress codes.

Michele Paradise, model:
Zandra Rhodes discovered me.
I was her muse for eighteen years.
I did fittings and catwalk shows and
trips but I never really did photos.
I was never one of her poster girls.
I had started modelling in 1979
and she was doing a trunk show
at Bloomingdale's in Washington
DC. The show was full of her big
'chocolate box' dresses, those big
crinolines. I remember there was
a lot of spinning in the show.

I was a good showgirl. I had
a good walk and I was a quick
changer. That's how I made sure
I got more outfits. I was a
frustrated actress. On the catwalk
I loved the applause, the heat
of the audience and the instant
gratification. Catwalks used to
be six feet high and fifty feet long
and it was amazing, a real show!

There is a similarity between Zandra
and me. She saw that in me and
invited me to London. I felt very
comfortable in London. My look
is very strong. I am not a blue-
eyed blonde Cheryl Tiegs type.
I guess I was the Erin O'Connor
of my day. I was always a catwalk
girl. Mostly I found photographic
modelling boring and, to be
honest, I'm not that photogenic.
The times it worked, it was like
the pictures we did together. You
saw that androgynous element
that I had, and played with it, and
it really worked. You knew how to
get the best out of me. I felt very
connected to it. I was in my element
on that shoot. I like to play a role
and have a motivation that I can
act out. You had a narrative in your
shoot and it was a challenge, but
I built on that. I'm kind of horsey-
looking too, so that worked. It was
like, 'this feels right'. It's obvious
when you look at the pictures.

I knew that if I was ever going to
be in a magazine that it would be
a magazine like *BLITZ*. I needed
someone to create an environment
around me and not try to fit me
into the magazine. People didn't
really understand my look. A few
did. Zandra did. Thierry Mugler did.
Adel Rootstein did, who made a
mannequin of me. And you did.

I left America because it was very
homogenised. The US prescribes
to the sheep mentality. I felt
strangled by it. I came to London
at the end of the punk era. London
was more open-minded. In the US
I was considered extraordinary
with my big red permed hair and
lots of make-up. Here nobody
really looked twice. Here I could
reinvent myself. You could be an
individual here. Imagine when I met
Zandra for the first time with her
pink hair and things stuck on her
face. I was from Baltimore, which
was never ever edgy.

BLITZ was one of the first
magazines to take that look from
the street and put it into a format,
to applaud it so others could be
inspired. You put things together
in a personal way. Real fashion was
on the streets, and I was part of it.
I loved those times. It was the best
time to be a model. We collectively
made it happen and it wasn't a
business.

In those pictures, you captured
an essence that not a lot of
people saw, that not a lot of other
photographers captured. These
photographs are such a nice
reminder of another time.

I adored model Michele Paradise. I had originally met
her when working for Zandra Rhodes. She was the ultimate
catwalk model, who could throw poses that were a reminder
of the halcyon days of *haute couture*. She had the most
marvellous profile that harked back to Diana Vreeland.
She was astonishing. She was not trendy but I felt that she
was just the model for this story. We shot it in a stable near
Hyde Park. The look was vaguely historical, as designers
were showing lots of cape coats and rich layers. I like how
the photographs have a still, painterly mood. Perhaps
I suggested Pete reference old paintings by Constable.
Michele was a thoroughbred among models. Still is.

Clothes horses

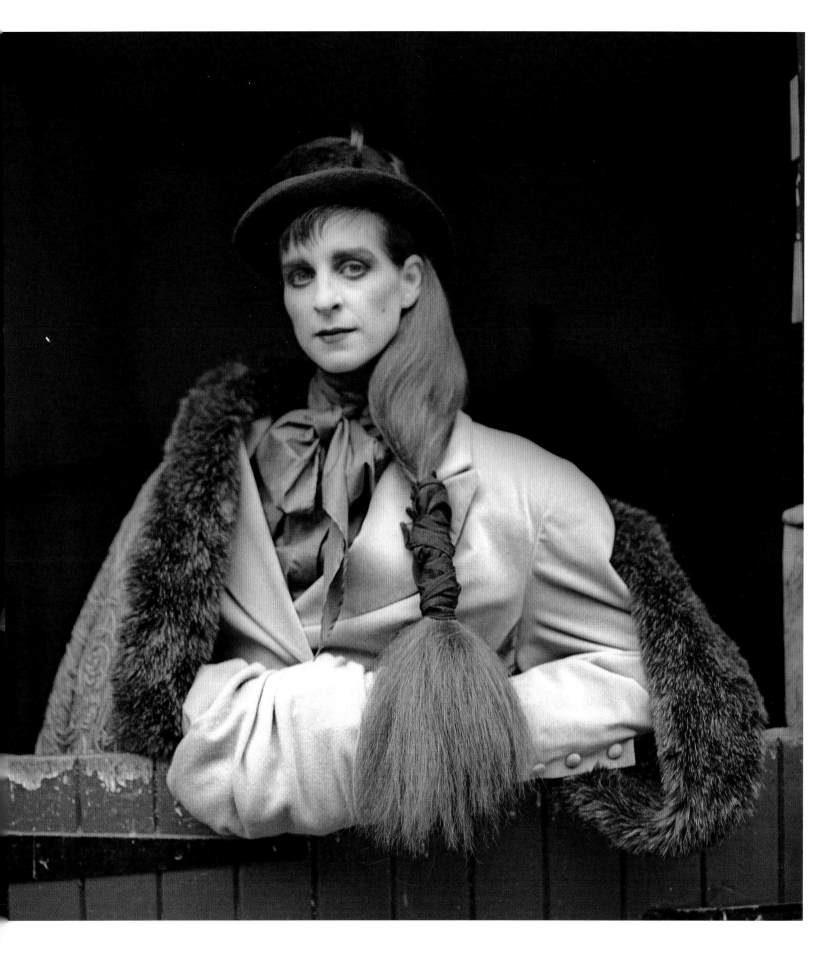

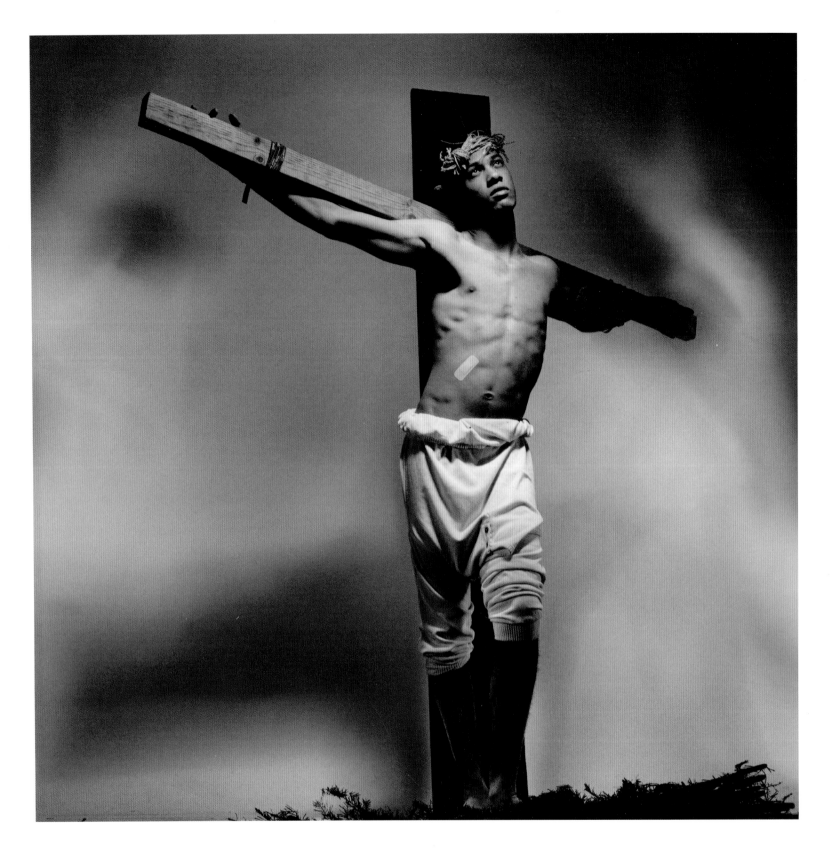

Photographer: Peter Ashworth

Models: Mark Lawrence,
Anna Paolozzi

Make-up: Debbie Bunn

Hair: Fraser Francis at Schumi

Clothes: Judy Blame, Stephanie
Cooper, Sue Clowes

Peter Ashworth, photographer:
Mark portrayed the fashion-crucified man, shot from a low viewpoint, standing semi-naked in the wilderness. I used a strong searing light on the background, as if in a storm. I knew this was going to be a provocative image, but it was beautifully done and was not intended as an insult to religion, but as an ironic twist to the clichéd image of Christ on the cross. There were lots of threads to the picture, and it showed religion and fashion entwined. There is tenderness in the place of pain, black instead of white, and the twisted Hermès ribbon replacing the cold nail. Anna was the ultimate earth mother. I was not involved in casting – at that point of my career I had not dealt with model agencies for any of my shoots, as I was specialising in music and street style.

Anna Paolozzi, model:
I was told I might be on the Christmas cover as the Virgin Mary, but the bloke who was Jesus was used instead. The shoot was all day. I went on the tube and came back on the tube and there was no lunch. The dress I wore was lovely. It was fitted and we couldn't do it up round my bust, so I wore a corset underneath. I doubt very much the Virgin Mary would have liked that. The halo was genius, designed by Judy Blame, and was made out of spoons, forks and whisks.

Did we plan to do a religious inspired story because Christmas was looming? If so, our religious festivals got mixed up (as one writer to the letters page pointed out). Knowing our wayward way of thinking, it might have been part of the plan to simply stir things up. Whatever the reasons, I'm still proud of our audacious use of sacred iconology. Reactions certainly varied. The letters page was filled with rants from 'Offended of Torquay' but my intention was never to be sacrilegious; during my upbringing I attended church three times every Sunday. Instead, I wanted to rework for a new generation these powerful images of Christ and the Madonna that had themselves been reinterpreted down the centuries. One reader praised: 'It is a revolutionary presentation of Christ as being a man of the East and not the West ... a reassessment of Christ who has so far been presented to us as being exclusively white and European.'

Stephanie Cooper, designer:
BLITZ was one of the few publications around at the time that rebelled against preconceptions of contemporary fashion, and questioned and explored social convention so innovatively. Your beautifully anarchic aesthetic was a beacon for a new generation of fashion designers fresh out of college, and hoping one day to be selected for the pages of BLITZ fashion editorials. The magazine's pages pushed, kicked and tormented fashion forward at a wonderfully alarming rate, disregarding trends or even wearability. It educated and inspired, broke rules and smashed boundaries. You helped create a new fashion language in which anything was possible. Fashion was my religion and BLITZ became my bible.

At that time, London Fashion Week was held in the cavernous Olympia exhibition hall. I was playing with the grown-ups, showing for the first time on my own. I was thrilled when you told me you liked my small collection. I admired your vision. You would use an established or unknown designer, a vintage piece, an obscure item of clothing or something that wasn't even a piece of clothing at all, so long as it achieved the look you wanted. It wasn't about selling clothes or promoting labels, it was about the possibilities of what fashion could be.

Vogue Fashion Editor Liz Tilberis chose a similar dress from the same collection for the 'British Fashion Now' editorial of February 1986, in which she styled Uma Thurman as Marie Antoinette in shepherdess mode. Anna Paolozzi looked incredible as the Virgin Mary. The image was irreverent, subversive, contentious, offensive, and as creative as it was controversial. This shoot was incredibly important.

BLITZ started a revolution that took things to a different level from which you could never go back again. I'm hugely proud that it's one of your favourite photographs. It's still one of the highlights out of everything that has happened to me.

Christian, model:
I remember shooting for a cover proposal for BLITZ with Mark Lewis, as an ethnic Jesus Christ, but unfortunately a cover with a similar theme with Mark Lawrence as a black Jesus was published that same week. But eventually my other flatmate, Susan, managed to get that coveted cover (October 1986 issue).

Princess Julia, model:
These pictures have got a classicism as well. Did you get your mates in because you knew you could make them do more or less anything you wanted?

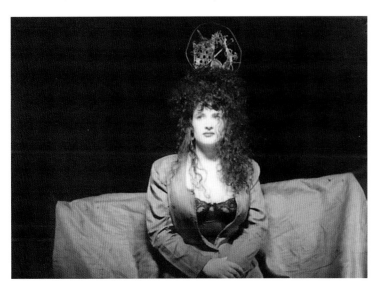

Immaculate

BLITZ #37
December/January
1985/86

Photographer: Gill Campbell

Model: Martine Houghton
at Marco Rasala

Make-up and Hair:
William Faulkner

Clothes: Stephen Jones, The Hat Shop, Tracey Jacob

Gill Campbell, photographer:
For me, my fashion work was verging on a style similar to still life. I loved to light. Even if the subject was chaotic, there was always a calmness and clarity to my work. I think that was why we worked so well together. I especially loved to work in black and white. Because of the limitations of budget, we never shot masses of film, thus there wasn't hours spent on editing. But that suited my style well. I wanted every shot to be perfect.

Martine Houghton, model:
I'm drawn to fashion, art and drama. My mum used to drag me to the theatre. The theatricality of your work is what attracted me. It was about the look, totally. I love this picture. I have a rule that if you see a picture and you don't recognise yourself then it's a good photograph. I remember at times feeling I wanted to tear everything off and walk out. I didn't really know what the future held.

Stephen Jones, milliner:
So much of what *Vogue* and *Harper's* and *Tatler* represented were one person saying, 'This is the way you are supposed to look and the reason you are supposed to look like that is because I'm telling you so'. In the '80s these new style magazines introduced the idea that fashion was there to enable you to express yourself. That didn't come from fashion designers. It showcased the whole idea of customising something whatever that may be – Keith Haring painting on his own clothes or you putting two hats on or doing a really strong look and wearing it everyday.

What people do not realise is that in those days the *Daily Telegraph* had half a black and white page for fashion once a fortnight. *i-D*, *The Face*, *Smash Hits* (to a certain extent) and *BLITZ* really created a new media. It was a big revolution for visuals. It was the beginning of the 'Designer Decade'. When you look back at early copies of *Vogue* from the 1930s and 1940s, they were also very much about ideas, but in the '80s there were a whole load of fashion magazines that treated fashion just as a runway picture, or re-styled it for the reader – but that certainly wasn't for us. What style magazines (because that's what they were called then) invented was that mix of image, typography, narrative and everything all blended together as one.

Carol Brown, make-up artist:
So many colours and products that we take for granted weren't available then. I used to go to an art supplies shop, L. Cornelissen & Son, in Covent Garden, to buy pure pigments to mash up with lipsticks or Vaseline, or I'd use Caran D'Ache coloured pencils. I remember struggling to make a vibrant lime-green eye shadow. Theatrical make-up from Charles H. Fox was useful, but it was important to keep everything very matte because of the strong tungsten lights usually used – and we were shooting on film, so there was no Photoshop. Retouching was done by hand, and was way over-budget for most jobs. I remember seeing MAC make-up for the first time around the late '80s, when a Canadian make-up artist was working in London, and had brought it over in her kit. It had been launched in Toronto by a make-up artist in 1984. Everybody in London was desperate for it because it was so matte. Honestly, I was often making mistakes through inexperience, but I was bold, and enthused by the eccentricity of the girls.

Sometimes it was just an opportunity to take pictures of a favourite model. Martine was a constant on the pages and in my life. This photograph is an exquisite portrait capturing her weird beauty. The black polo was *au courant* with the cool crowd who liked its intelligentsia beatnik associations. It made a useful anonymous backdrop. Stylistic tricks like doubling up the safety pins (a nod to punk) and the hats became a thing for me. I had seen photographs of Bolivian peasant women with hats piled high on their heads in *National Geographic* magazine. I have often returned to this look.

Millinery two step

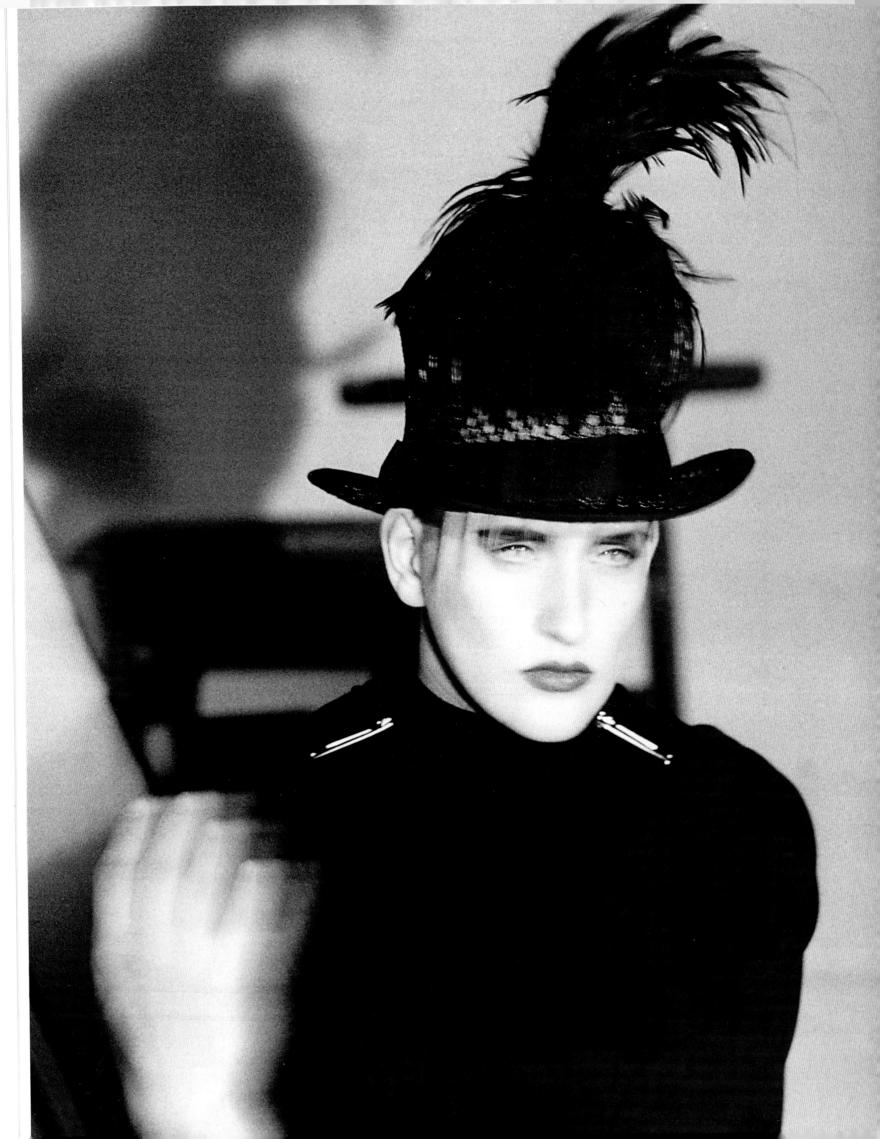

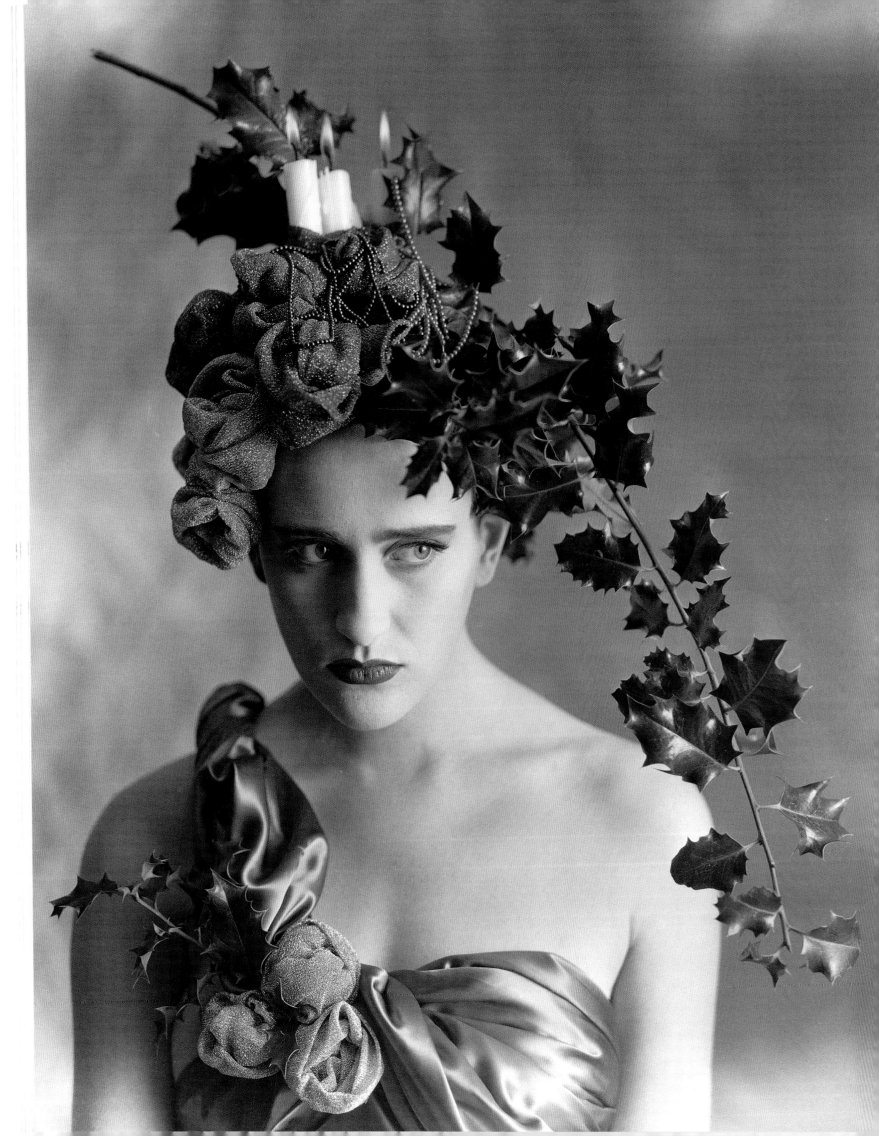

Martine Houghton, model:
For *BLITZ* and *i-D* I was given a young, trendy look, but for other magazines I was often portrayed as a glam woman. Both were putting on a look. There were a lot of ball gowns. The candles on the head became a bit of a theme.

I was always very self-conscious and very, very shy. I did a shoot with Robert Erdmann on a beach dressed like a twenties riviera flapper, and people walking by would stop and stare and make comments. But I did get into it. I used to get a lot of trouble because I looked so like a boy, and I used to wear Dr. Martens and a leather jacket. I can remember coming back from a shoot where I had been wearing nail polish and this bloke giving me stick, really laying into me on the tube, and nobody doing anything. That happened a lot.

Robert Ogilvie, photographer:
That was the first proper shoot we did, and actually it was the first time I ever really used a 5 x 4 camera properly. I borrowed it from my college, and talk about pot luck. It was a slow, old-fashioned process, and it shows in the quality of the image when you compare it to the pictures I took on the Hasselblad camera. Her pose is hugely fixed, and I love that because for me it draws on all those original portraitists, whose subjects would stand in the studio with a clamp behind their head. What's so beautiful about 5 x 4 is you're in the dark with a cloth over your head and it's actually quite hard to compose an image, as the image appears upside-down in the camera.

Martine was absolutely amazing to work with. I'd never really worked with a model. I was doing a degree in photography, so what was interesting for me was looking at all the construction of meaning. At the time, half of me thought that fashion was a bad thing, so balancing those aspects of myself and turning up at college with these kinds of pictures was all very strange, but I knew very little and was really learning on my feet. I think it was several years after that that I felt like I was beginning to learn my craft; but back then I was never quite sure how things worked.

Louise Constad, make-up artist:
The Ghosts of Christmas Past, Present and Future was the brief. It was your Christmas card and you gave a wodge to everyone for doing it. Everybody was credited because it was for free. Credits were the only currency we had. You always let loose in a really creative way. Those roses were actually Lurex ankle socks.

Paul Bernstock and Thelma Speirs, designers, Bernstock Speirs:
Because you studied fashion design, you would often create and customise garments for your shoots, which gave your work a unique dimension.

This picture was originally created as a Christmas card. I asked Martine to model, along with her sister Caroline and Hilde Smith. They were supposed to be the three Ghosts of Christmas. I bought a length of satin from Berwick Street market and draped and pinned it around Martine. Although I now feel guilty about the things I asked her to do, she never once complained, even with wax dripping down her back. She looks exquisite in this photograph. She has the same pure beauty of an Irving Penn model.

Photographer: Robert Ogilvie

Model: Martine Houghton at Marco Rasala

Make-up: Louise Constad

Clothes: Berwick Street Market

Photographer: Mark Lewis

Models: Rick Giles, Michael Rathbone at Marco Rasala

Grooming: Stephanie Jenkins

Clothes: Crolla

L to R: Michael, Rick

The Raj becomes the rage

Mark Lewis, photographer:
You would arrive at our flat in a black cab overflowing with bin liners, often on your own, always on time, and rarely flustered. You'd sit on the bed, needle and cotton in hand, as there was always something to be added or improved on the garment we were photographing. There was no money for studio hire, or rather we chose to spend it on Polaroid film, so guests who were staying in our (Stephanie's and my) flat were evacuated for the day, the bed pushed to the side, and a shooting space cleared. Hair and make-up was done in the bedroom. Everyone always seemed pleased to be working with us. It was a very friendly atmosphere with lots of cups of tea and whatever could be mustered for lunch.

I must say, it was and still is the best working relationship I've ever had with a fashion editor. There was an implicit trust in what we could achieve together, with not much fuss and angst, from the selection of models to the final choice of image and layout.

Georgina Godley, designer, Crolla:
I absolutely wouldn't have minded that you turned the trousers into a turban. I was probably wearing mine as a turban too. It was an era of unadulterated creativity. The words *commercial* or *accessible* were not in our vocabulary. Those words were for dull and boring Americans. The more crazy we got, the more buyers came to us. Of course, like all excess, it couldn't last. Almost overnight *more is more* became *less is less*; enter the All White collection by Rifat Ozbek, Azzedeine Alaïa, and a clean palette. Suddenly the gold thread, paisley, ikats and florals were relegated to the sofa. By the summer of 1986, my collection was made from pure white Lycra and I couldn't look at a pattern again.

Crolla was founded in 1981 at a strange time of extreme austerity and absurd affluence. It closed in 1988, having supplied outrageous Savile-Row-on-LSD tailoring to rock stars, celebrity artists, trustafarians and yuppies.

Crolla was the wild child of two art students, myself and Scott Crolla. Young London was all about taking risks and creating something out of nothing through passion and ambition. I was surrounded by the salvage artistry of Tom Dixon and André Dubreuil. There was the first rap club in London, called the Language Lab, and endless warehouse parties. We were both serious clubbers.

Crolla was a brand that caught the imagination of a new generation of 'Boho Affluents' who had grown up on punk and the Blitz club, with a desire to live it large at the Embassy club, Annabel's, Tramp, the Titanic. Club kids and self-created artists like Leigh Bowery, Rachel Auburn, Stephen Jones, Judy Blame and Crolla, amongst others, received Japanese support following the London Goes To Tokyo trip in 1984. Money came in the form of sponsorship and licensing deals. The Japanese were the best patrons, respecting and buying pure fashion from top to toe. It was a godsend. The Americans pared it down, the French ignored it unless it actively crossed the Channel, and the English only celebrated a home-grown designer if they had made it elsewhere first.

When we opened Crolla the manufacturing industry was almost belly-up, so this offered an opportunity to make short runs of great quality garments, work with top mills at knock-down prices, and find bankrupted stock of incredible fabrics from traders all over England. We wanted Crolla to hark back to the heady days of glamour that reflected the ever-increasing multi-culturalism in music, dress code and populace. And always quality. Luxury was new and desirable, and for young hot-blooded opportunists in the City, who traded by day and danced by night, it was accessible.

An influx of Arabs funded a new level of extravagance. How else did clubs like The Embassy thrive? How else could penniless artists, young models, cross-dressers and eccentric, dedicated partygoers support their habits without the sponsorship of outsiders who wished to wine and dine them at their expense? We got into every club, every art opening and every event for free. Were we so beautiful and special that our company was worth buying? To this day I don't know who paid for all those parties and nightclub frenzies, but when I say 'we', I mean a whole generation of Londoners dressed out of the pages of *BLITZ* magazine.

We never slept, we worked incredibly hard, and ideas bred ideas because no one stood in our way. We were incredibly lucky. Scott and I opened our store in 1981 as total unknowns, and by 1983 we were selling worldwide. I met wonderful people who are still firm friends and who still share the same value system. Never compromise, stay true to yourself and enjoy yourself. I can't stay up all night any more, but I can still eat, drink and breathe fashion. I work mostly with young people now, who are the same age I was in the early '80s. They are re-visiting all the looks we did, but with their own spin. I learn something new and exciting every day and hope never to lose that passion that filled our hearts and, in my case, drove the sewing machine.

By the time this shoot was published, I had left Crolla to set up my own label, but maintained a creative direction role.

On my first trip to New York, I was lucky to be given a guided tour of Diana Vreeland's Royal Costumes of India show at The Metropolitan Museum of Art's Costume Institute by the wonderfully bonkers Simon Doonan, Barneys' Ambassador-at-Large, window dresser supremo and amusing author, who had landed the enviable job of assisting Vreeland. I was totally entranced by the lavishly decorative display and went mad for India. Here, Crolla trousers became turbans. To mis-quote the Country and Western adage: *The higher the turban, the closer to Ganesh.*

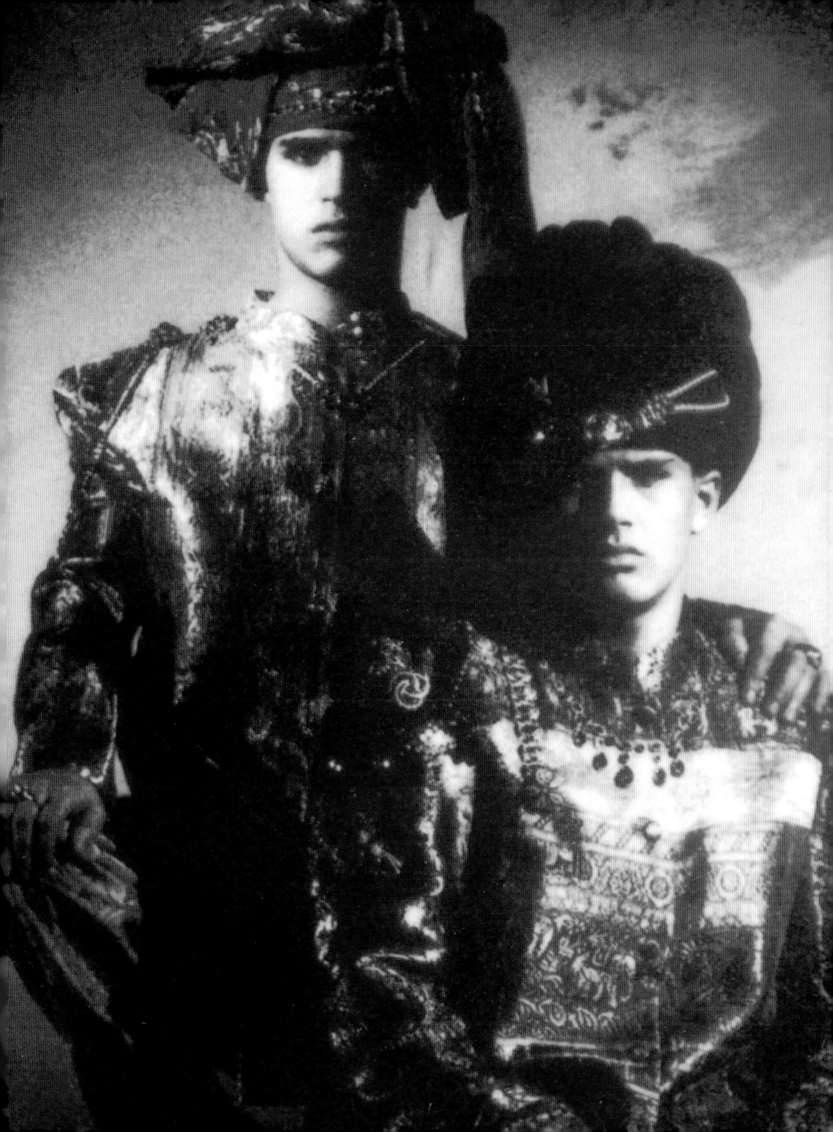

106 Beng

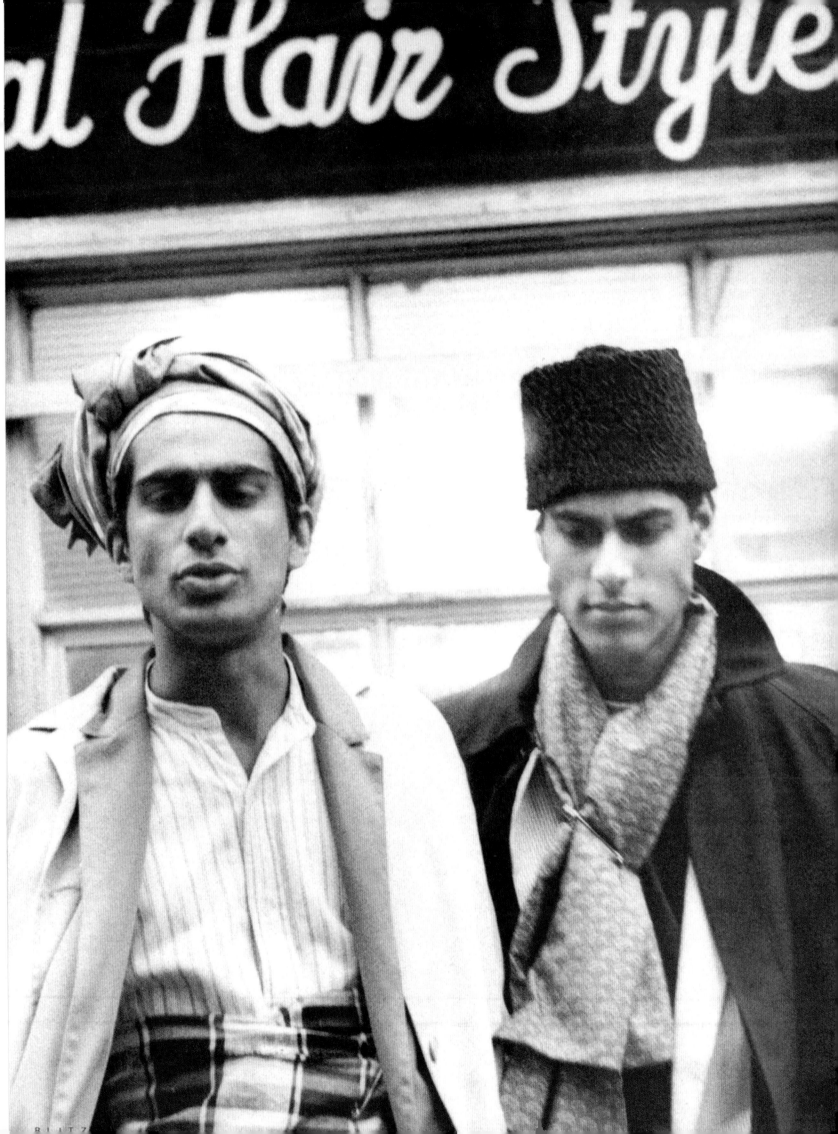

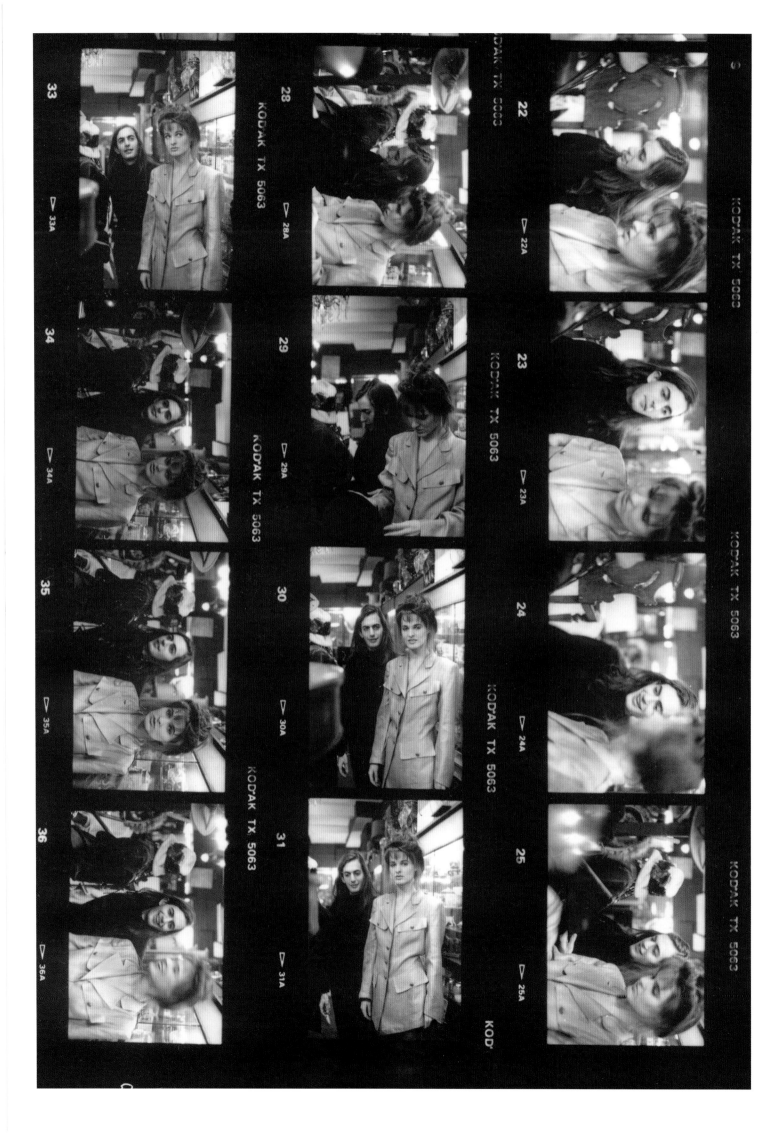

PEOPLE
MARC JACOBS

On our first night in New York, Pete and I decided we had to stay at the notorious Chelsea Hotel, the home of celebrity junkies and out-and-out crazies. It was an experience that neither of us will forget, but it pretty much cleaned out our funds. A friend told us about John Badum, who was always happy to accommodate freaky waifs and strays from London (many contributors to this book have acknowledged that they were lucky to share his hospitality). So we boarded with him for the remainder of the trip. John was charming, entertaining and generous (in every sense) and trailed us to all the happening parties and clubs in New York, introducing us to the city's alternative scenesters. One of these was a young designer and club kid, Marc Jacobs, who John raved about with such gusto that we had no choice but to meet him. Jacobs had not long graduated from Parsons School of Fashion and was designing sweaters for Charivari and sportswear for Sketchbook. So, on a Sunday morning (we were returning to London later that day) Jacobs duly showed up with a model wearing one of his designs. To photograph the pair we simply went next door to the antique store. I chatted with the designer and then flew home. In *BLITZ* he mused: 'I feel it's horrible for young people to get locked into anything, to be immovable. My look changes from season to season. I'm still figuring out what I want to be.' Who knew that Jacobs would become such a big deal? John did. He knew everybody, and treated everyone like stars.

Photographer: Pete Moss

Marc Jacobs, designer:
There's nothing I love more than youth and beauty. I think they're the same word at the end of the day anyway. The energy of youth, the purity, the freedom and the excitement. I had such a good time as a young person and I've continued to have a good time, and I love people who get up to the plate and just do it. So whether it's The Strokes or an artist, writer, or whatever, I always find that so stimulating and I guess, without even planning it, I surround myself with people who really love that same thing, who love that same energy. And it's not about creating something *avant garde* or new that no one's ever seen before, it's about constantly celebrating the same energy and the same youth. Whatever way it manifests itself is fine, but it is a constant re-celebration of what turns us on, which is youth, energy, vitality, freedom.

I was a club kid for way too long, but now I live vicariously through whatever we're working on. I stopped doing all of that at some point. Sometimes I miss it. For the show we used a group called The Stuck-Ups and it so reminded me of music I used to listen to. I was glad that it continues to inspire me, but it's also inspired a bunch of new people who didn't live through it the first time, but who kind of get the essence of it; maybe the style without the substance, but it doesn't matter. D'you know what I mean?

Instead of regretting it, or having guilt or shame or whatever about all those horrible things I did back then, and the way I dressed, and how I behaved, and what I did and who I did, instead I just think 'wow, that was so great'. And the fact that I can continue to draw on it – and not in this kind of pining for the past way, but again, just constantly celebrating that that energy is still relevant ... yeah.

At Marc Jacobs and Louis Vuitton we often play with European references – this season there were references to Bodymap and Vivienne Westwood, and I love that. I'm the American in Paris so I'm more apt to refer to Chanel, but as interpreted by Adolpho, so I play these games.

I used to think that American design was wearable clothing, and European design was decorative. I could put things into neat little boxes and say American design is all about practicality and functionality, and even though it can be expressed in luxury fabrics, you could always sit on the floor in it; whereas the European attitude was clothing as works of art – form first and function second. But it's just so unnecessary to define it that way, because really all those things don't matter anymore. I don't really mind bows that don't hold things together but are just applied on something, whereas that could have driven me crazy in a fundamentalist, purist kind of way when I was starting to work.

You can see a simple floor-length cashmere dress from an American designer, and you can see a feathered headdress with a sequinned bra and knickers on a French catwalk, and both of them are pure fantasy because real women don't wear either. They just don't. They are both completely unwearable and undesirable by most women. I think American designers are just as full of fantasy as European; it's just not the cliché of what fantasy is. I've played this game so many late nights with a bunch of gay boys, where they all say what they would wear if they were women. They all talk about how they would wear beige and black or whatever, and none of them would ever get laid. You have the one straight boy who says, 'I would wear Ungaro,' and he'd be the only one who'd score. I can't even tell you how many times I've had this discussion, way back, a long time ago in my career with people who were working at Calvin, and they'd say, 'Oh no, I'd never wear nail polish, I'd never wear any make-up', and I'd be like, 'Yeah, and you'd grow up with no friends and you'd never get married and you'd never get laid.'

Photographer: Pete Moss

Model: Pallas Citroen

Make-up: Kim Jacob at Pin-up

Clothes: Mark & Syrie, Ravel

Pete Moss, photographer:
Pallas in a beer mat robe, smoking a fag in the Northumberland Arms in Charlotte Street that was run by a mate's mum and dad. She had that French New Wave influenced film starlet look, and the whole shoot was an homage to that era in a way. I was very inspired by filmic stuff and that's why I liked using locations rather than studios. The beer mat robe was such a simple idea. Humorous, but also really beautiful.

Pallas Citroen, model:
Mark & Syrie. Whatever happened to them? The beer towel jacket was quite ghastly. I remember thinking that I must look like some tart sat in a pub. A lot of what we were doing did require role playing rather than being yourself.

I was discovered when I was fourteen by Terence Donovan but my Mum wouldn't let me do it. Then when I was at university, the photographer Adrian Peacock stopped me in the street and asked to take some pictures. He took them to Premier Elite, who signed me up, but I got into a lot of trouble there. I was quite naughty. I didn't understand the premise of being a model. There was a very old-school thing of 'be seen and not heard'. I got on well with the owner Carole White, who took me to clubs like Annabel's, which was so not me. I was a member of the Young Communist party. I got sent on the ubiquitous trip to Japan, which turned out to be a disaster. I went with my boyfriend, who was a musician. Japan was a culture shock. If you were a model, you could get free meals at the top floor restaurant of the hotel; we got really drunk one night and were caught going up and down in the elevator half naked. We got arrested and spent twelve days in prison. I was actually in chains, like in the 1930s, sitting in a metal cage. We eventually got released because we said we were getting married.

Mark and Syrie were two young London designers bursting with typically British bravado. Their approach was anarchic and irreverent. Their designs utilised the mundane, cheap and cheerful. Tourist tea towels, table-cloth gingham, carpet remnants, and even promotional pub beer towels. It seemed obvious to take the jacket down their local in Soho. Pallas had some of the best legs in the business, so was the perfect choice to pose on a barstool. I interviewed the designers. I am not sure if Syrie was actually present at the interview or whether Mark acted as their mouthpiece (he was notoriously unafraid to speak his mind). Following the publication, I received a hand-written five-page stream-of-consciousness tirade. I think, in essence, it was a thank you note, although to this day I am still not sure.

The beer towel jacket back where it belongs

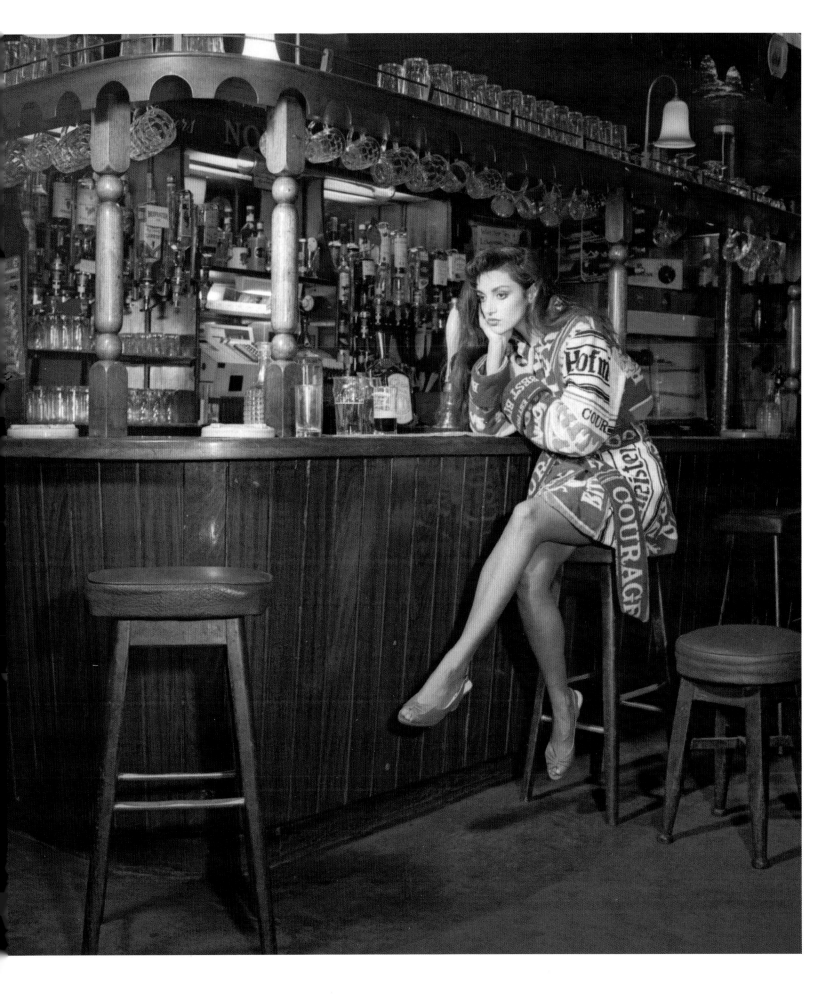

A little outrage never did anyone any harm. Essentially, once again, this was a knitwear story. I have always had a thing for knitwear, perhaps kick-started by my mum, who was always knitting some kind of jumper for me and my siblings. This featured oversized knits by Martin Kidman for Joseph, John Galliano and Workers For Freedom. I used the sweaters to envelop Sibylle, who became part Russian doll, part Madonna. I do not remember what I stuffed up her sweater to give the impression of a pregnant belly. Her innocent, cherubic face was the perfect choice when puffing on a pipe – perhaps the ultimate taboo for any mum-to-be.

I didn't see these images as provocative at all. They were quite dreamy actually. It was funny being the pregnant Madonna. It was like, 'Oh, yeah, why not?' I didn't see evil in what we were doing. It was just making a fashion statement. Pregnant. Yeah. Smoking. Why not? A pipe as well. I showed these pictures to my son and he said, 'Do you have another baby somewhere?' It was a pillow, I think.

We were like a family having fun. We were like children playing and telling stories. We were lucky to be working in fashion, so we could make up stories all the time and not just on the pages. Every Friday and Saturday night was another story. My goodness, the time we took to put a look together; the hours of preparation before we went out. I would never go out without [making] the effort.

Pregnant pause

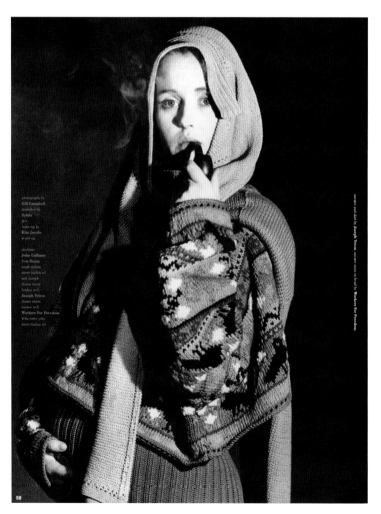

Gill Campbell, photographer:
I loved Sibylle. This is my second favourite shoot, with the pipe, wonderfully controversial. I have a Polaroid somewhere of us practising for this shot. You weren't sure that pillows were going to work well for the bump, so I put all the jumpers on and we tried out a variety of stuffings. I will try and find the Polaroid.

Sibylle de Saint Phalle, model:
A significant moment for me was when you had me twirl down a catwalk at London Fashion Week looking like a nun, in a black and white dress and a pair of Jesus sandals to *The Sound Of Music*. I think the designer was Dutch, tall and pretty [Barbara de Vries].

Then I was photographed in *BLITZ* as the pregnant Madonna. That was John's [Galliano] first knitwear collection. He had literally just finished them, and some weren't even stitched together yet. There was a guy who was the link between the factory and John, organising production, and his name was Adrian Joffe, who went on to be Mr Comme des Garçons. They were beautiful pieces of knitwear. Such gorgeous colours.

Kim Jacob, make-up artist:
Collaborating together was inspirational, and creative freedom was always embraced. As a make-up artist you gave me freedom, and at the same time we had fun. I am not sure, in this world driven by sales and commercial values, that happens anymore. Being able to enjoy the success of *BLITZ* enabled my career to flourish and grow. It enabled me to become an international make-up artist, working on many advertising campaigns and editorials worldwide. As there were so few great publications in the '80s, it was a privilege to work for *BLITZ*, and with a talented art director like yourself. Time has shown that we have both survived this crazy, sometimes fickle business.

Photographer: Gill Campbell

Model: Sibylle de Saint Phalle

Make-up: Kim Jacob at Pin-up

Clothes: John Galliano, Joseph, Workers For Freedom

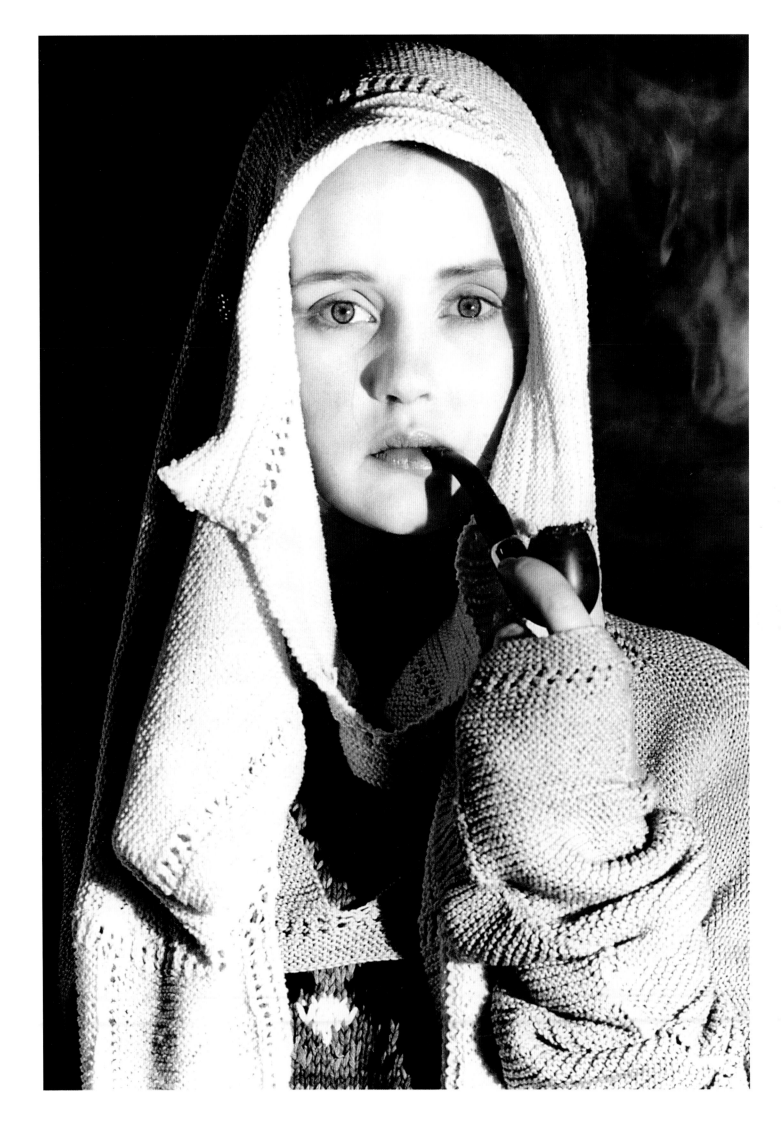

Faking it

During my tenure at *BLITZ*, certain collaborators were a constant; none more so than Eric Bergère, the designer-in-chief at Hermès in Paris. Bergère's makeover of the old fashion house made the label desirable among young, *avant garde* Londoners, who enjoyed the humour and heritage being offered in the new designs. Of course, the label was spectacularly expensive and out of our reach, so it was not surprising that high street labels like Pink Soda created an affordable version. Pink Soda's colourful baroque print scarves were an instant hit, but instead of just photographing them, I got my trusty right-hand lady, Darryl, to stitch some together to make a tailored jacket (worthy of the label) and hip boxer shorts (a nod to Nick Kamen). The shoot, by Carl Bengtsson, also included a portrait of Bergère, taken by Robert Ogilvie at the Paris HQ. This image made the cover. Far from being annoyed by our rip-off versions of their designs, Bergère and the Hermès team congratulated us our modern interpretation.

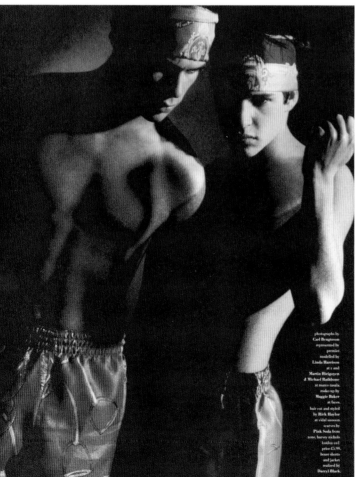

L to R: Martin, Michael

Photographer: Carl Bengtsson

Models: Linda Harrison at Z, Martin Hirogoyen and Michael Rathbone at Marco Rasala

Make-up: Maggie Baker

Hair: Rick Haylor for Vidal Sassoon

Clothes: Pink Soda

Eric Bergère, designer:
Again, this was a fresh rediscovery of Hermès. I think that Jean-Louis Dumas was an exceptional president of the company. His past as an artist, musician and illustrator gave him a really open-minded point of view. He was a visionary for his brand, his house.

Stephen Linard, designer:
I guess we started that thing with Hermès, Chanel and Gucci. It was a real moment, and then it faded away until Tom Ford did his thing. Before we started wearing it, it was all old ladies and Middle Eastern customers. The punk rockers suddenly had money, so we decided to wear those labels but style them in a way that they weren't meant to be worn. I think I made some bondage trousers out of Hermès silk scarves. That was how we were going to wear it, not how they wanted us to wear it, with a cardigan and slacks. You probably gave them ideas with those pictures you did.

Barry Kamen, model:
The way she's holding that photograph on her shoulder, that attitude is so you, that's *BLITZ*. This image is *über*-powerful. Acknowledging fashion, turning it upside down – literally – and going through a hell of a process to make the picture. But it's all about attitude, when you come down to it. The casting of the girl, the precision of the hair and make-up and then the complete irreverence of the way it's put together. That really is you. And it's still a nod to the heritage of the brand because there is no moment of taking the piss. It's completely reverent, yet at the same time it's saying, 'This is new, this is where we are, this is now'. This image for me is completely wow!

Moose Ali Khan:
Martin was the most intelligent model out of all of us.

Darryl Black, fashion assistant:
You could slot these pictures in anywhere in time, really. It wasn't linked with what was going on around, was it? It was from your crazy head. So much work and hours of thought went into the pictures, and making things. I think we were organised, especially with the shoots, but we had some hum-dingers. I had to be on the ball. I was definitely challenged. This must have been the first time I worked with scarves. The inspiration continued as I still make clothes from vintage silk scarves. I always loved our re-purposing projects and am still obsessed with it. Being eco-conscious, in my life and business, remains my overriding and abiding passion, and it's very exciting that the fashion world is now finally beginning to catch on.

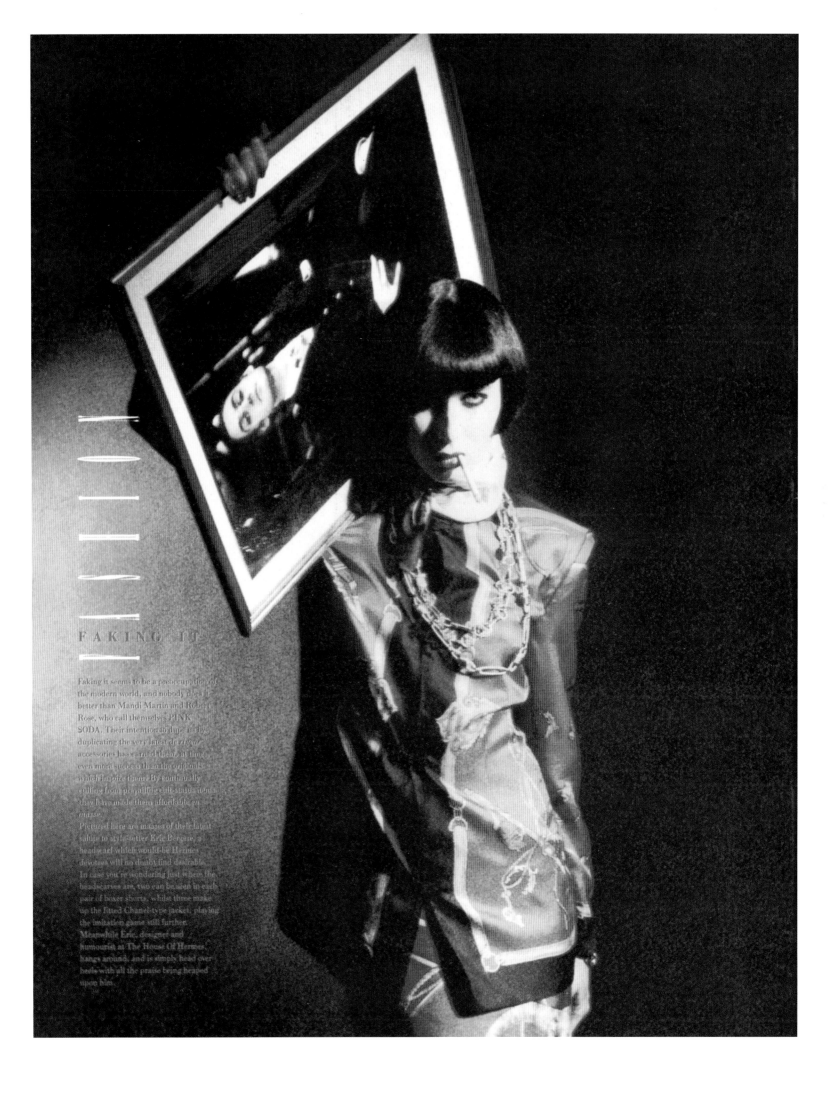

FAKING IT

Faking it seems to be a preoccupation of the modern world, and nobody does it better than Mandi Martin and Robert Rose, who call themselves PINK SODA. Their intention to duplicate by duplicating the very latest *de rigeur* accessories has earned them, at times, even more success than the originals which inspire them. By continually calling from prevailing elite status icons they have made them affordable, *en masse*.

Pictured here are images of their latest salute to stylesetter Eric Bergère, a headscarf which would-be Hermès devotees will no doubt find desirable. In case you're wondering just where the headscarves are, two can be seen in each pair of boxer shorts, whilst three make up the fitted Chanel-type jacket, playing the imitation game still further. Meanwhile Eric, designer and humourist at The House Of Hermès, hangs around, and is simply head over heels with all the praise being heaped upon him.

Ziggi Golding, model agent, founder of Z:
The bizarre imagery was actually our world. The mainstream world hadn't cottoned on to that yet, but *BLITZ* not only represented that, it pushed the boundaries too. There were designers like House of Beauty and Culture, John Galliano and John Flett. We took the models to John Galliano's studio and I remember the two Johns and Amanda [Harlech] teaching them to walk. Mostly I remember lots of wine. We were all interlinked and sharing the same mindset. *BLITZ* gave designers like Gaultier and Galliano a platform to show their clothes and their fantasies. Your pages provide a vital record of that time.

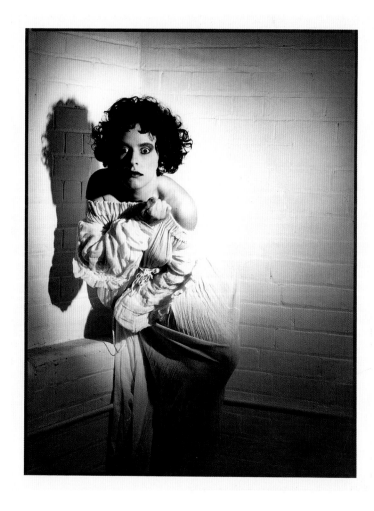

I am not sure if this photograph was shot to be used on the subscriptions page, or whether we made the picture and it was seized upon by art director Jeremy for that purpose. I loved the muslin Regency-style dresses that Galliano had shown on his catwalk, wetted to his models' bodies (a particularly victim-ish fad at the turn of the nineteenth century). They felt quite madhouse, and the fabric referenced Westwood's *Destroy* shirts. Hilde was a marvellous actress, so was happy to play the demented diva. We ran the strap line: 'Hilde awoke one morning to find her clothes were talking to her'.

Debbie Dannell, hairdresser:
She looks so silent movie. Her face is telling the whole story. Old films were really important and a massive influence. I would study Bette Davis movies. The hair sets, the make-up. We would go to all-night John Waters screenings. We definitely nicked stuff from that but it was always about glamour. I remember you made me a cream dress with gold eyelets around the hem, which was really tight, and I wore it to a party and a fight broke out and it split right up the back. And you said, "That dress isn't for fighting in". I never went out in anything less than a four-inch heel. It was all about the ritual of getting dressed to go out. Straight boys and gay boys and girls.

We still feel very passionate about what we do. I always go in early on a job to check out the lighting. It's so important. Where's the key light going to be? I guess it is very old school but it makes a difference.

Nick Knight, photographer:
John [Galliano] and later Lee [McQueen] are the artists of our generation who communicated the finer things of life much more than any contemporary artists, which is why I have stayed in the world of fashion. Being that type of person, seeing what other people don't see, more things affect you visually, mentally, emotionally, and you use those things when you are shooting.

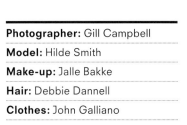

Photographer: Gill Campbell

Model: Hilde Smith

Make-up: Jalle Bakke

Hair: Debbie Dannell

Clothes: John Galliano

Subscriptions

BLITZ #40
April 1986

The 1980s saw the emergence of the designer label. It seemed like everything had to have a designer tag, right down to a bottle of water. These labels came to have their own currency, a snob value shopping list for the newly emerged fashion victim. I was fascinated and disturbed that people would buy anything with a label attached. Calvin Klein stamped his name over and over on his underpants (although this was before Marky Mark wore his jeans low and his CK pants high), while Jean Paul Gaultier literally tagged his jackets on the outside. Although the former was bare-faced in its egotism and the latter more discreet, both allowed the wearer to parade their purchase power. So, how about just wearing the label or posing in the packaging? The shoot featured a headband of Comme des Garçons labels and a Chanel No. 5 perfume bottle earring, realised by jeweller Lisa Vandy. Stephen Jones made a hat from an Hermès box and ribbons.

Head shots

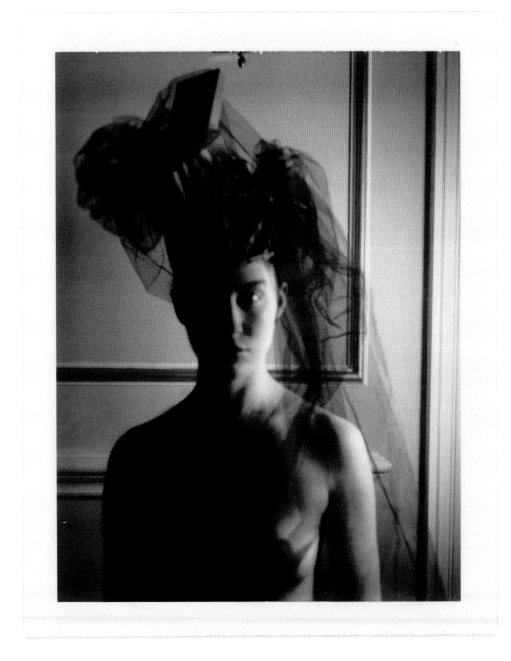

Stephen Jones, milliner:
I like the box-coming-out-of-a-box-coming-out-of-a-box thing. Nowadays we know all about Hermès because they have big publicity campaigns, so we know Christophe Lemaire or Gaultier or Margiela is the designer, but back then Hermès was so exclusive. It was extremely grand and completely inaccessible, so I would have loved the opportunity to work with the label.

Barry Kamen, model:
What differentiated you and BLITZ was that you were brave enough or foolish enough (however you look at it) to embrace that high fashion side; to embrace Hermès, Chanel and the like, and not put an enormous distance between that and the street. What i-D was doing, what The Face was doing, was much more street and sporty, and only featured a tiny element of this, whereas you came in from that fashion direction. It set you apart. It's like you were saying, 'No, we are decadent. We are coming from the English eccentrics thing (not the brand) and we're also coming from that international dandyism thing, but that is still the street.' You started from the top and filtered down, whereas a lot of people started from the street and went up. Now I can see how much more in touch you were – this need for labels. You were actually saying, 'Here's the label. Here's the fashion. I'm not ashamed of fashion. Here it is!' But you were also being the rebel and bringing a healthy dose of cynicism. The Face was a bit too hoity-toity to admit they loved a bit of fashion when they actually did. We all loved a bit of fashion, which is why I had so much to do with you and Stevie and David and Leigh and people like that.

Louise Constad, make-up artist:
Wearing the labels themselves. Buying the brand not the clothes. I didn't realise how forward-thinking that was. These were in my folio for a long time. I was really proud of them. I didn't think what we were doing was bizarre at the time. I was so up my own arse when it came to fashion that I thought I knew so much better than everybody else. I just felt I belonged, and it was just right.

Photographer: Wong
Model: Lynda Bridges at Premier
Make-up: Louise Constad
Hair: Louise Constad
Clothes: Hermès, Stephen Jones

Martine Sitbon was one of a new breed of French designers that we were smitten with. Her designs drew inspiration from the historical as much as the modern; imagery that we old New Romantics were already familiar with. Our worlds collided and we have remained friends ever since. Martine epitomised Parisian cool; a latter day beatnik poet, working fabric in place of words. Along with her partner, art director Marc Ascoli, they were the ultimate power couple for the post-Power Dressing generation.

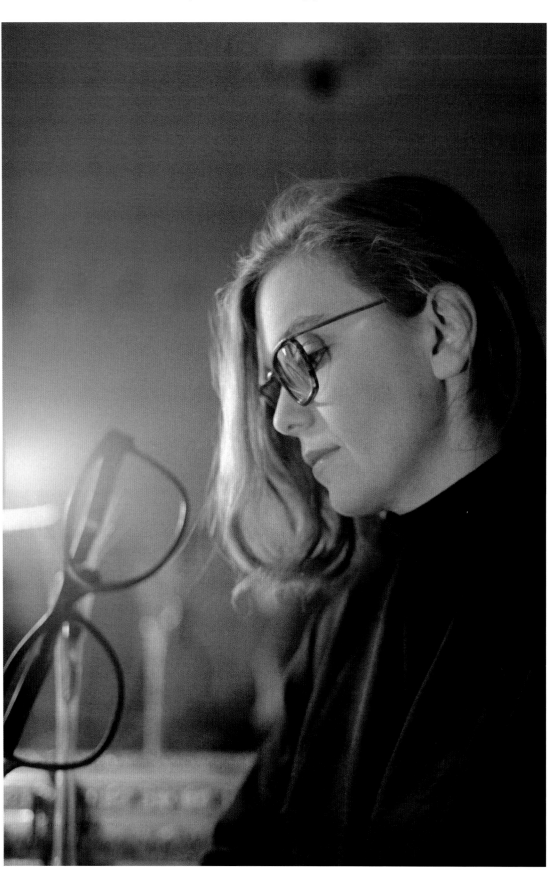

Photographer: Robert Ogilvie

Martine Sitbon, designer:
BLITZ magazine truly reflected a very particular atmosphere in London at that time: the creativity was overflowing. This was quite stimulating for us Parisians. It gave us energy and a pulse. Each issue of *BLITZ* covered so many different pop artists, movements, happenings; it was fun yet always very informative. We had no internet at the time, so magazines were very important to us. *BLITZ* was a celebration of fashion, music and art with no censorship. It symbolised freedom of expression; it always felt genuine and free, unlike many jaded publications nowadays, and probably because fashion wasn't such a big industry yet.

French journalists would often say that I was a Parisian designer with British energy. I would regularly go to London because I felt in tune with the movers and shakers working there. You were one of the first journalists that featured me in the UK. When I look at the portrait that you and Robert took of me, it evokes both tenderness and a little irreverence. You can tell from the picture that you were amused by my style and designs. You always described them in a very sharp way because you understood my references and my universe. This is why I felt so comfortable when you interviewed me.

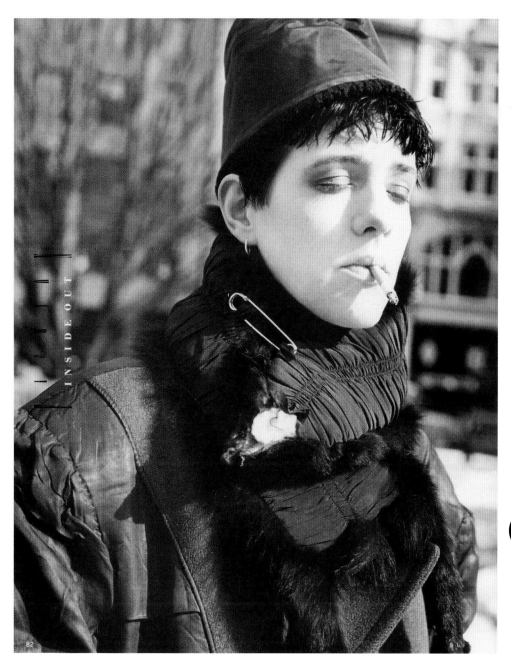

Marc Ascoli, art director:
This image is my favourite because I think it captures a sort of freedom and very particular emotion. It reflects the atmosphere of that time that often combined violence with poetry and romanticism. This shot is very different from the polished ones we are used to seeing in magazines now. I also always love the androgyny of your pictures, which are still very fresh to look at today.

Johnny Rozsa, photographer:
We had the freedom to be creative, but we created the opportunities. It was Punk meets New Romantic, and you can't really get better than that. It was incredibly brave.

Inside out

Photographer: Iain R. Webb
Model: Caroline Houghton

This was my first attempt at photography, under the watchful eye of Pete Moss. I loved Caroline's look, which was pure *demi-monde*. The location was Golden Square, just outside the office on a crisp winter day. We only did three photographs, and the concept and styling were very simple: I used clothes that I found at home (the stockist was credited as 'Back of the Wardrobe') and simply turned them inside out. The story had queer beginnings. I had read about a group of homosexuals in 1950s San Francisco who identified themselves by turning their jackets inside out but, honestly, I just liked the way the tatty, worn-out linings looked. In another picture, the coat loop on the back of the collar resembled Jean Paul Gaultier's trademark tag. This was a do-it-yourself version. I love Caroline's closed eyes — it was a sunny day and she was smoking. I was happy years later to see the photograph pinned to the inspiration mood board of designer, Martine Sitbon.

BLITZ #40
April 1986

I went to Paris to interview Jean Paul Gaultier. This was a pretty big deal for me, as the designer was emerging as the poster boy of the *avant garde*. He was a sartorial hero for young Brits who found his unique brand of satirical fashion and stylish sense of humour intoxicating. His clothes were a brilliant combination of rebellious street style and old school *haute couture*, something I felt totally in tune with. He looked to the future but had a healthy respect for history. I was eager to meet him, if a little scared. We hit it off from the start and soon realised we had much more in common than our bleached blond haircuts. The studio shot was a no-brainer: Mimi and Stephen sharing one wide trouser leg.

Jean Paul Gaultier

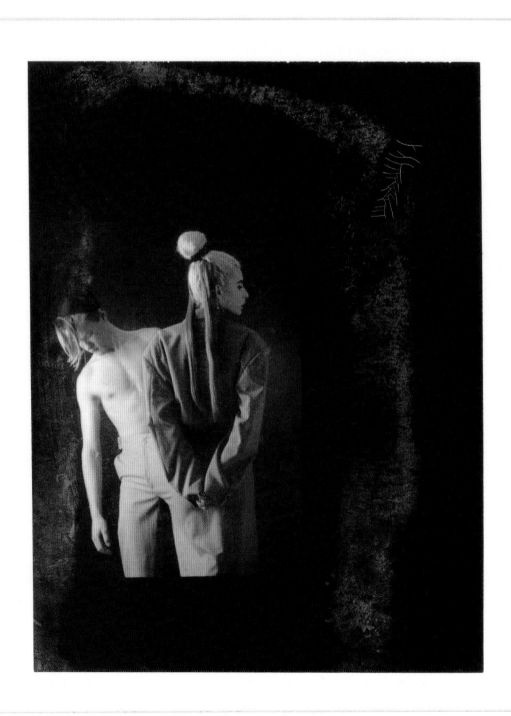

Robert Ogilvie, photographer:
It was a bit of a moment for everybody, I think. The first time I'd photographed someone very famous. I took pictures while you were talking. I like the pictures far more now than I liked them at the time.

Jean Paul was loving it. I was pretty terrified. I had this little window of opportunity to make the picture. It was quite full-on but he was hugely accommodating. He looked at BLITZ and loved what you were doing. He loved the interview and the pictures and wanted the originals, so he asked if we would go back and be his guests in Paris.

I had something very specific in mind when I took that portrait, as I was doing a college project using the same photographs. I like these images because he's so calm-looking, and normally he's so cheeky. He was so full of life. Even in his relaxed moments that still came through. I wanted them to look like police mug shots, so for my project I used his label in front.

Amanda Cazalet, model:
He was called the terrible child of fashion. His whole ethos was along the same lines. There was a great meeting of attitudes and pooling of ideas. The work dovetailed. I guess it was kind of inevitable that I would work with him. The first time I met him, I had been working in Milan and was coming back to London on the plane, and I could see this guy with peroxide hair kept staring at me. At the baggage collection he approached me and said, "Are you Amanda Cazalet? I'm Jean Paul Gaultier." Luckily I had heard of him. He said he'd seen my work and really liked it, and would I like to go to Paris and do his shows. The rest is history.

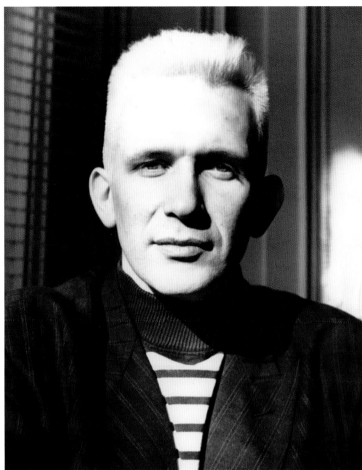

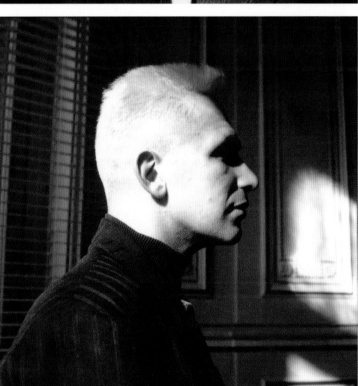

Photographer: Gill Campbell

Models: Mimi Potworowska at Z, Stephen Clasper at Marco Rasala

Make-up: Maggie Baker

Hair: Sally Francomb

Clothes: Jean Paul Gaultier

Portraits: Robert Ogilvie

Jean Paul Gaultier, designer:
All I ever wanted to do was make a show. Not a collection, a show. It was all I knew about from the TV, from the newspapers. Everything I learned, I learned from the journalists. What they said then was the bible. Also, I was looking at *Elle*, which was not just covering the *haute couture* but also showing how you could take a vest and wear it like this or like that. So I really wanted to do a show, but we had no money and in France it's not like in England, because the spirit is more free in London. You are not ashamed of selling your clothes in Portobello Road. In Paris you had to be more serious.

My first show was a total catastrophe. I was not ready at all. Nothing was planned, the clothes were not so good, they were not so well made; and then the show was scheduled at the same time as Emmanuelle Khanh, who was the top star in Paris. So nobody came, only friends and the oldest journalists in France who wanted cocktails, and there were no cocktails. So the music starts (I can remember there was one bit from Stanley Kubrick's *A Clockwork Orange*) and it was like a disaster. I didn't know which clothes to give to the models.

The first show was terrible, with only three or four patterns and a lot of variations. It was just the time when fashion was becoming very loose, so I made everything very tight. It was like jumping into a swimming pool and you don't know how to swim. Somebody tries to tell you how to, but you have to do it yourself. We still had no money so I was eating spaghetti at my relatives' and then sleeping on a friend's floor. The second one was not at all a success either. I couldn't find the shoes for the models, so I put socks on them but no shoes. The third one, more journalists came, but I didn't sell at all. It was only after the fourth collection in 1977 that people started to talk about me.

At that time I had nothing to lose, but after you have a little success there has to be another one, and it has to be a little bigger.

I think my first version of the trouser-skirt was a little too long. I think men prefer to show their legs, so now I make one that is shorter and more like a kilt. It's more sexy. Maybe that was my mistake before.

I enjoyed the interview we made and I remember I wrote to you and asked for a copy of the wonderful photographs. Bravo Robert!

Martine Baronti, photographer:
To make a living I was a designer employed by Nina Ricci in Paris. I later moved into photography, working with several magazines including *City* and *Tempo*. The model Leslie Winer had a flat above mine, so we did a shoot with Bodymap for *Jill* Magazine.

I came to London alone with a camera and one little lamp. I didn't have much money, but the GDP measures everything except what makes life worth living. I was rich in inspiration and poetry and was socially safe at least. You gave me a chance, as did Lynne Franks, who was my agent. I was doing portraits, catalogues, editorial and advertising, and styling for videos.

BLITZ is mentioned in my 1985 diary, on Friday 8th, week 44. It also mentions Ray Petri, who told me I was an art director. I'd had previous interviews with Terry Jones in *i-D* magazine and Robin Derrick at *The Face* magazine. I telephoned *BLITZ* to show my book and there you were: calm and concentrated with a distant attitude. With your wild, torn blue jeans, you were like some kind of bird. I remember I left my keys at your office so had to spend the night in a hotel for Pakistani workmen. You later phoned me and commissioned this story. I felt brave and scared at the same time.

We had an easy-going relationship and were inspired by each other's differences. You managed to let me be myself. We both loved story-telling and playing with paradox. You selected the fashion and models and edited the shots I had made. The process was fast and efficient. The Tamzin shoot was done at Faroe Studios, which was run by artists in west Kensington. The unit we shot in belonged to David Ross, and it was a large space with great natural light. I used his paintings as a background. The natural light worked beautifully, but I had to work fast as it was a very cold winter day. I loved the Lewis Carroll reference and the jewelled frock. The make-up was doll-like and Tamzin captured the spontaneity of the games little girls play.

BLITZ was a mirror for my taste for the *avant garde* and my attitude in life. Our objectives were not to play the game in a straight, conventional way. It was wonderful. You were a gift to me, as was London.

Tamzin Davis, model:
It's been great looking at these pictures, some of which I've never seen; others, like the furs and sequin dress, have been on show in my grandparents' house for years. I did a little reminiscing with my Uncle Greg, but the actual shoot is still pretty blurry. I was about eight or so? The studio was quite industrial. Wasn't it an artists' studio? I didn't have a clue where we were. Before putting on the sequinned dress, I remember getting mascara in my eye and thinking I was going to get in trouble for ruining the make-up artist's work.

I did feel quite strange wearing the fox furs, which I guess is not surprising, as I went on to be a bit of animal activist. But I always loved dressing up and posing, and this shoot allowed me to wear glamorous, grown-up clothes, which I'm sure pretty much every young girl would love to have done.

It was only later that I really understood how iconic *BLITZ* magazine was in the '80s. I certainly look back at these images as being some of my favourites, especially the one of me in the sequinned dress.

Dream child

A little girl dressing up in glamorous, grown-up clothes provokes powerful emotions. This story was all about fantasy. We dressed Tamzin, who was the niece of my flatmate, Gregory Davis, in a full-length Conran gown that drowned her in sequins, and an old lace dress that we covered in fabric flowers. The styling used symbols of girly glamour — sparkle, flowers and furs. Martine and I wanted a story that was dreamy, but at the same time a little unnerving. The accompanying text referred to *Alice In Wonderland*, and the pictures do have a trippy quality. We made every effort to make Tamzin feel comfortable in the bizarre situation. The story was printed in black and white, and the colour image only came to light when Martine unearthed a sheet of transparencies. I do not know why we didn't use it originally, as the colour is exquisite.

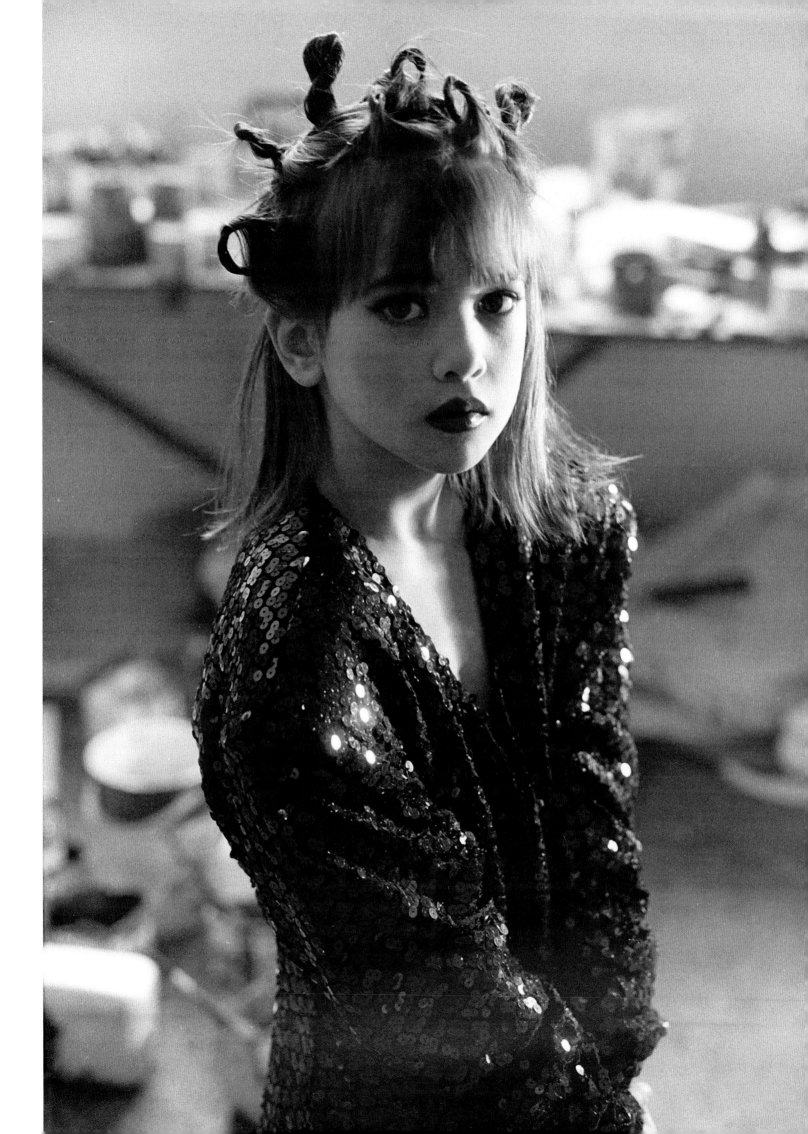

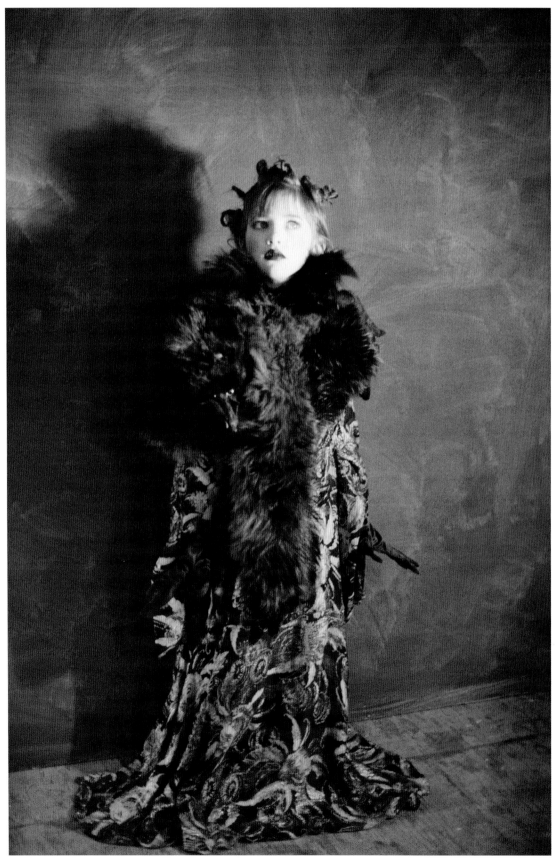

Photographer: Martine Baronti
Model: Tamzin Davis
Make-up: Jalle Bakke
Hair: Jalle Bakke
Clothes: Jasper Conran,
Clignancourt flea market

Jasper Conran, designer:
This is fabulous. At that time
stylists were doing incredible
things, and along with the
photographers there was an
amazing hub of extremely creative
people, who were making fashion
more out of a genuine passion
than in the hope of making money.
We were not business-minded at
all, but that made London much
more wonderful. It's a great
lesson. It's not about money but
about the process, and having
the opportunity to work with
fabulous people. Remember
how close everyone was? The
stylists, the photographers, the
models – we were like family. Even
other designers, like Bodymap.
Remember how we'd party
together?

Debbie Dannell, hairdresser:
Tamzin is like a little Lolita, but
we looked at it in a fashiony way.
That was our naïvety I guess.
None of us would have thought
it was sexual. So what if she was
wearing make-up? That story was
all about innocence, and actually
really enriching. We were pushing
the boundaries and doing what
we wanted. It wasn't being done
to be controversial.

Ken Flanagan, model:
Jeff was so friendly, and doing a shoot with my wife was cool. I remember having to clutch her breasts in one of the shots, and the fact that it seemed perfectly OK says a lot about how relaxed and natural the whole shoot was. This was definitely my favourite shoot. My picture being taken meant a lot more to my agents than it did to me. I was just keen not to let anyone down. Being a male model was not how I saw myself, so the novelty of being asked to be photographed, or even being paid for it, never diminished. My mum loves it now when she digs out the old tear sheets and I think I only really enjoyed it for myself on this shoot where I got to be with Sherry. That was special.

Sherry Lamden, model:
What this shoot reminds me of most is how, at that time, it was possible to do a shoot like that; to just go ahead and make a story about us just being together. That was testament to the freedom of ideas that you and the magazine shared. Jeffrey and you worked very closely on the feel of the shoot, Jeffrey wanting to capture the 'love's young dream' mood, as we had just got married. We were typical twenty-year-olds, very certain and confident we would be in love forever! *BLITZ* and *i-D* at the time were celebrating their own culture, and making momentary superstars of people like us within it. We were so flattered by the story, and were enshrined as a couple by it. Looking at the pictures now is like looking at my wedding photos.

Photographer: Jeffrey Rothstein

Models: Ken Flanagan at Marco Rasala, Sherry Flanagan (now Lamden) at Premier

Clothes: Romeo Gigli

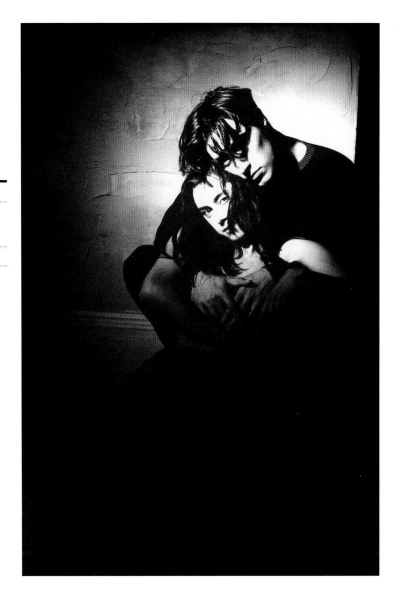

You should have seen everyone's face when I walked in with him

I had a massive crush on Ken Flanagan. But then again, who didn't? The premise was that Ken would be the ideal boyfriend or indeed husband; the kind of guy you want on your arm when you walk into a room or, better still, up the aisle. Sherry Lamden was the lucky girl who snagged him. They were a perfect couple of laid-back Londoners. This was what romance looked like. I don't recall the clothes, mostly because you could barely see them in the pictures. I remember I wanted the clothes to merge into the background, but I was a bit peeved with Jeffrey for almost obliterating them in the shadows. Ironic really. They do make stunning portraits — and a nice memento for Ken and Sherry, who sadly did split up.

BLITZ #41
May 1986

In his tiny showroom, designer Rifat Ozbek showed an exquisite collection dedicated to the dance. His models wore feathered *Swan Lake* headbands and 'point' shoes by Manolo Blahnik. When I was a teenager I had wanted to be a ballet dancer, and had cajoled my Mum into knitting me the kind of cropped sweaters that dancers wore off-duty. I added these to jersey dresses from Ozbek and English Eccentrics. I love how David Hiscock's artistic technique makes the image look painterly. The cat's-eye make-up, part Margot Fonteyn, part Soo Catwoman, was a genius touch, and Kal's poise and posture (I think she had trained in dance) was just right.

Photographer: David Hiscock

Model: Kal at Premier

Make-up: Ellis Faas at Jackie Castellano

Clothes: Rifat Ozbek, Manolo Blahnik, Jonathan Aston, Betty Webb

Ballet—hoo

David Hiscock, photographer:
My post-production technique was prompted by the fact that we shot in the same place a lot, so it was a way of taking the images away from the environment. I used to shoot things knowing that I would work on the prints, which is why the Polaroid you've got with the ladder in the background is interesting – I wouldn't have bothered cropping it out because I knew I was going to get rid of it later. I didn't shoot 35mm much; it was always two and a quarter. We got given a whole lot of Polaroid film and a processing machine for 35mm, with a windy handle, which was pretty new then. A lot of the time I would project images on the wall and re-photograph them.

Rifat Ozbek, designer:
The Ballet collection was shown on three models who changed behind a screen, and we had a little ghetto blaster and some tapes. It was all very unprofessional and naïve, but genuine, enthusiastic and non-jaded. It was like a 'ready-to-couture' show in the style of the little private salon shows of yesteryear, with only twenty or so guests at each showing. People liked it. They felt looked-after and special, but it was done purely for financial reasons. It was the only way we could afford to do a show.

The Ballet collection came about because I was friendly with Rudolf Nureyev's boyfriend, Robert Tracy. We hung out, and he took me to a lot of contemporary ballet by Merce Cunningham and the New York City Ballet. Then the Mexican collection was inspired by a holiday with Todd Oldham. There was another collection inspired by a visit to the Native American Museum in New York. There was always something to inspire me.

I belonged to that period when Karl Lagerfeld (who was designing at Chloé) and Yves Saint Laurent were doing different looks each season. Then you had someone like Armani who just kept doing the same beige things season after season. My fashion was all about theatricality and character. My designs were colourful and exciting. I liked to do themes. I was inspired by different things each season. And then I went from look to look to look…

Manolo Blahnik, shoe designer:
Rifat asked me to design a shoe for his collection. He said, 'I love, love, love the *Ballets Russes*', so I said, 'Anna Pavlova or Nijinski?' I think it was more Nijinski. I did something like a ballerina's point shoe, rounded but with a flattened end. It had a *Directoire* look with the criss-cross ribbons. I made that shoe in a beautiful silk satin and in suede, navy or black. Rifat designed these Jean Muir-ish jersey dresses that were very Martha Graham. I think this was one of his most ravishing collections and I adore this photograph. I am very happy that you chose a pair of my shoes for this picture. It is so atmospheric. The hair is perfect and I love the tights. I love stripey tights and socks, I always wear stripey socks myself. This photograph evokes incredible memories of the time I spent with the wonderful Tina Chow. Everything we did then was to express ourselves. We did it because we loved it and nobody thought about selling anything. Do you remember Cindy White used to work with Rifat to merchandise the collection, and he'd just say, 'But I want to do this! I want to do that!' He never thought about whether the things he was designing would sell or not.

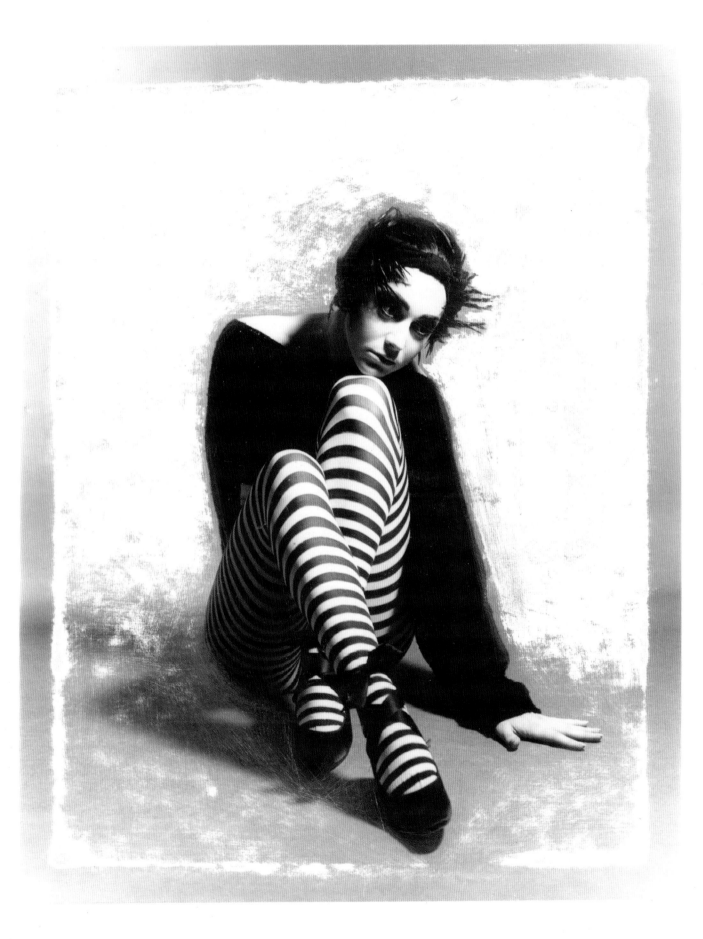

Vivienne Westwood, designer:
At the time we spoke, I think I was ambitious to be acknowledged for what I had done. But I have always cared more about all the other things I want to do. I always cared about injustice and suffering, and that involved me learning and understanding more about the world, so it was always, 'When I've finished this pair of trousers I can read my book.' The great thing is the credibility I've got now, as my fashion has given me a voice, so now I can try to do something about climate change and human rights. Also, I use the fashion as a medium, so the fashion and all the things I want to do are coming together.

The truth is, I have never really been interested in magazines; but I am of course pleased when someone shows me a lovely photo, and I am pleased with the work we do with Juergen Teller. So, thank you for all your past enthusiasm. All your work in the past seems important to you, and I am happy to be part of your memories.

I was never interested in the club scene either. I loved dancing but the only clubs I liked were the ones you could talk to people in, and where it was bright enough to see people. That's why I liked Louise's, small and packed as it was.

I thought punk was so exciting that I went to see Grace Coddington at *Vogue* with my samples in a suitcase, whilst my King's Road shop was closed, and before the launch of our punk fashion. She was embarrassed, and told me to go to *RITZ* magazine. She was holding a bondage boot and I was nonplussed that she didn't even say she liked the design. She was wearing a copy of my striped mohair sweaters at the time. Later, I thought that the photo of Soo Catwoman, which appeared on the cover of *Anarchy* magazine, ought to have been on the cover of *Vogue*. Certainly by then, punk had a big influence. *Vogue* had changed enormously three months later, even the hairstyles were wild. Everything has changed today; it's hard to think now that punk was shocking. Now, anything goes.

Marysia Woreniecka, PR:
I think we met professionally when you were also writing for *Over 21* magazine. I was representing Vivienne Westwood. She had taken me on when they started to do fashion shows and I worked on her first show, the Pirate collection at the Pillar Hall. Later she did the Nostalgia of Mud collection, which we took to Paris, and put on a show in Angelina's Tea Rooms. I remember sleeping in the hotel room under her 'paddicoats'. Vivienne called them paddicoats instead of petticoats.

It was interesting, because in Paris all these major establishment people were excited by Vivienne and wrote about her in a sophisticated way; not sensationalist, but seriously intellectualising her and her work.

British *Vogue* was very supportive too. I remember I used to represent Edina Ronay, and one day I took Liz Tilberis from *Vogue* to see her in her showroom in Chelsea. When we had finished I took Liz to see Vivienne's World's End shop. It was still quite terrifying on the King's Road – it was not long after all the fighting between teds and punks, and all the shop windows getting smashed every weekend. She was nervous but I told her not to worry. We walked in and she was amazed by the place. *Vogue* gave us great coverage, but I think Liz was a bit annoyed because Grace [Coddington] took over the story.

The Face, i-D and *BLITZ* were magazines that not only represented what was going on, they actually defined what was going on. These magazines were actually driving what was happening. It all happened pretty fast. I remember thinking that British *Vogue* were tentatively treading on something, a scene that had been ignored by them until then, until it was made important by these magazines covering it. They definitely wouldn't have done it one their own.

It is hard to quantify just how influential Vivienne Westwood has been in British fashion and, by default, globally. Her unfettered imagination and shameless bravado rocked the establishment and has provided endless inspiration down the years. Without Westwood there would be no Galliano. I had first interviewed the designer when I was a snotty fashion student and she was a bleached blonde punk wearing tartan bondage. This time around, she was happy to come to the *BLITZ* office and, as usual, stayed longer than originally planned. I have interviewed Vivienne on many occasions over the years and she has always been remarkably generous with her time, and never fails to entrance or seduce. She is a most remarkable woman.

Vivienne Westwood

Photographer:
Benjamin Westwood

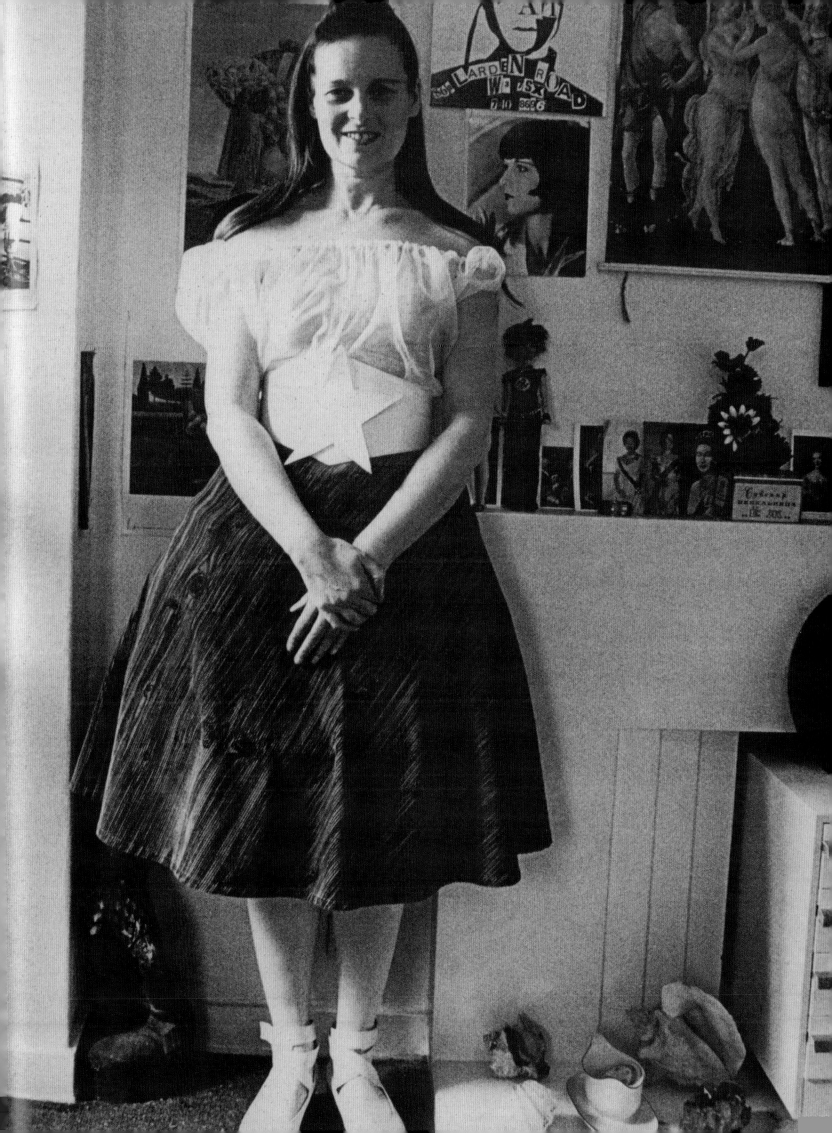

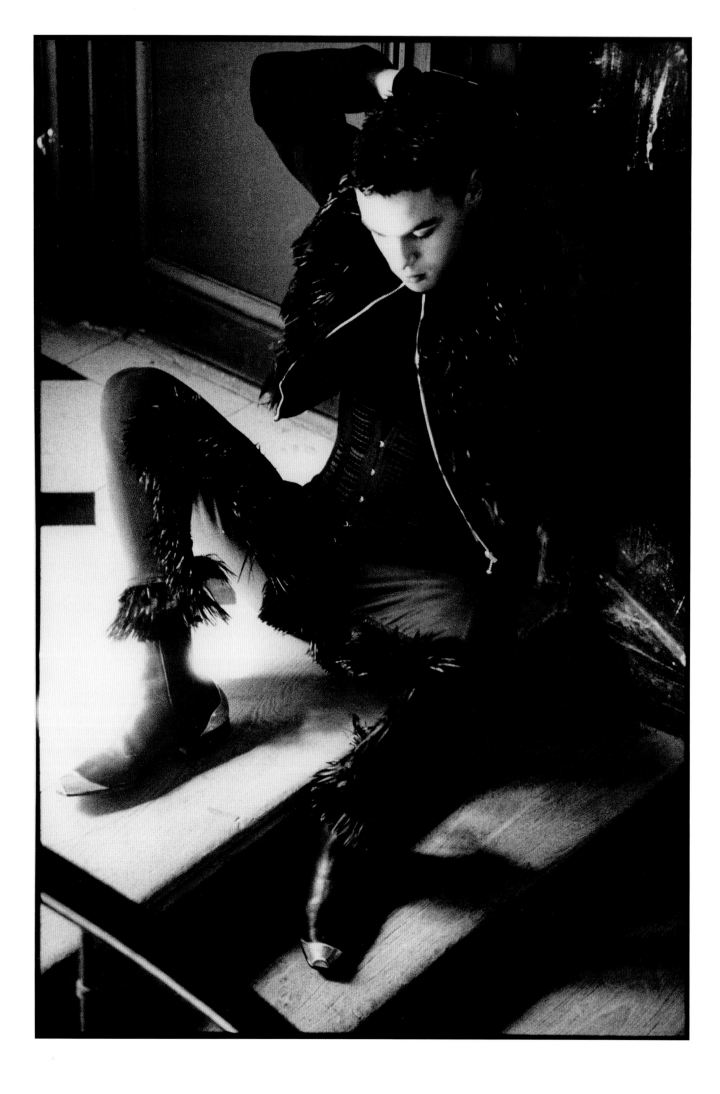

BLITZ #42
June 1986

Photographer: Robert Ogilvie

Model: Rudolf

Clothes: Jean Paul Gaultier

Future Legend

This shoot totally emphasises the spontaneity that was at the heart of what we were doing. Everything just fitted together. The boy, the designer, the clothes, the location. It's a beautiful portrait of Rudolf, a photograph that just happens to have clothes in it. A totally *BLITZ* image.

Robert Ogilvie, photographer:
So we went back to Paris to see Jean Paul Gaultier and he told you to pick something from his collection, and you picked a sweater. I think you bottled it, and didn't go for a leather coat. So he had all these wild clothes, and Rudolf was there, and fortunately I had a camera, so it just seemed to make sense to do a shoot. That was on the stairwell just outside his *atelier*. I remember people were walking past, and I think in one of the pictures there's someone walking through the shot. It was natural light from a window, with no fill or anything. I still wonder what was going on in his head at that point. Was he German? He looked like a kind of strutting bird. What strikes me is how masculine he is in that outfit, wearing something like that. He's even wearing a girdle. He was really fascinating, wasn't he?

It's like he's left the party. He's dressed for a party and he's on his own on the stairs, just thinking.

We were inspired by the images we saw where we lived, on council estates and in tower blocks, people sitting on the stairs, drunk or drugged up. But you do immediately think Paris when you see that floor. It's not the Hackney borough, or under the Westway. But we could have shot a London version of that on your old estate.

Jean Paul Gaultier, designer:
I never tried to be anti-establishment or to shock. I think there are still critics who find me like that, so maybe I am still a little shocking. When I did my first corset dress and underwear as outerwear some people thought I was joking.

I think my clothes were completely wearable, but people were shocked by them at the start. I was making classical clothes but with new proportions, and mixing them in a new way. In the first collection I made conical bras out of straw place mats. It was because when I was little I found a beautiful pink satin corset in my grandmother's wardrobe.

When people said 'you cannot do that because it is not chic', I used to think, 'how boring, how stupid'. Sexuality is always taboo, but for me it's completely natural, and nobody has anything to be ashamed about. Sexuality is part of life so it's in my collection. A girl wears a corset dress because she feels confident in herself. I think there are a thousand ways to be sexy. In my collections I like to show that there is no frontier between good taste and bad taste, all that kind of stuff. I want to show that men can be feminine and women can be very strong, but at the same time fragile.

I think it is important to push at the boundaries and barriers and to provoke, because truly I was shocked by some of the reactions of people in France. I was shocked by their attitude of always criticising people for being fashion victims. In England I found the contrary. In England, people like yourself were more open to ideas and seeing through the clothes. Everybody had a personality and wanted to express themselves. I gained more confidence going to London, because when I was there I was feeling freer. It gave me more confidence in what I was doing. I was happy that people in London liked what I was doing. I love the English.

BLITZ #42
June 1986

Photographer: Jane Hilton

Model: Hamish Bowles

Grooming: Gilda at Lynne Franks

Clothes: Stephen Linard,
Wayne Shiers for Stephen Linard,
Chanel, Butler & Wilson, Arcade,
Pink Soda, Jasper Conran

Hamish Bowles caused a sensation when he carried a Chanel handbag to London Fashion Week. The ladies of the front row almost fainted in shock. Always a good sport, Hamish posed for this shoot in one of his own Chanel jackets (he is a seasoned collector of *haute couture*) along with a knitted look-alike suit by Pink Soda, a company known for their designer homages. He also modelled a jacket by Stephen Linard, and a bottle of Coco. What Chanel herself would have made of it all is anyone's guess. I created the collage layout by colour-photocopying the transparencies, and simply cutting up the images and pasting them onto a sheet of A4 paper. This I handed to art director Jeremy Leslie, so that he could fit text around it. I don't think Jeremy was always so pleased with my maverick approach, but he was pretty cool about it.

Chanellie Queen

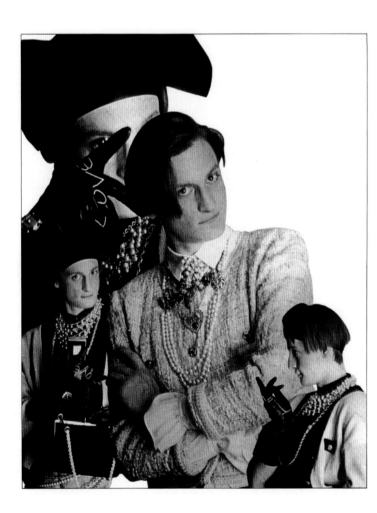

Jane Hilton, photographer:
It was all a bit scary, as you and Hamish seemed so iconic. I was young and very new. We met through photographer Gill Campbell, who I assisted. Either she was ill or not around, so you decided to try someone new. We shot it at Gill's studio so everything was familiar, and I was totally happy working with you because we'd done lots of shoots already; but I was still terrified. I had a big role to fill. A lot of responsibility. But you instantly calmed me down. You said it was a very straightforward shoot, explaining how you would piece the pictures together. Hamish was so up for it too. You'd already gee-ed him up. I don't know when he'd last worn a dress? I think it had been a while, so he was really up for it. He really enjoyed it. You were good friends too, so it all helped.

I was a bit terrified of Hamish. I thought he'd either love or hate me. But I remember Gill worrying about her shoots too. I thought the idea was totally bonkers but just went along with it – you must have known what you were doing, it would all make sense in the end ... and it did.

BLITZ had an amazing reputation at the time, so to be given this opportunity was huge. It wasn't just any old magazine. I was dead proud to see my pictures published in the magazine. I had finally made it. That's why I still have a copy of it. I don't have everything I did from back then. It was my first proper fashion shoot, and weirdly it was a mix of portraiture.

Hamish Bowles, model:
These pictures were your playful idea to amplify a fad I had at the time for dressing in Chanel (decades before Karl thought of menswear for the brand).

After all, didn't Coco build her career on appropriations from the wardrobes of her lovers, Boy Capel, Grand Duke Dmitri of Russia, and the Duke of Westminster (to name but three)? Why not shake the gender blender further still?

At the time I was the Junior Fashion Editor at *Harpers & Queen*, and my paltry salary meant that I had to be especially inventive with my clothes. However, thanks to Bernadette Rendall, the London PR for Chanel, I was invited to the thoroughly exclusive press sample sales, where I fought over accessibly priced treasures (many of them pre-Lagerfeld era; he had just joined the House) with the thoroughly groomed and immaculate Caroline Kellett, my counterpart at British *Vogue*.

My haul here included such gems as a brace of identical shantung jackets (one white, one black, which I wore as a twinset – one buttoned up, the other shrugged over the shoulders) and a classic quilted navy jersey bag slung on a gold chain.

Jasper Conran fuelled the trend with some faux 'Chanel for Men' pieces – and made me a pair of trousers cut from full circles of navy jersey to wear with a black raw silk jacket, with gold buttons placed *à la* Coco.

I brazenly wore these without a thought or a care to the Paris fashion shows, where cab drivers yelled obscenities, on the Manhattan subway (then very grungy and dangerous), where the thugs were dumbstruck, and to the London shows where Anna Wintour first clapped eyes on me thus attired.

I can never forget arriving at the Café de Paris in a pale pink fleck tweed Chanel skirt suit, worn over turn-of-the-century country gaiters that buttoned to the knee, just as Caroline Kellett, done up to the nines, swept in with a current beau she was clearly hoping to impress. She was wearing exactly the same suit, and I doubt she has forgiven me yet.

Johnny Rozsa, photographer:
That is unreal!

Barry Kamen, model:
What's he like?

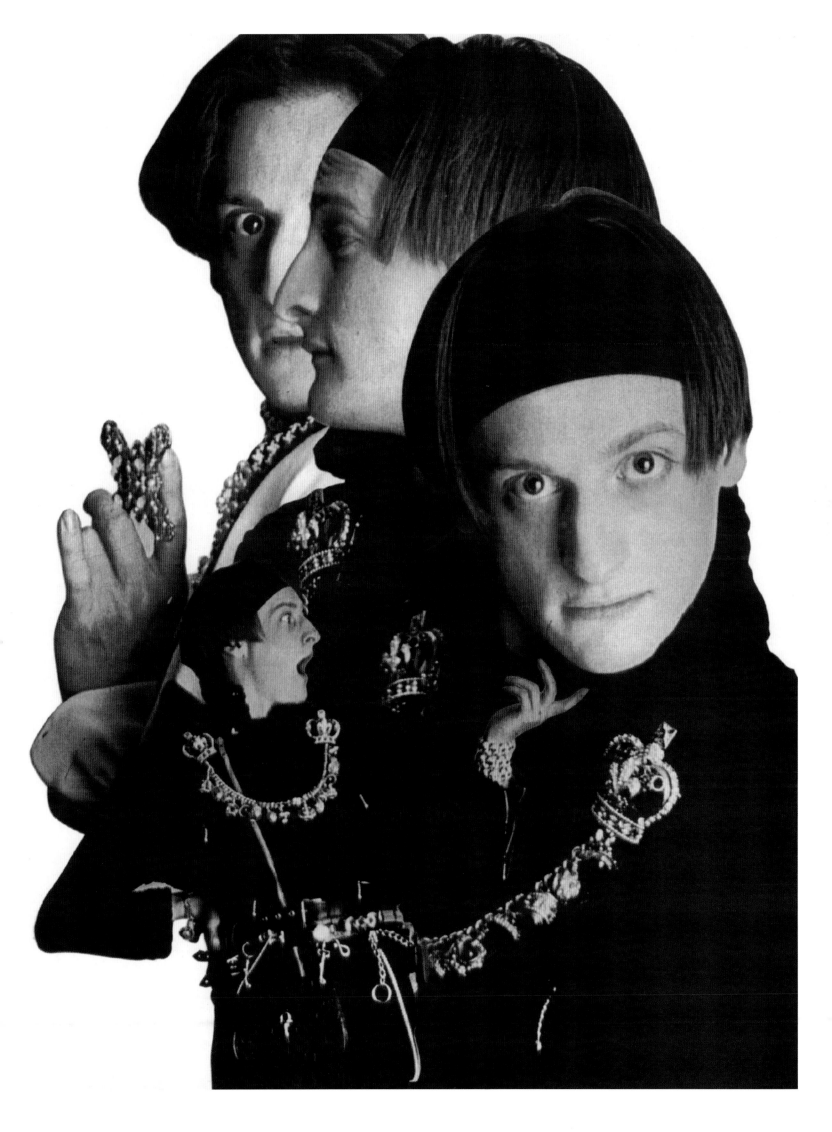

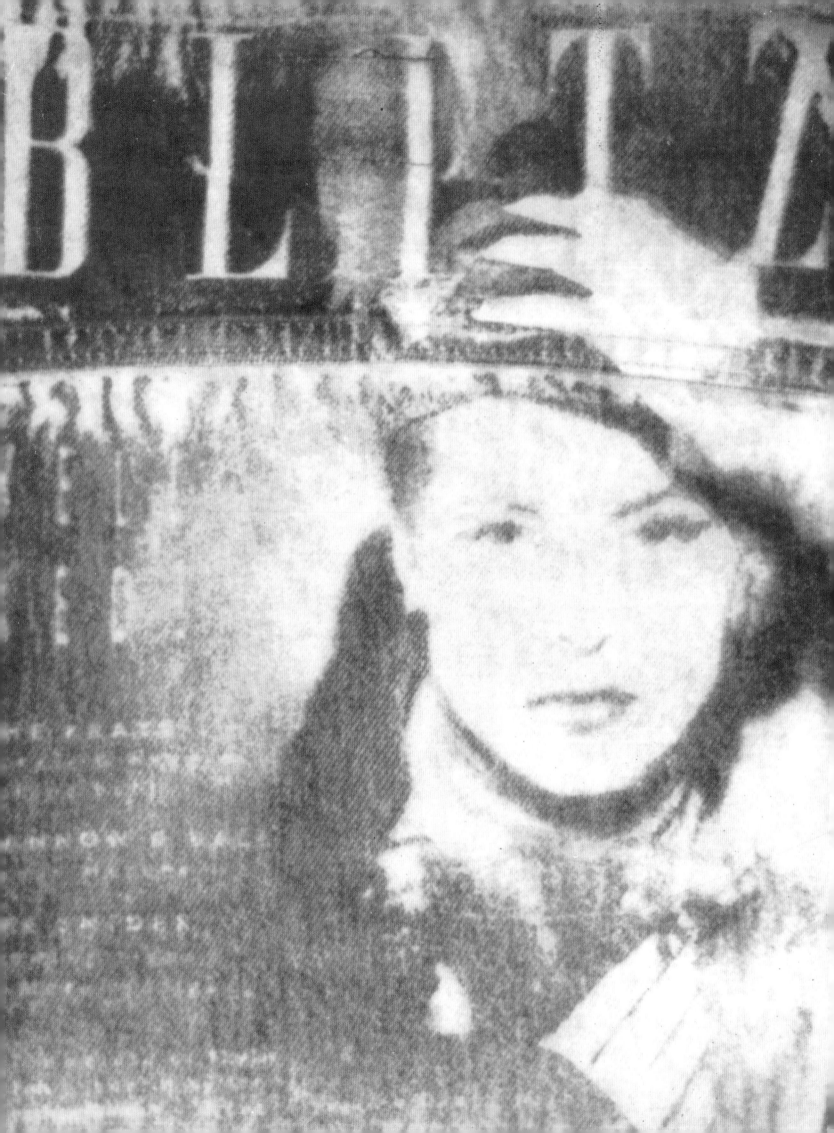

BLITZ Designer Denim Jacket

The *BLITZ* Designer Denim Jacket project was an editorial idea that just grew and grew. I wanted designers to customise the classic Levi's jacket. PR Peter Shilland and Marquita Bowen, who were marketing the Levi's brand, immediately saw the potential and became co-conspirators. I then called around a few friends – Mr Galliano, Mr Linard, Miss Muir – and with them on board everything just snowballed. Simon and Carey felt it was bigger than just a fashion story, and suddenly show producer and PR wizard Mikel Rosen was masterminding a live fashion show at the Albery Theatre in the heart of London's West End. This was staged on Sunday 15 June 1986, and comprised a stellar cast of models, actors, musicians, and Boy George! The event raised money for The Prince's Trust, as did the auction of the jackets at the Victoria and Albert Museum (V&A). This exhibition, displayed on blue mannequins by Kevin Arpino from Adel Rootstein, then transferred to the Musée des Arts Decoratifs at the Louvre in Paris. Barney's department store in New York took up the baton, presenting a version of the show that included Yves Saint Laurent and Andy Warhol. I promoted the project with surreal TV appearances on the BBC's *Breakfast Time* with Frank Bough, and a music show called *Solid Soul*, where the researcher was a chap called Jonathan Ross. Darryl and I created this unique jacket, cropped matador-style and bleach printed, with the cover featuring Maria Cornejo. At the Albery Theatre show, model Barry Kamen, who is also a brilliant illustrator, hung around backstage throughout the event capturing the madness and marvellous mayhem.

Maria Cornejo, designer, Richmond Cornejo:
Just to be in the magazine was great, so being on the cover, and then on the jacket, was really great. Your approach was different. There was always an interesting angle to things. You were bringing everybody together and capturing that energy. It was very reflective of what was going on.

Mikel Rosen, PR/show producer:
You asked Levi's to provide denim jackets and got designers to customise them, and suddenly it was, let's stage a show, let's get the designers to get celebrities to model them, let's get a charity to auction them and put on an exhibition at the V&A. This was just like the magazine and the way you worked. One idea became a hundred ideas in a minute.

I had my own PR agency but also produced fashion shows, so I was happy to take charge of the event at the Albery Theatre. The process was very organic. I asked Miss Muir if she would be in the show, she asked Daniel Day Lewis if he would model her jacket, and you asked him to read a piece you wrote about Miss Muir. It was like that daily. Gillian McVey at Paul Smith got Curiosity Killed The Cat to wear his jacket and perform. They sang *Misfit*, which seemed appropriate. Rifat got Tina Chow. Bodymap got Michael Clark, who danced with David Holah and Hilde Smith. John Galliano had a troupe of Morris dancers. Leigh Bowery modelled his own jacket. Pete Moss acted as announcer, and we decided to put you and Darryl in the show too, wheeling the jackets across the stage on a rail with one taken off as each scene went by.

On the day, nothing went to plan. No one arrived at the scheduled call times. There were not enough back-of-house assistants, so I was running from one side of the theatre to the other to get performers on stage. We were running in and out of the stage door looking to see if others were coming to rehearse, or just hanging out in the alley taking drugs. There was so much to do that from the start it felt like we were running out of time. The show itself was total chaos, confusion and complications. Backstage was full of celebrities, clothes horses and cartoon characters. The show started with the *Clockwork Orange*/Bowie intro, with the stage flooded in blue light. Everything was going to plan until suddenly I had no headset communication with the crew; nobody was doing what they were shown at rehearsals … and no Boy George! But we didn't have time to worry. We were too busy just doing it. And George did show up, and did his turn with model Vivienne Lynn. Then, applause, appreciation and the aftermath. The day after, the national press was filled with 'George on heroin' stories, but the *BLITZ* blue denim moment was the talk of the fashionable town.

Pete Moss, photographer:
During the Denim Jacket Show, I escorted Margaux Hemingway to the pub next door for a drink. She was a little confused as to what was going on, I think.

Illustration: Barry Kamen

BLITZ
CHARITY
SHOW
ALBERY
THEATRE
15/6/86

Eric Bergère, designer:
Luxurious but still discreet. A few Hermès scarves were quilted inside the jacket, and there was the addition of a dark green mink collar. Scarlett Cannon gave an edge to this *bourgeoise* verson of the jacket. Just perfect. The show was amazing and it was great to be able to share such a good time. It was the first time I had met many of my fellow fashion designers. I remember clearly the support of all of them, particularly John Galliano, who was a sweetheart.

Stephen Linard, designer:
It was great doing that project because my dad helped me with the jacket. He made a lot of the leather pieces that I added to it, and Lisa Vandy got a lot of the things silver-plated for me. It was the ultimate camping jacket for around town, and was lined in pink taffeta. When we did the show, the boys all had silk shorts on with bows on the back. It was a great show, a great night. It was a very, very hot day and we were drinking a lot of champagne. Because it involved Levi's, there was a lot of it. I got arrested that night in Trafalgar Square. I was wearing my gold cowboy suit. Then there was the auction at the V&A, and I think John Moore bought my jacket. When I took my Mum and Dad to see it, the knife and fork and spoon had gone off my jacket. I couldn't believe it. Half of it had gone missing. There was a rucksack on the back and a Chanel-type purse, and a silver-plated hip flask on the arm. That went too. It was a collaboration before they were called that. Now you can't get away from collaborations – I'm doing one now with Fred Perry. At that time I was doing my own collection and two ranges a year for Japan, so doing something like that was real fun.

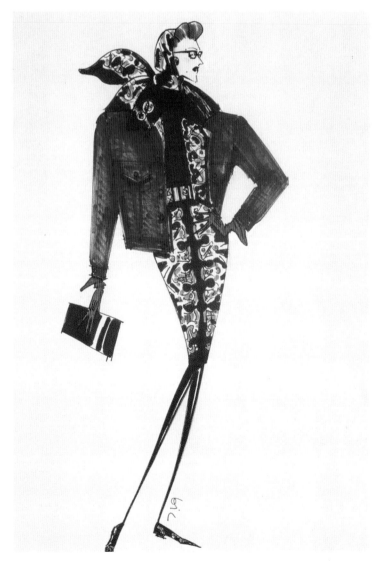

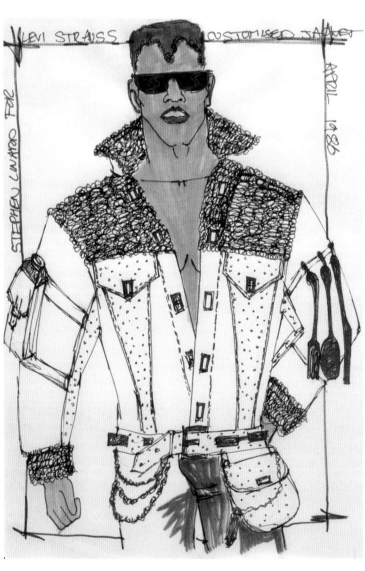

BLITZ DESIGNER
DENIM JACKET

Jasper Conran, designer:
Do you remember how much fun this was? We did it because you asked us to. It wasn't demanded. We knew we'd have fun doing it. The truth is that we didn't really have a clue what we were doing. No idea. I used to spend my time in factories in Dalston. That was the day-to-day reality. Yves Saint Laurent wasn't having to do that, was he?

Rifat Ozbek, designer:
The Hussars jacket was my first thought, because I was doing a lot of military pieces at that time: coats and jackets with frogging and stuff. I picked up that jacket in the bazaar in Istanbul. Tina [Chow] wore it in the show. I certainly do remember that show. It was fantastic. Tina and Leigh and so many have all gone now. It's unbearable.

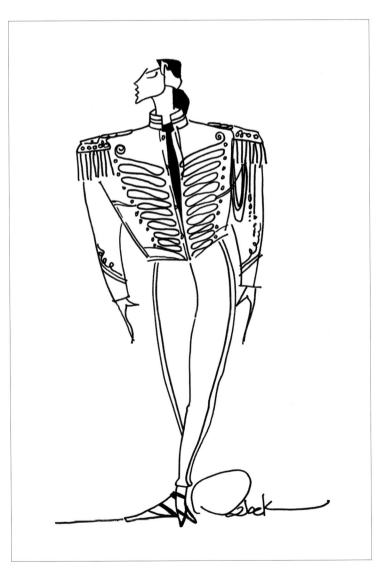

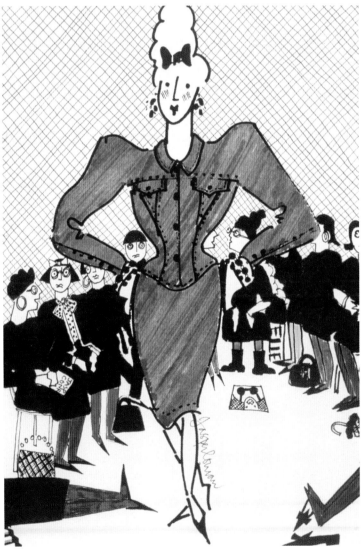

Maria Cornejo, designer, Richmond Cornejo:
I clearly remember us cutting the jacket in half and putting a long tube of jersey into the middle, but I don't think we made it to the show because at that time we were always travelling to Japan. I was only in London half the time. My interns say it seemed like a great time to be part of, and it was. There was such an energy. The music scene as well. We were all part of the whole scene. And there was lots of cross-collaboration. We didn't make any money but we had a lot of fun. The interns now come with a total business plan. Some people had it totally figured out and were happy to do the corporate thing. You were never corporate.

Photographer: David Hiscock

Models: Isobel Deeley at Look, David Paul at Models 1

Make-up and Hair: Louise Constad

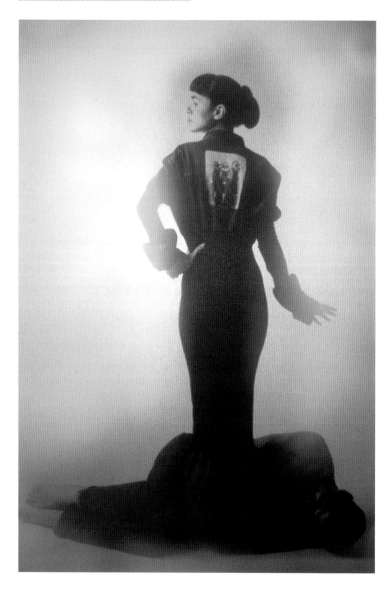

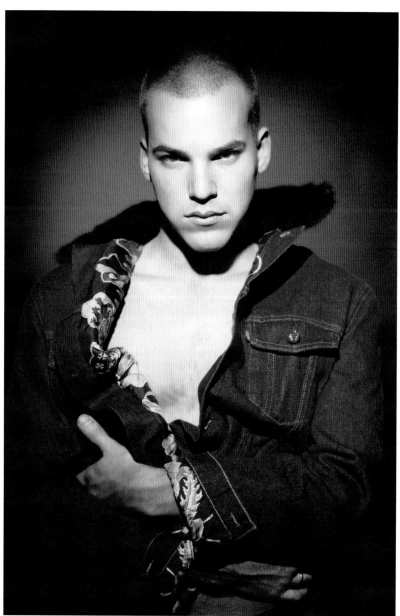

Photographer: Mark Lewis

Model: Jaime Travezan

Jaime Travezan, model:
You got me to wear crazy clothes. They were crazy looks, but I loved them. I was booked to do a shoot with Mark Lewis, and his studio was in the East End, and the other model was Martine. I got lost and she says that when I arrived about an hour late, you asked where had I come from, and I answered, "Peru". She said that's when she knew we would be friends. In those days I would never go further east than Holborn. These days I never go west.

BLITZ DESIGNER
DENIM JACKET

Photographer: David Hiscock

Models: David Paul at
Models 1, Isobel Deeley at Look

Make-up and Hair:
Louise Constad

David Hiscock, photographer:
I was always contained by
the rectangular frame of the
photograph, and I was always
fighting against that. Of course,
when I worked on it I wasn't
thinking about the outside bits,
but that became a language in
its own right for my work later, so
that was the beginning for all that
scratchy stuff, I think. I didn't care
for the pristine image, I never did,
which is why I like the Polaroid
with the ladder in the background
more than the treated images.

Katharine Hamnett, designer:
I am glad we studded it with VOTE
and the CND symbol. Using our
vote to bring peace is still the only
way we will ever achieve it.

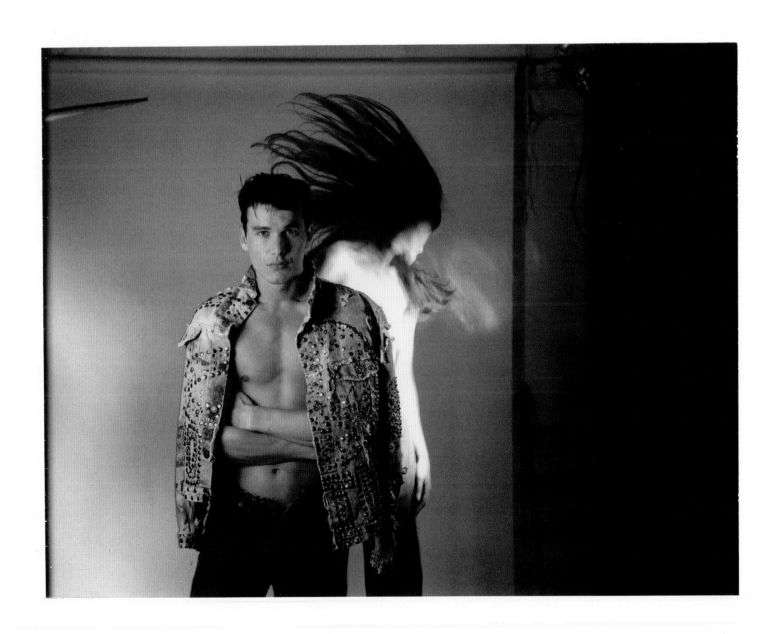

Albery Theatre 15.06.86

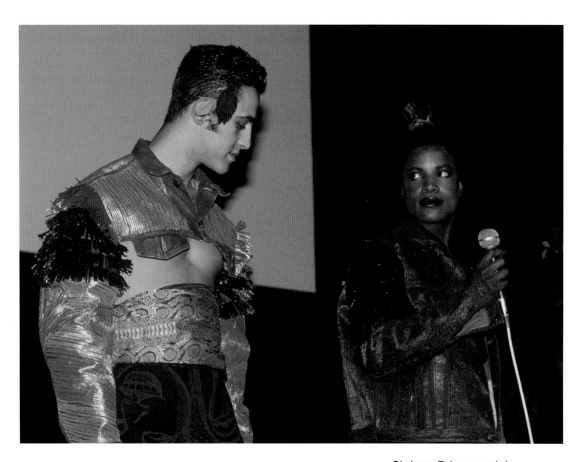

Photographer: Unknown

Models: Christos Tolera, June Montana (of Brilliant)

Christos Tolera, model:
I remember my resistance to the Lycra, but you begged me to wear those matador shorts. It's strange, but I always credit that day with changing my attitude to how I might be perceived by my mates, and I realised that it was all a performance and that I didn't have to identify with the look, but just make it work. The flower behind the ear was a last-minute touch to embrace the personal surrender that I'd secretly made. The other thing I remember was seeing Miranda Richardson backstage and thinking how much I fancied her. I was introduced to her but I don't think I made an impression in my too-easily-misread attire. I never saw her again.

Paul Bernstock and Thelma Speirs, designers, Bernstock Speirs:
You would often ask us to make special pieces for your shoots, which we were always happy to do as it pushed us to take our work in an unexpected direction. The Designer Denim Jackets project was an amazing showcase of talent. The calibre and mix of the designers, artists, models and musicians that were involved is a testament to the respect that you had gained from the creative community. We were excited to be included and decided that we wanted to create something that had a 'street couture' sensibility. We covered the jacket in indigo-dyed glossy raffia, which we stitched flat so that it became integral to the denim, and then added thick bands of fringing to add volume and drama.

June from Brilliant was a great model for the outfit, as she had amazing style and presence, and carried it off magnificently. We saw her as a modern version of the amazing black models that Yves Saint Laurent used in his *couture* shows in the 1970s. We also created a cropped version for Christos and Christopher, who we saw as sexy Puerto Rican hustlers wooing June.

We were always inspired by Warhol's Factory, and loved the idea that our studio also be a social space. We often threw parties where anyone who wanted to have a good time was welcome. Most of London's creatives partied there at some time, including John Galliano, Leigh Bowery, John Flett, Jeremy Healy, Judy Blame, Rachel Auburn, Stevie Stewart and David Holah.

In 1983 Paul opened White Trash with Dencil Williams, a Saturday night dance club in Piccadilly. It was open for three years and became an important part of the London scene. Regulars included Boy George, Paul Weller, George Michael, Sade, Michael & Gerlinde Costiff, Rifat Ozbek and Michael Clark, as well as visits from David Bowie, Mick Jagger, Matt Dillon, Thierry Mugler, Norma Kamali, David LaChapelle and Michael Roberts.

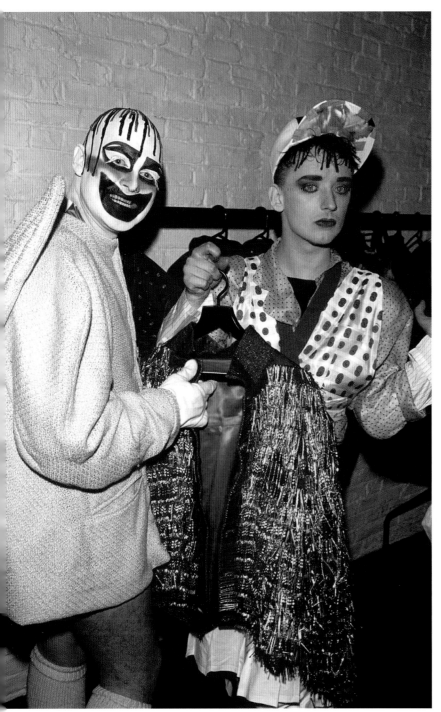

L to R: Leigh, Boy George

Photographer: Brendan Beirne/
Rex Features
Models: Leigh Bowery,
Boy George

I asked old friend Boy George to appear on stage with model Vivienne Lynn, who I had featured way back in issue 11 (May 1983). She would be wearing the *BLITZ* jacket. He readily agreed, but until the very last minute we were not sure if George would turn up. The show fell right in the middle of his 'Heroin Hell' scandal, with TV presenters begging him to turn himself in to the police. So what did George do? Instead of keeping a low profile he appeared on stage at a West End theatre. I have always been grateful for his loyalty. At that time he could have easily stayed holed up at home in Hampstead, but he kept his promise and performed wonderfully, emerging on stage from behind a recent issue on which he was the cover star. He is a natural star and, along with Leigh Bowery, encapsulated the magazine's celebration of unique style. The audience delighted in their antics.

Vivienne Westwood, designer:
I was proud of my jacket. I like to take traditional things and push them into the future and I wanted to give myself a plug, so I used my own logo on the back – the flying orb; it's an example of a traditional English motif, but with the Saturn ring around it to make it futuristic. I lit it up because I like the spirit of competition, which naturally comes when artists have the chance to directly employ their own hand to give their best. I did my best, and when I finished I was sure that no one would have a better jacket than mine. Leigh Bowery covered his jacket with fringes made from thousands of golden hair clips. I thought that was really good.

Judy Blame, designer:
Leigh Bowery was punk rock on his own! He didn't need a whole movement around him, and to watch that man work and be a friend of his was a massive inspiration to my life. I could tell you every person that inspired me but, you know, we'd still be here at four o'clock in the morning. I'd like to say Leigh Bowery and Diana Vreeland together though.

Lynne Franks, PR:
The scene now is very unspontaneous. In PR you have a budget, you get some young girls in to connect with the bloggers, you get quasi-celebs to wear your clothes at a party sponsored by Red Bull. They get their photo taken. It's so formulaic. It's so contrived. I would go absolutely mad! It's not creative in the same way. It was a wonderful, outrageous time. I remember being on a shoot for *Stern* magazine and Leigh [Bowery] was part of it and Rachel [Auburn] and those guys, and Leigh came out of the dressing room covered in gold paint with this huge gold erection. It was wild and silly. It was fun.

Louise Constad, make-up artist:
Meeting Leigh Bowery was lovely. He was such a sweet man. He turned up with all his safety pins and finished it off on the shoot. I went home after the shoot and cut up my jean jacket. I've still got it. I completely remade it, and that was what it was all about.

BLITZ DESIGNER
DENIM JACKET

Designer: Joseph

Models: Paul Coster, Adam Perry, Wade Tolera at Models 1, John Rawlinson at at Nevs, Jenny Howarth

Paul Coster, model:
How could I forget it? It was in that really amazing old theatre. There was me and Adam Perry and John Rawlinson and we had those big motorbikes. There was no rehearsal, and when we had to push those motorbikes on stage I got stuck in the doorway. I was in my pants holding up this motorbike. And then we had to throw Joseph perfume samples into the audience, and I hit a woman right in the face. I was on stage with my kit off in front of a theatre full of people. It was amazing.

Designer: Paul Smith

Models: Ben Volpeliere Pierrot and Curiosity Killed The Cat

Paul Smith, designer:
I remember with great fondness the collaboration I made with you, customising a Levi's jacket. Projects like this are quite commonplace now but in 1986 it was quite a unique thing to do. In a way this sums up *BLITZ* – very adventurous, edgy, and always pushing new boundaries.

Designer: Stephen Jones

Models: Jane Spencer at Z, Nick Heyward

Stephen Jones, milliner:
I always enjoyed being asked to make things, whether it was an Hermès hatbox or a pink wig. It was never just something from the collection. You'd always ask me to do something special, which culminated in the Levi's denim jacket project. That was as far as that could go. And I was always pleased to be included.

Joseph

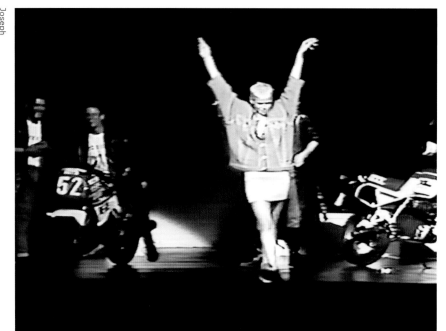

Paul Smith

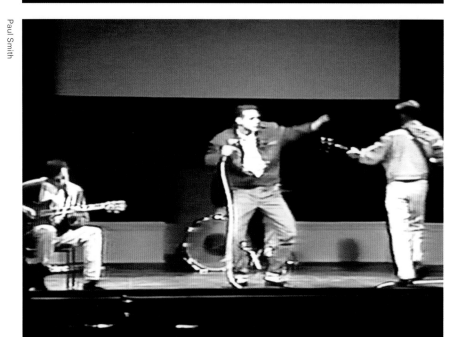

Stephen Jones

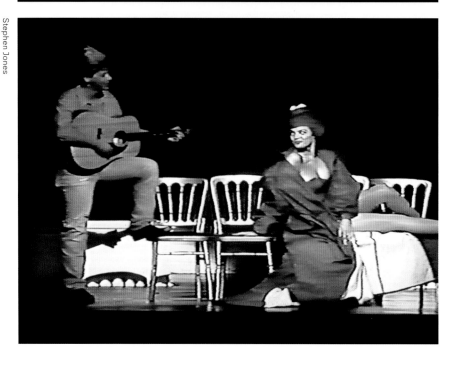

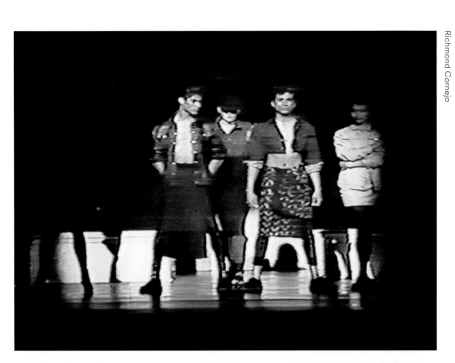

Richmond Cornejo

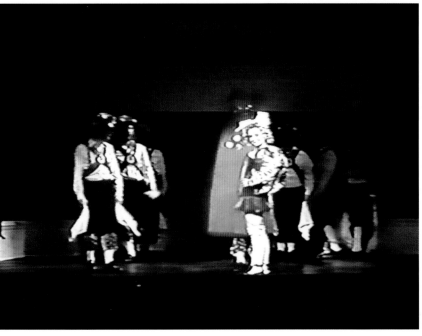

John Galliano

Designer: Richmond Cornejo

Models: Chazz, Moose, Pallas at Z, Leah at Premier, Akure at Models 1, Jenny Howarth

Moose Ali Khan, model:
We were in leggings and skirts all the time. It was about a year before I wore a suit in a show. In Paris I did all the Japanese and freaky *avant garde* designers and I wanted my agents to send me to Dior and Saint Laurent, but they said it wasn't my style. It was a real struggle, as we wanted to make some money as well. So I snuck myself into one of those classic designer's castings and got the job. There was a big transition when Chazz and I went from doing only *avant garde* to eventually only doing classic stuff.

The show was really exciting, everybody was there. We had such fun with Richmond Cornejo. They were really creative. If Richmond Cornejo hadn't done those skirts and stuff, then Gaultier probably wouldn't have done the things he did. I can remember going to see Gaultier and getting the night bus over to Paris and having the appointment to see him, and then we're in the show and, 'Wow, how did that happen?' We got to do so many bizarre things that we never ever dreamed we'd be doing.

Chazz Khan, model:
And it still looks really strong, doesn't it? It still looks 'out there'. I did a show for St Martin's recently and these looks have gone full circle. There are still versions of what was going on. The kids now are referencing our history.

Designer: John Galliano

Models: Sibylle de Saint Phalle at Z, The Enfield Morris Men

Sibylle de Saint Phalle, model:
I remember very little that day, but then I think we were very drunk. I know I was very embarrassed about dancing with all those old men. I was wearing John's jacket with velvety shorts, and I thought I looked like an elf.

The reason I started modelling was to pay the rent. I didn't really like it. I wasn't really extrovert enough to feel comfortable in front of the camera. I never wanted to be a professional model. I was the shorty model before Kate Moss. But all the memories are happy ones. We made everything into a creative experience, even making a cup of tea. We always made an effort. We were all hanging out together, always planning something or other. That might be a photo session or a trip to a museum or a night out. But we always dressed up.

Barneys, New York 10.11.86

Simon Doonan, Creative Ambassador-at-Large, Barneys New York:

BLITZ goes to NYC. In 1986 I went to work at Barneys in New York, where the new expanded women's department store was just about to open. We needed to plan a groovy event around the Fall unveiling. I had heard all about the legendary *BLITZ* Denim Jacket event through my room-mate Robert Forrest, who worked for Rifat Ozbek, and we decided to partner with *BLITZ* and create an American version with more than eighty jackets. Designers included Andy Warhol, Basquiat, Gaultier, Valentino, Blahnik, Sprouse, Haring and basically everyone on Earth. I bought the Alaïa jacket, the best one, and gave it to my London pal Gill Valenzuela. She still wears it.

The models paraded down the circular Andrée Putman staircase. They were quite drunk and utterly fab: Iman, Diane Brill, Nell Campbell, Teri Toye, Edwige and everyone who was groovy at that particular New York moment. Madonna, who had just become the most famous girl in the world, modelled a jacket designed by her artist pal Martin Burgoyne. He was dying of AIDS (the whole event was an AIDS fund-raiser) and was visibly disfigured with Kaposi sarcoma. Madge stayed close to him all night and held his hand. It was very touching, and when people say mean things about her, I always tell them this story. Remember, this was back when lots of people thought you could catch AIDS from kissing.

On a lighter note, John Galliano, who was an emerging genius, came to the event with Susanne Bartsch and Leigh Bowery's New York pal John Badum (RIP Betty!). After knocking back several cocktails, John enlivened the evening by borrowing B52 Kate Pierson's massive red beehive wig. We were all so young and fancy free, back then.

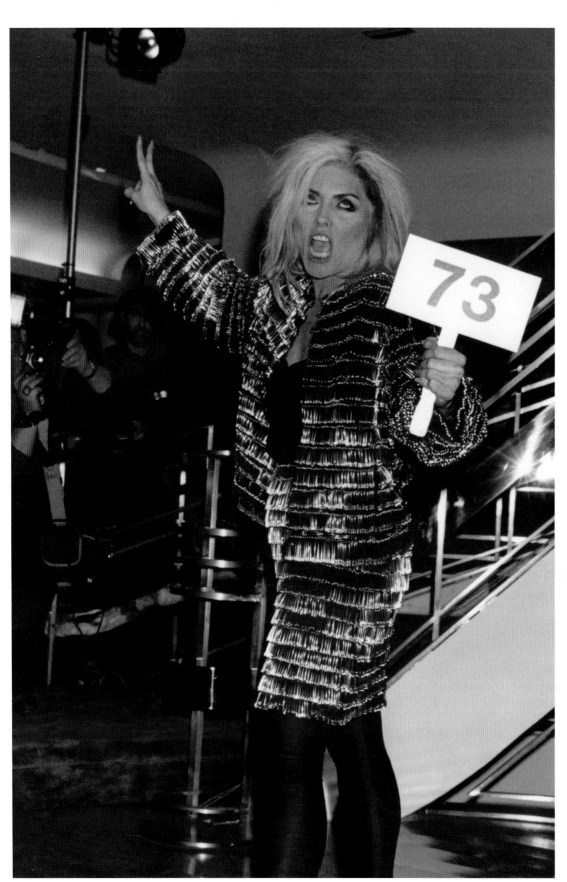

Photographer: Unknown
Model: Debbie Harry

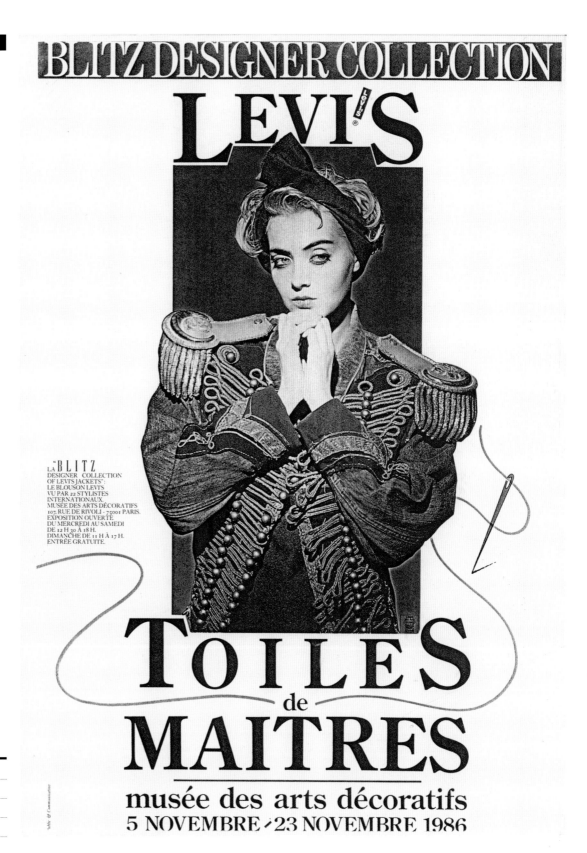

Photographer: Mark Lewis

Model: Zazie

Make-up: Stephanie Jenkins

Hair: Unknown

To say that the scale of the *BLITZ* Designer Denim Jacket project surprised me is an understatement. I could not have believed that what I thought was a simple idea would grow into such an international fashion event. To have the display transfer from the V&A (where during its three month run it was visited by two thousand people a day) to the Louvre in Paris (the spiritual home of fashion) was completely mind-blowing. I love this Xeroxed flyer that was done to publicise the event because it reminded me of the flyers for punk gigs.

Colour, pattern, frills, furs and a face full of make-up. This shoot was a tribute to flashy, trashy Americana. Patricia Fields meets tourist chic. Part Pop Art, part eye-popping. Felix was great at playing the movie star diva, ducking the paparazzi flash. The story was shot on Polaroid because its throw-away instant format provided the perfect metaphor for meteoric fame. We pieced the story together as we went along, doing a layout as the pictures popped out of the camera. I asked Julia Fodor to do the make-up. I loved the garish looks she was pushing herself, so was confident she could create something fitting. I love the dynamic mood of these images, even though they were shot in Pete's bedroom. I was adamant that we could blow up the Polaroids large scale. Little did I know that one of the images would be used for the cover. The result is part papped celebrity, part faded film star.

Pete Moss, photographer:
This was a very fun shoot, not least because of Princess Julia doing the make-up. I was a bit scared of her actually. Felix was perfect and it just seemed like layers and layers of pattern and texture and glitz, all extremely ahead of its time. I am sure Madonna saw this shoot and it seeped in there somehow.

Princess Julia, model/make-up artist:
Did I do the make-up on that? Oh, wow! I was a bit of a crap make-up artist. I did my own make-up and was quite good at doing drag make-up. I should have carried on really and pursued that as a career. These looks were really ahead of the fashion fireball. The scarf on the head is very *Grey Gardens*. The model is sensational. You must have felt you were doing something different from the mainstream, like *19*, or *Vogue* even. When you were working at *BLITZ* were you more or less allowed to do whatever you wanted?

Carole White, model agent, co-founder of Premier Model Management:
I started my own agency, Premier, in 1981 so I was pretty busy with that, even though I still had time to go to clubs and to play poker, which I loved. I always beat all the men. I drove my Citroën all around London, parked badly and got lots of tickets, which I never paid. You can't do that anymore. My lifestyle back then was definitely 'work hard and play hard'. *BLITZ* was very cutting edge, so we all wanted our models to be in it. It was different, and I think the styling was incredibly strong. It does not seem dated, even now. The imagery that you played around with was extremely radical and the shoots produced incredibly powerful pages. You were the hot new thing, so I had to ask you to design and style our model book, as Premier has always needed to reinvent itself through style and graphics. Of course, you came up with the goods and designed two wonderful books for us. I still have them and I think the style has never dated – lovely and strong. Just what I like.

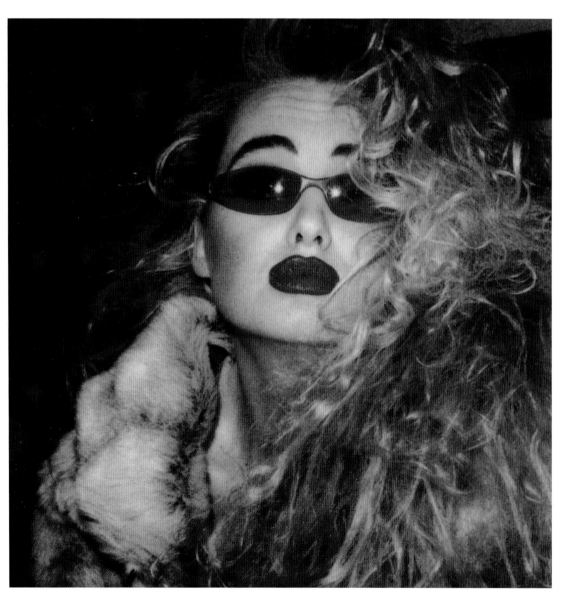

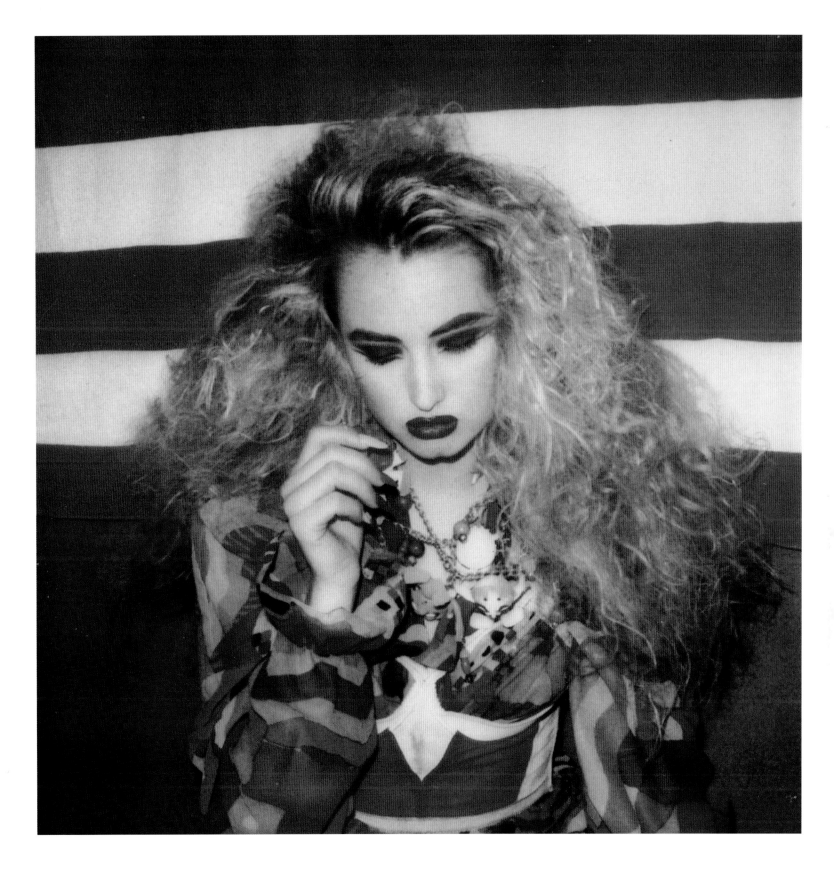

So you want vulgar

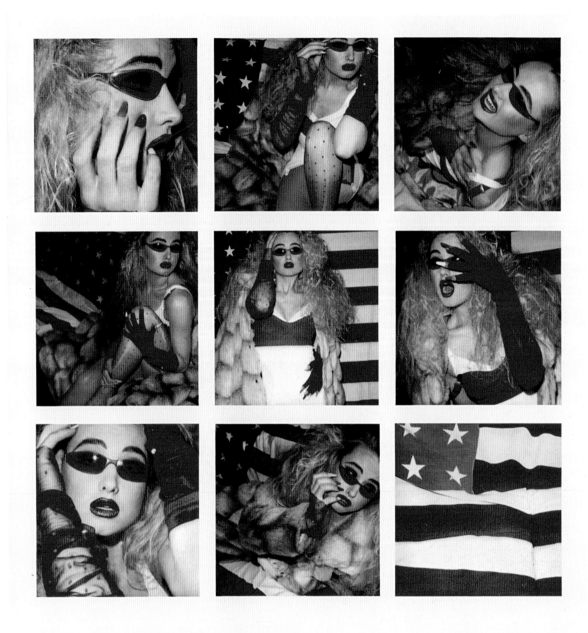

Photographer: Pete Moss

Model: Felix at Premier

Make-up: Princess Julia
using Barry M

Hair: Debbie Horgan for
Daniel Galvin

Clothes: Benedetto, Playtex,
Erickson Beamon, Darryl Black,
Demob, Cornelia James, Elle

WilliWear was a colourful, fun brand of clothing designed by the equally colourful and fun Willi Smith. I used his designs often in the magazine, so when he visited London his PR asked if I would like to interview him, which I did. Robert came along to photograph him. When the profile was published in the magazine, Willi sent me a note saying how much he had enjoyed the experience and how happy he was with the results: 'It's a pleasure to read something that's really me.' Tragically, he died within the year, another victim of the terrible AIDS scourge that was starting to tear through the fashion community. I got a call from his PR asking if I would write an obituary for Willi to be published in *The Guardian* newspaper. I had never written anything like it before, trying to encapsulate a person's life in a few hundred words. Sadly I have written several since.

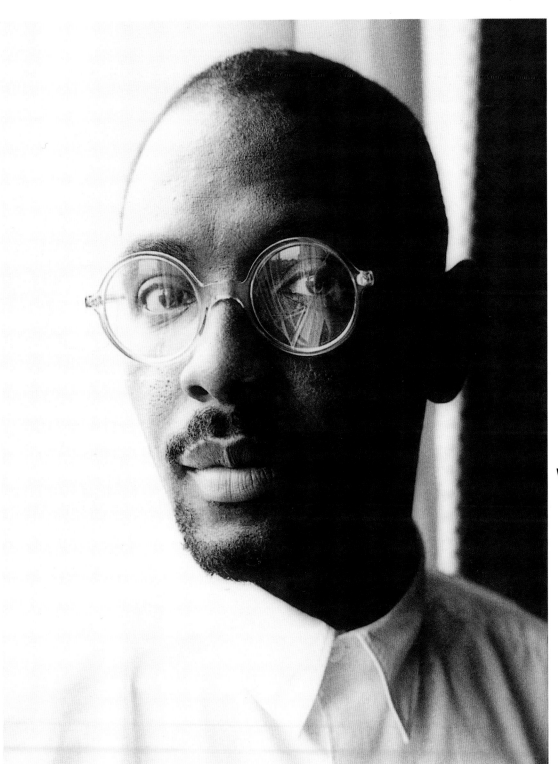

Marysia Woreniecka, PR:
At 19 I went to work for PR Jean Bennett, and half-way through I started freelancing, representing my own clients. Then in 1978, at 22 years old, I decided that I had to start my own PR company because I was getting too old, and if I didn't do it then I'd lose the chance. Everybody was starting their own businesses; it's the same as right now, I guess. I worked out of my flat. My very first client was Jasper Conran. I also represented a company called Miz that was owned by Tanya Sarne and Jane Whiteside, and I looked after Meenys on the King's Road. My best friend, Nicky Marks, was running WilliWear, so we all hung out together. After my flat I had a tiny office in Hanover Square, then moved to Marylebone and then to Chelsea. My boyfriend was in the music business and had an office in Chelsea Manor Studios on Flood Street. I was in the basement but eventually went upstairs as the business grew. By 1983, I'd done all my clubbing. I had my own business and I was living with somebody. All very grown up.

Willi!

Photographer: Robert Ogilvie

L to R: Paul, Adam

Nick Ferrand, photographer:
We shot the guys on a white background in the studio. I can't remember if it was Albion Studios or not. Then we selected the shots and had them printed on 10"x 8" paper. I cut them out and positioned and glued them on the backgrounds cut from travel posters. I then photographed the montage again on a rostrum.

Paul Coster, model:
My friend Mark at Top Models suggested I should do modelling. I was quite an ugly kid so everybody laughed. But I was learning to do upholstery in Shoreditch so I just went for it. I went to Models 1 when Davina McCall was a booker there, and she took me on. I didn't think I'd get in; my friend said to start at the best agency and you may get into one of the lower ones, but I got in. She gave me my first break. And Dick and José. They were great.

I was more worried about holding hands with Adam than I was about standing there with fish stuck down my pants. He was a builder and I was an upholsterer, so it didn't feel right. But I had already worked with photographer Robert Erdmann for *i-D*, and they had made me up like a queen in Speedos, a wig and platforms, and got me walking up and down in Soho with builders

whistling. I was horrified. It was one of my first jobs, but those pictures launched me, and I went on to do all the magazines like *L'Uomo Vogue*. You never knew where things would lead, so I learned to trust the stylist and the photographer. I trusted you. You knew what you were doing. You knew it would look good. You were trying to create something special.

Really, I'm just a puppet. It's the same on a film. You can ask my opinion and I can tell you what I think, but you're the director. You're the boss. Nakedness is all part of the job. If you can't do that you shouldn't be modelling. It was a great step for me when I went from modelling to acting; it really brought me out of myself. And with acting you get asked to do far worse things.

If you'd have done those pictures on location, it wouldn't have worked. Those dodgy backgrounds make it work. They remind me of the screens behind a car chase in a B-movie. Those pictures are lovely, brilliant, and the graininess is great. It all works.

Photographer: Nick Ferrand

Models: Paul Coster, Adam Perry at Models 1

Clothes: Nikos, Val Piriou , Malcolm Poynter

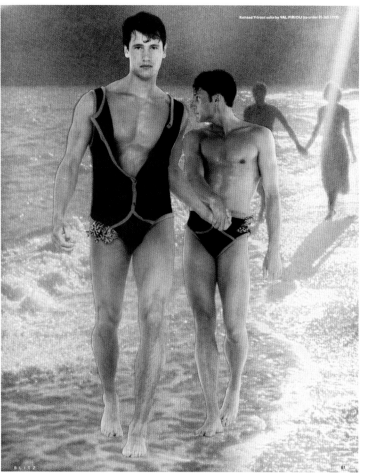

L to R: Paul, Adam

Beach bums

There were few men's magazines that dealt with fashion. We presented a new way of looking at men. Designers were offering fancy underwear, from the body-conscious homoerotic styles of Nikos, to the nostalgic knitted all-in-ones of Val Piriou. As we did not have a budget for a trip to some faraway location, we decided to collage the images of Paul and Adam onto exotic pictures gleaned from local travel agents. The fish accessories were all designed by artist Malcolm Poynter. This was the beginning of the men's fashion and grooming explosion.

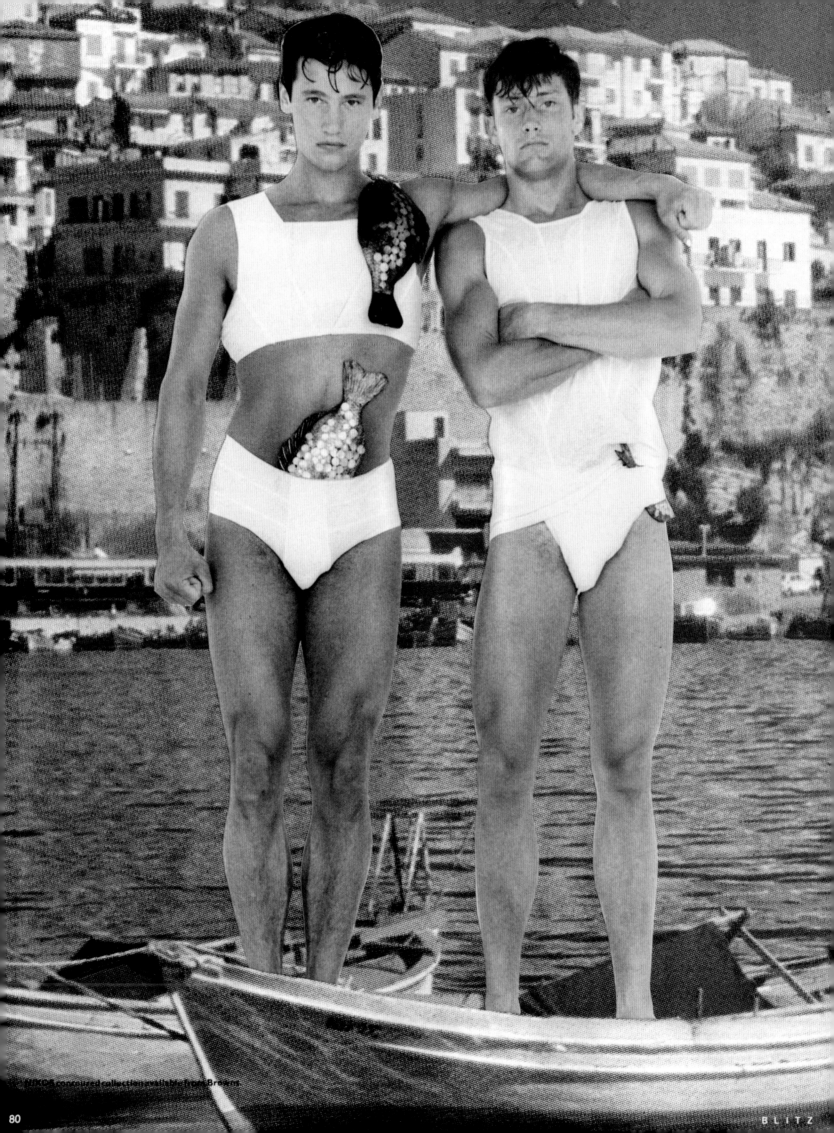

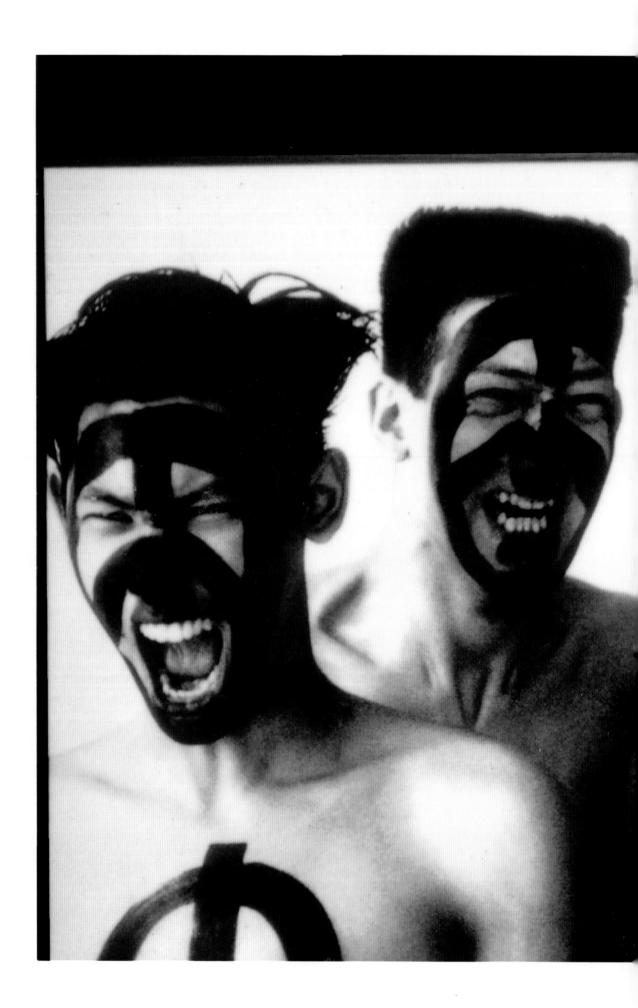

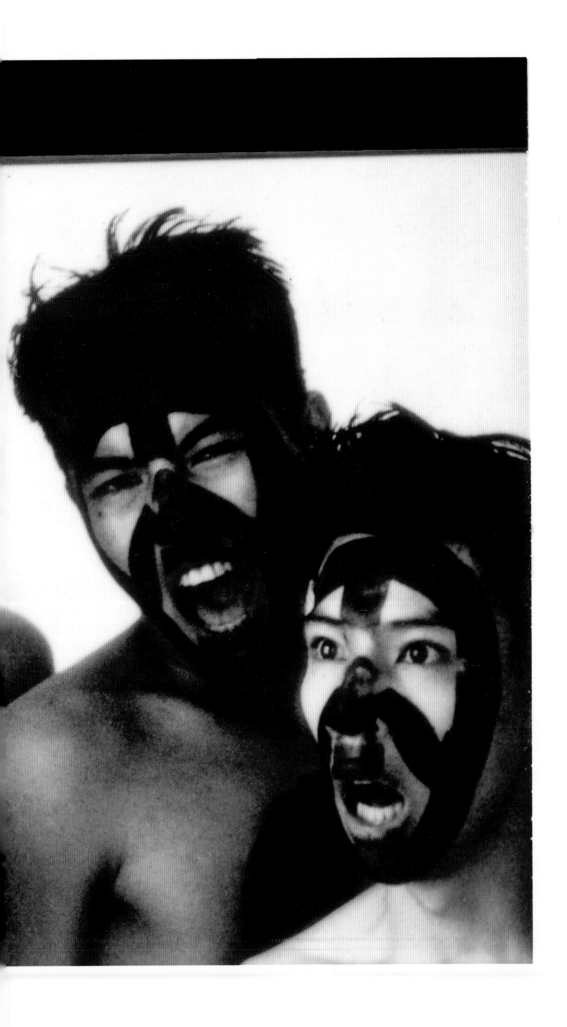

Mark Lewis, photographer:
I remember going into *Marie Claire* in Paris and showing them this story. I was pretty proud of that shoot and they were absolutely horrified, and it was then that I realised that we were quite radical, and how conservative the rest of the fashion world was – and how I would struggle to fit into the world of fashion.

Christian Nguyen, model:
As I used to live with Mark's sister, I would model for test shoots and projects for his personal portfolio. He was keen on using non-stereotypical models. Being friends with Mark and his make-up artist wife, Stephanie Jenkins, we developed a great working chemistry. There was always a relaxed atmosphere during the shoots. I also knew two of the other models Daniel and Duke (aka Jeffrey), who was my flatmate. The styling was very dark. I remember wearing a crown of dead black roses. The hand-painted T-shirt reminded me of Katharine Hamnett's slogan messages. It's such a powerful image. The photo of us screaming really visually describes the horror of a nuclear strike. I didn't realise how iconic this shoot would become as a reflection of the '80s. I was already pleased to be part of it, but have been delighted to see that the picture keeps reappearing in *Vogue Italia*, *Elle* and the book *Excess: Fashion and Underground in the '80s*.

Barry Kamen, model:
Who wrote that on the T-shirt? That's so you. It looks like Sid Vicious writing on his skin.

Mark Moore, model:
I think it was Darryl who asked if I'd do the photo shoot. I remember thinking, 'Finally someone with vision has discovered me.' People were always being discovered in nightclubs and whisked away to Japan or New York to model. It was perfectly normal really. For months I had been expecting Fellini to stroll into town and put me in his latest movie, but somehow it never happened. But this was it. I had made the big time.

The concept was all war paint, anti-nuclear, *Blade Runner* and Asian dudes. We all lived in fear of being nuked by Russia back then, as well as the earth crashing into the sun. On the shoot I felt like a fish out of water. The other guys seemed so relaxed. Were they real models? They certainly looked like real models. I felt very unattractive next to them. Then we were told we had to appear topless. I was nervous enough modelling fully clothed on my first big photo shoot and now I had to appear semi-naked displaying my skinny torso to the world. I could feel the doom setting in. Luckily the photographer was such a gentle and patient person that he put everyone at ease.

The finished photos were fantastic and my friends looked at me with a new sense of pride when the magazine came out. I was a *bona fide* supermodel. Gradually more photo shoots started to happen just as my DJ career was taking off: *i-D* magazine, *The Face* and more. When I formed my band S'Express, there would be a photo shoot every other day, but I took it all in my stride thanks to the basic training I received on this *BLITZ* shoot. Happy times indeed, and yes, we were out clubbing every night. How we ever got up in time to see daylight still puzzles me to this day.

Princess Julia, model:
It's such a contemporary image. It's so now. Do you know the stylist Matthew Josephs? He's amazing and he looks a bit like this boy. These are all the images he's inspired by.

Rick Haylor, hairdresser:
It was about making a statement, breaking the rules. Now stylists are forever being told that 'you can't put my clothes with somebody else's clothes', whether it's Prada, Marc or Givenchy. It's not giving people the opportunity to be stylists. You were basically saying, 'Don't buy the clothes' – not the best way to build a career in the fashion industry. But you were being honest and pure, and that statement in itself ended up getting you the jobs. You believed in what you were doing. We were all really excited about what we were doing. *BLITZ* gave us a vehicle that allowed us to be creative even if we weren't making money. None of us started off wanting to make money. I would rather have earned nothing and done something special than make loads of money and do something shit. I tell my girls: 'You're going to be working for a very long time, so if you do something with that passion, it will sustain you.' You loved what you were doing and you shared that enthusiasm.

Hiro

The story was prompted by the pervasive threat of nuclear war. I was totally seduced by the film *Blade Runner* and its doom-laden, future-world landscape, a hybrid of the technotronic vibe of urban Japan and the raggle-taggle shabbiness of post-punk realism. The photographs showcased neo-couture accessories by jewellery designer Judy Blame and shoe designer John Moore, who created unique pieces from salvage. The models wore bondage trousers and draped robes, barefoot with black roses in their even blacker hair. The mood was purposefully menacing, yet spiritual. During the shoot I scrawled on a white T-shirt in black paint: 'WE'RE NOT HERE TO SELL CLOTHES' (see frontispiece). For me, this photograph encapsulates my entire ethos in one image.

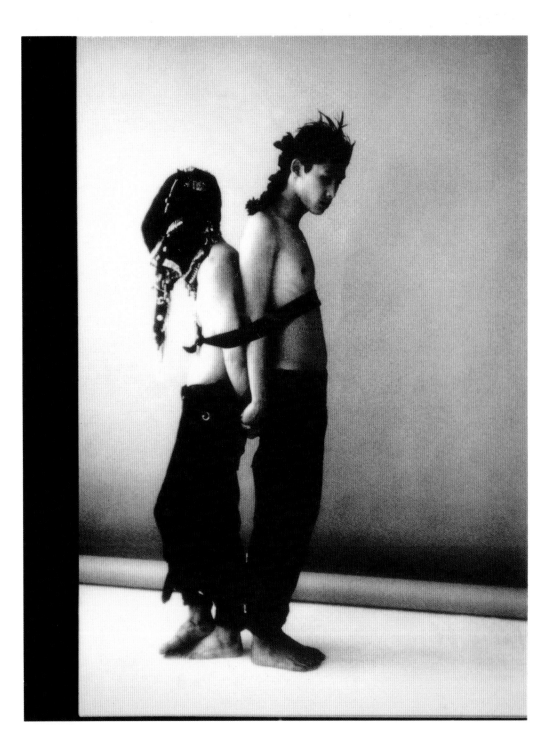

L to R: Christian, Duke

Photographer: Mark Lewis

Models: Duke, Daniel at Z, Hiro at Marco Rasala, Mark Moore, Christian

Clothes: Seditionaries, Judy Blame, Sara Sturgeon, Yohji Yamamoto, Paul Craig, Comme des Garçons, John Moore

No nukes is good news

In 1986 the Inner London Education Authority merged London's art, design, fashion and media schools together as the London Institute (now known as University of the Arts London). To celebrate, it hosted a fashion show at the glamorous headquarters of the Greater London Council on the banks of the Thames, showcasing a 'Best of...' line-up of graduating designers. Among them was Kumars Moghtader from the London College of Fashion, whose work became the featured collection that accompanied my review of the event. I liked his glam baroque moment.

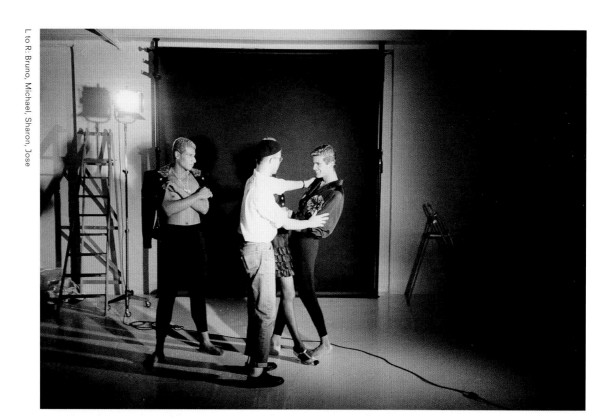

L to R: Bruno, Michael, Sharon, Jose

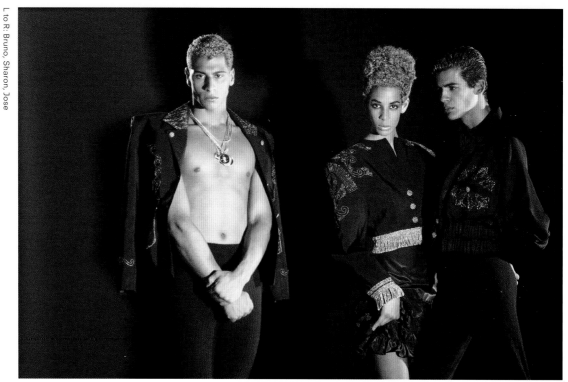

L to R: Bruno, Sharon, Jose

Second time around (in more ways than one)

Michael Daks, photographer:
I left Wolverhampton Art College in 1981 and spent a year in my hometown of Southport running my own studio, shooting model tests for Liverpool and Manchester agencies and building my portfolio. I was already reading *BLITZ*, *i-D* and *The Face* when I moved to London in 1982. I was a club kid, hanging out at the Wag, Café de Paris and especially Taboo, and then getting the night bus back to Camberwell. I was lucky enough to meet the most interesting characters on the scene – Leigh Bowery, Ray Petri, Boy George, Duggie Fields et al.

I had a small studio on New Cavendish Street in Marylebone, underneath a trendy hair salon. If I wasn't shooting or showing my book, I'd hang out at the Soho Brasserie on Old Compton Street doing some serious networking, or at The Groucho Club, Fred's or The Zanzibar.

I had already shot portraits for *BLITZ* before we met. I was pleasantly surprised that you liked my colour photography because most clients preferred the black and white. Your first commission was an ethnic story. At that time I was mostly shooting at my friend Nick Ferrand's Albion Studios. It was much bigger than my own and had great daylight. John Galliano used to rent a corner and was often there drawing or sewing.

This story was shot at Albion. The models were Brazilian. For some reason I shot black clothes against a black background but backlit them so they would stand out. I really liked the embroidered gold brocade, and had hairstylist Paul spray their hair to match. Fortunately, it washed out. Seeing the photograph of me on set directing the models reminds me of my own shoot wardrobe – a white Hamnett shirt, original Levi 501s, black Dr. Martens shoes, white socks and, of course, a beret! I got a huge kick out of seeing my work in print. I still do.

Photographer: Michael Daks

Model: Sharon Dolphin at Z, Bruno Soares and Jose Enriques at Marco Rasala

Make-up: Regina at Lynne Franks

Hair: Paul Kennington for Joshua Galvin

Clothes: Kumars Moghtader

Kumars Moghtader, designer:
In the summer of 1986 I graduated at the London College of Fashion, the end of four years of studying fashion, having previously attended Great Yarmouth College of Art. It was an exciting time to be a student living in London. Having spent hours deciding 'the look', we'd spend our nights at clubs like Taboo, Ascension and Kinky Gerlinky, high on all the inspiration and creativity around us. Then we were up, after four hours of sleep, all bright eyed and bushy-tailed and ready for the new day.

1986 was a special year, as the merging of the art schools meant we would present our final collections at our regular end-of-year fashion show and also at a second show alongside the more prestigious Central Saint Martin's, one of the leading design schools in the world.

It was intimidating, but an opportunity to share the media attention that CSM garnered. My collection had already received a very positive reaction, but I held no expectation of standing out amongst the students from the revered college (that, incidentally, I had initially applied to but was not accepted at, following a dismal interview).

I could barely believe the great response I got that night, and was even more amazed to get a call from you asking to feature the collection in *BLITZ* as your pick of the graduate fashion shows. It felt like I had won the lottery.

The piece was so much more than I had imagined. A whole spread and so beautifully styled. I loved that one of the men was so casually and confidently wearing one of my tailored women's jackets, without forsaking any masculinity. The image was so true to the spirit of fashion of the time and, in some ways, timeless.

After seeing the issue, Keith Spicer, who ran Bazaar men's boutique on South Molton Street, contacted me. They stocked the likes of Gaultier, Galliano, Judy Blame and Christopher Nemeth, and he wanted to sell my clothes too. It was an opportunity that, grateful as I was, forced me take the plunge into a world that I was not yet ready for. With hindsight, I should have used this valuable coverage to gain experience working with a more established designer.

With no backing, I spent a couple of years working day and night on small collections and commissioned designs. In the meantime, a love for vintage Barbie dolls had me doing freelance work for Hasbro on their Sindy doll, which desperately needed a makeover from homely girl to modern '80s teen. Soon, Hasbro asked me to join them full-time and I jumped right in.

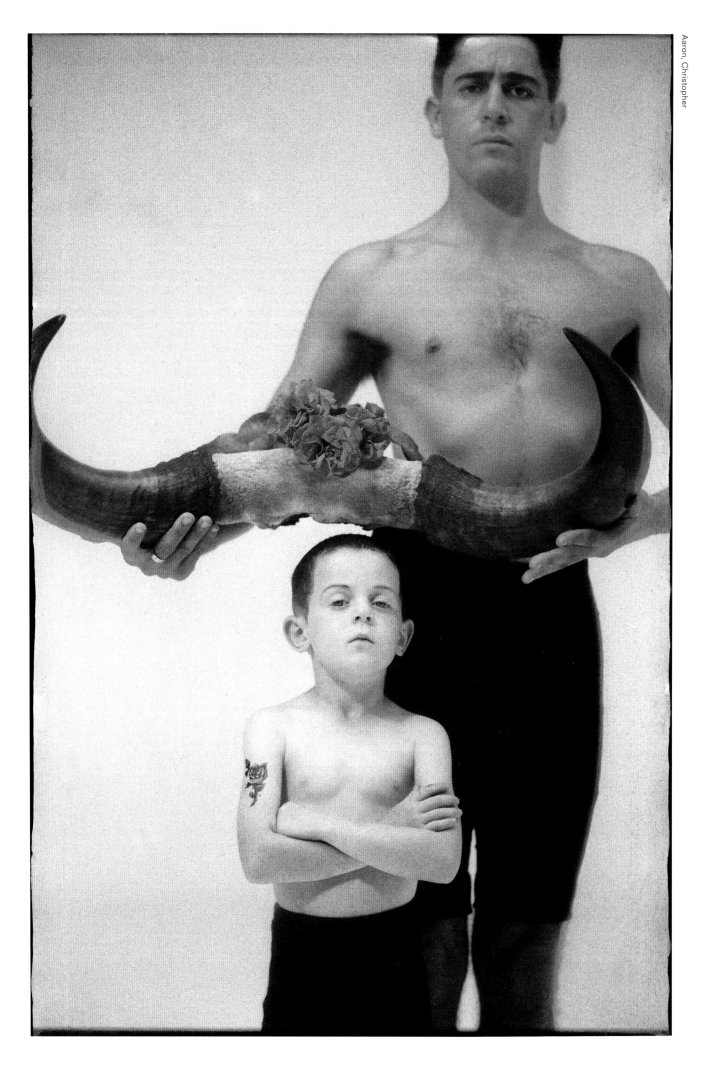

BLITZ #45
September 1986

Photographer: Willem Odendaal

Models: Megan at Premier, Christopher at Askews, Davide at Z, Aaron Dryland

Make-up: Maggie Baker

Hair: Debbie Dannell for Edmonds salon

Clothes: Moschino, Cornucopia, David Fielden, Trevor Hill for John Flett, Samco, Condor Cycles, Joe Casely-Hayford, Darryl Black, Jasper Conran

Willem Odendaal, photographer:
Every time we worked together on a *BLITZ* fashion spread it was a great challenge – seeing what you were imagining, creating strong images that would reflect my vision, and, at the same time, capturing the spirit of the ideas that you had laid in front of me. The little matador boy has always been one of my favourite images. I have never lost your *BLITZ* spirit. In a way it stuck with me, and always sneaked in to the photographs I took for other magazines.

You jump-started my career as a photographer and I have always been grateful for that. You gave me the opportunity of a lifetime. Before they liked me in the Netherlands, you liked me first.

Debbie Dannell, hairdresser:
It was completely rebellious, against fashion and what a fashion shoot was supposed to be. It was against what was out there. We weren't wearing fashion. Some of the stuff, we made. It was all made up.

Johnny Rozsa, photographer:
I think we looked at everything and found inspiration everywhere. I worked at a shop called Nostalgia, so I was traipsing up and down Portobello and buying thirties or forties dresses, or twenties beaded dresses, or Victorian stuff. I really knew my references – it was a history of fashion, in a way. I didn't learn it or go to college, but I got that from working in the shop, and then Friday night we'd go to a film. We knew who Ava Gardner or Rita Hayworth were. I didn't know who Marie Antoinette really was, but I knew that she had her hair all piled up, or I knew a Japanese reference. Visual or historical or cultural references were key.

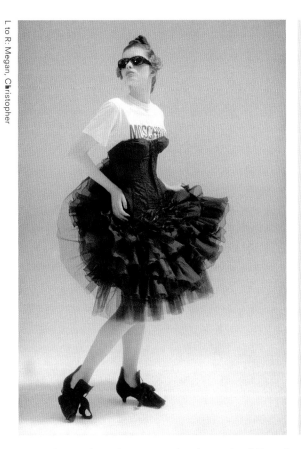

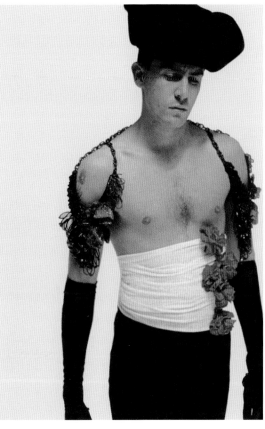

L to R: Megan, Christopher

Barry Kamen, model:
We were all interested in film, art, music and rebellion, but we used clothes to tell the story. And the idea of doing a campaign, or trying to get a tear sheet that would please Miuccia Prada or somebody, would just not figure.

On a Saturday afternoon I had watched *Pandora and the Flying Dutchman*, the 1951 movie starring Ava Gardner and James Mason, on TV. On Monday morning I went into the office and said, 'Let's do a Spanish story'. I wrapped the boy's waist with bandages and pinned on red roses to resemble blood (the heroic gored matador). A Jasper Conran red taffeta ballgown skirt became a toreador's cape. Darryl attached hundreds of tiny gold safety pins to a pair of black Lycra cycling shorts and we sprayed the hairdresser's nephew's hair black and gave him a fake tattoo. Picasso-esque *Toros* were painted on the boy's chest, while Megan modelled a Moschino T-shirt under her corset, and a blindfold accessorised with a tulle petticoat as a mantilla. Think Spain!

Spanish stroll

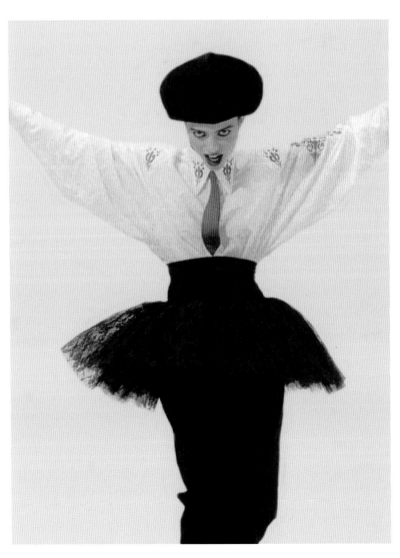

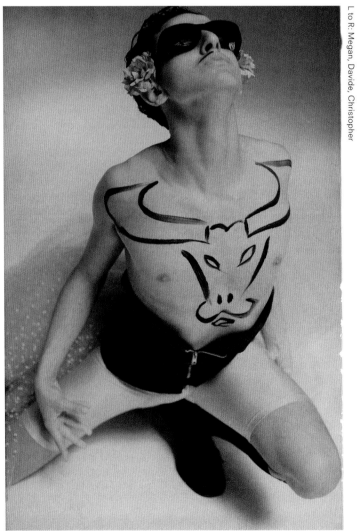

L to R: Megan, Davide, Christopher

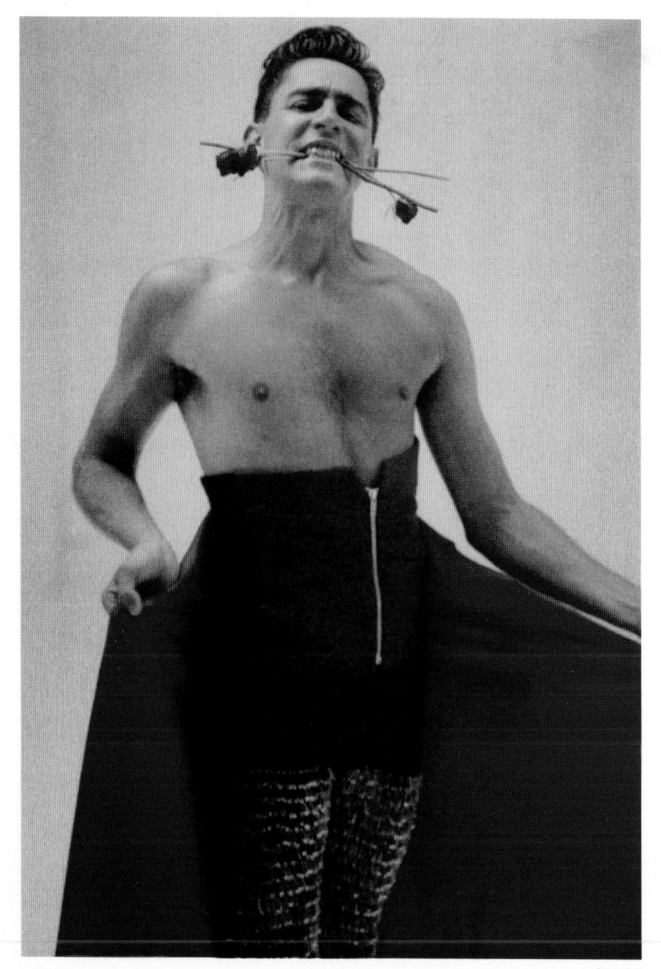

Safety pinned shorts realised by **DARRYL BLACK.**
Zip front corset by **JOE CASELY HAYFORD.**
Red taffeta skirt by **JASPER CONRAN** 37 beauchamp place london sw3.
Sword kindly loaned by **TONI KINMAN.**

This story was another production with a cast of models, some old favourites and some new faces. I guess this was another knitwear story, although the emphasis was less direct, and also included sheepskin coats and anoraks that were children's size, and worn on the boys' heads. People have asked if they were supposed to be superhero capes, like a child would wear in the playground, but actually I had seen a young father carrying his son's coat the same way. Maybe he wanted to appear like a superhero to his little boy? The shoot also included knitted squares that my Dad had stitched up, which I fixed to the models with masking tape. I also wrapped some of the models with blue and white striped paper bags that I had ripped apart. I have no idea where that particular style statement came from, but I love the end result.

Skinny ribs

Michael Woolley, photographer:
I always did my own thing. My plan was just to make images, and hope that people would like them and use them as they wanted. You were very good at that; you reacted as I wanted. I was never part of any particular movement, but was always able to click with those different movements without becoming part of a scene. I think this afforded me longevity and an international career; more so than many of my contemporaries that started out at the same time. It was always a pleasure working with you, often eye-opening and eye-watering at times, but I was along for the ride. I was very grateful to be a part of it.

It was an interesting look. Your dad knitted those squares, didn't he? Where did those ideas come from? I always wondered how much you were working off the top of your head and how much was planned. Being one of my first published jobs, I was in between being scared and amused with the whole idea. At the same time, I thought it looked great so I decided to make the most of it. We shot it simply and very graphically because there was a lot going on. I was quite nervous, so it was a cautious decision to keep it very simple. I didn't want to overegg the pudding. If I shot this story now I'd probably do it on location. The casting is very strong, especially the men. I'm pretty sure the style magazines just wouldn't use a story like this anymore. They are so accountable to the advertisers now.

I wasn't really hung up on wanting to screw the models, which seemed to be the motivation for a lot of other photographers to get into the business. I took a more artistic approach. In the long run this gave me an identifiable point of view. I definitely ploughed my own furrow. It took me in an interesting direction that other people weren't doing, although sometimes I was seen as over-precious. What I did at that time kept me alive for things that followed.

Simon Ringrose, model:
I was doing whatever work came up: editorial, advertising and shows. I suppose the big difference with BLITZ was that it generally wasn't selling anything; it was more about being different, and challenging the way we look at fashion. For me, not being from a fashion background but enjoying all things alternative and art-related, I felt proud of what I helped achieve with BLITZ. It was very much your thing, but everyone involved was encouraged to have an input. We were helping to make some art, if that doesn't sound too poncey. But the bottom line is, we all had fun and a good laugh, as most of your ideas were pretty out there. BLITZ was very serious about what it did, but you had to look at it with your tongue firmly in your cheek, and always with a pinch of salt. I had a crazy four years immersed in the world of fashion and I still wonder what it was all about. Nice arm-warmers.

Barry Kamen, model:
Who made those knitted squares? Taped on. That's brilliant. This is really beautiful styling. The big sleeves, that's beautiful. They are totally like paintings. When you took a picture of Simon, you were taking a picture of someone who was thinking, and so often models are not thinking, they are posing. With Simon you could always see there was something going on, he wasn't just an empty vessel.

Photographer: Michael Woolley

Models: Ian, Andrew Burn at Marco Rasala, Simon Ringrose, Laurence James Thomas and Robert Bennett at Z, Susi Vaughan

Make-up: Beth Satchat

Hair: Beth Satchat, using hairpieces from Hair Raisers

Clothes: Benetton, BHS, Katharine Hamnett, Reldan, John Rocha, Reg

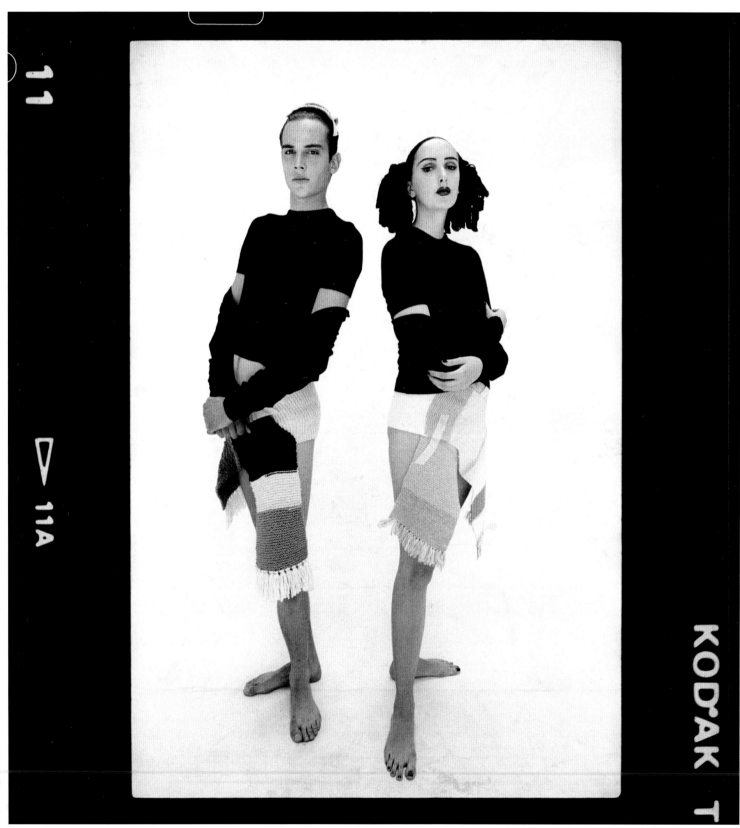

L to R: Simon, Susi.

L to R: Andrew, Simon, Lawrence James

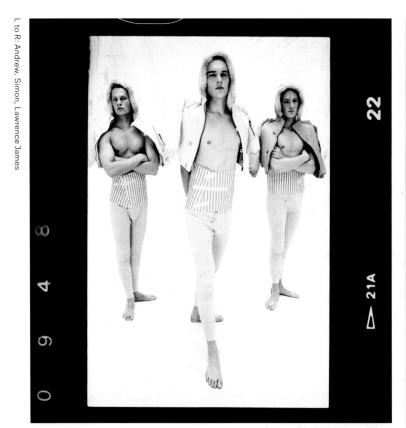

22 ▷ 21A

Ian

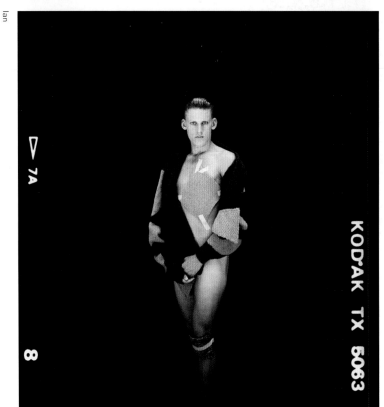

▷ 7A 8

KODAK TX 5063

KODAK TX 5063

Simon, Andrew

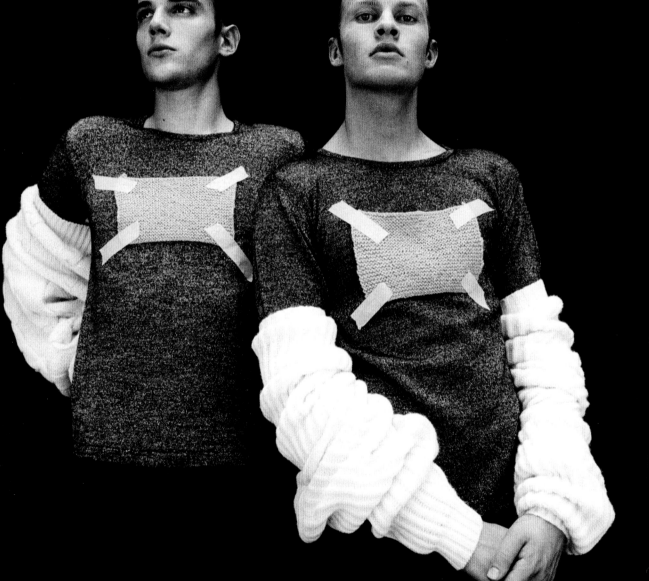

Shady character

Photographer: Pete Moss

Model: Sharon Dolphin at Z

Clothes: Vivienne Westwood, Stephen Jones

Pete Moss, photographer: London was very much an open city then; one didn't need permission, it seems, to shoot anywhere. I remember shooting this story at the back of the Bank of England at night, with a petrol generator and set of 'red head' lights. We simply parked our cars right next to the shoot and fired up the generator, which was really noisy. We didn't ask permission and amazingly no one asked what we were doing. I can't see that happening now. This was such an inspired idea of yours, and really nice to shoot, as it was so formally and so conceptually spot-on. I think this is one of the best shoots we did. Sharon was excellent.

Stephen Jones, milliner: I love that shoot and I love that hat too. It was in my collection, a very traditional jersey glove in a taupe colour, hand sewn together. It was made for me by Cornelia James in the department that made hats for the Queen. That was also the year that Philip [Treacy] was working for me.

Even though *BLITZ* catered for an arty readership, I was always getting letters that complained, 'We can't see the clothes properly'. This sparked me to do a shoot where there would be no clothes to see, only the shadows they cast. Thankfully, that particular season, silhouettes were especially exaggerated, so worked well with this concept. The model, Sharon, was wonderfully bendy, with expressive limbs. Ever the professional, she changed in the car, parked up on the pavement. I really like the elongated Westwood mini-crini image and the Stephen Jones glove hat, with its overtones of Schiaparelli's surrealist hats.

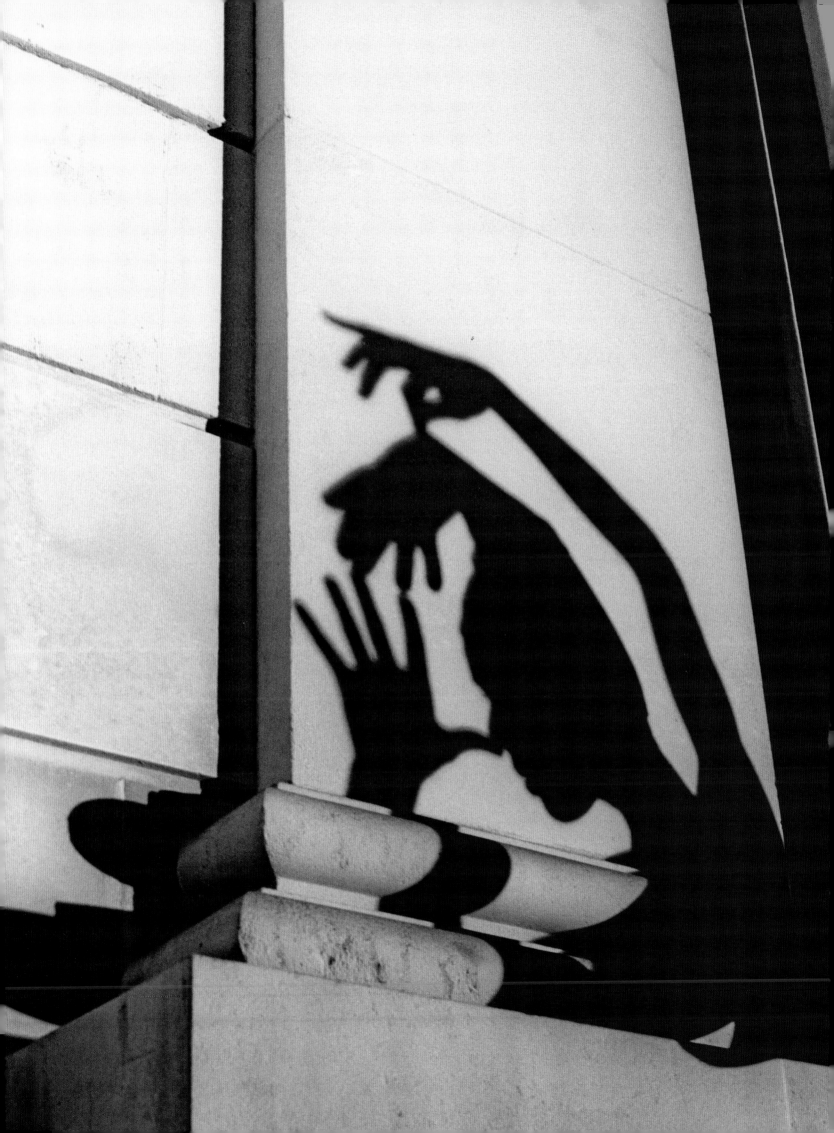

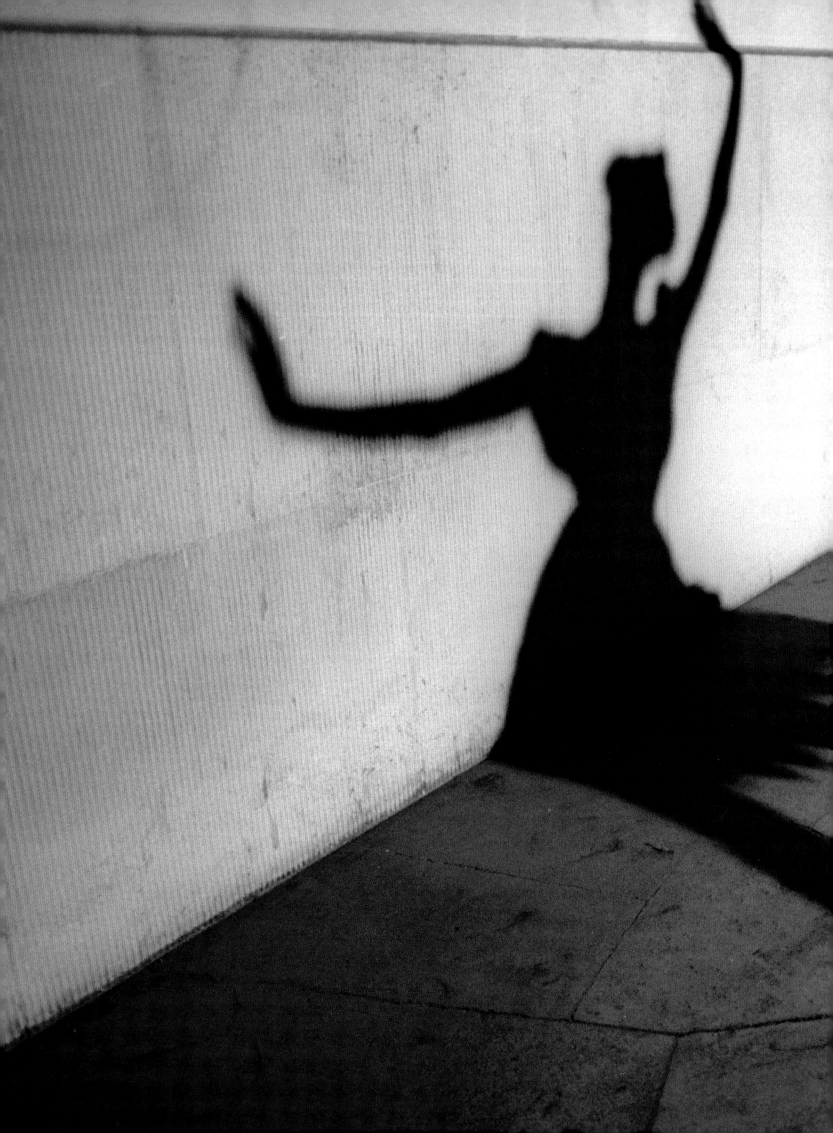

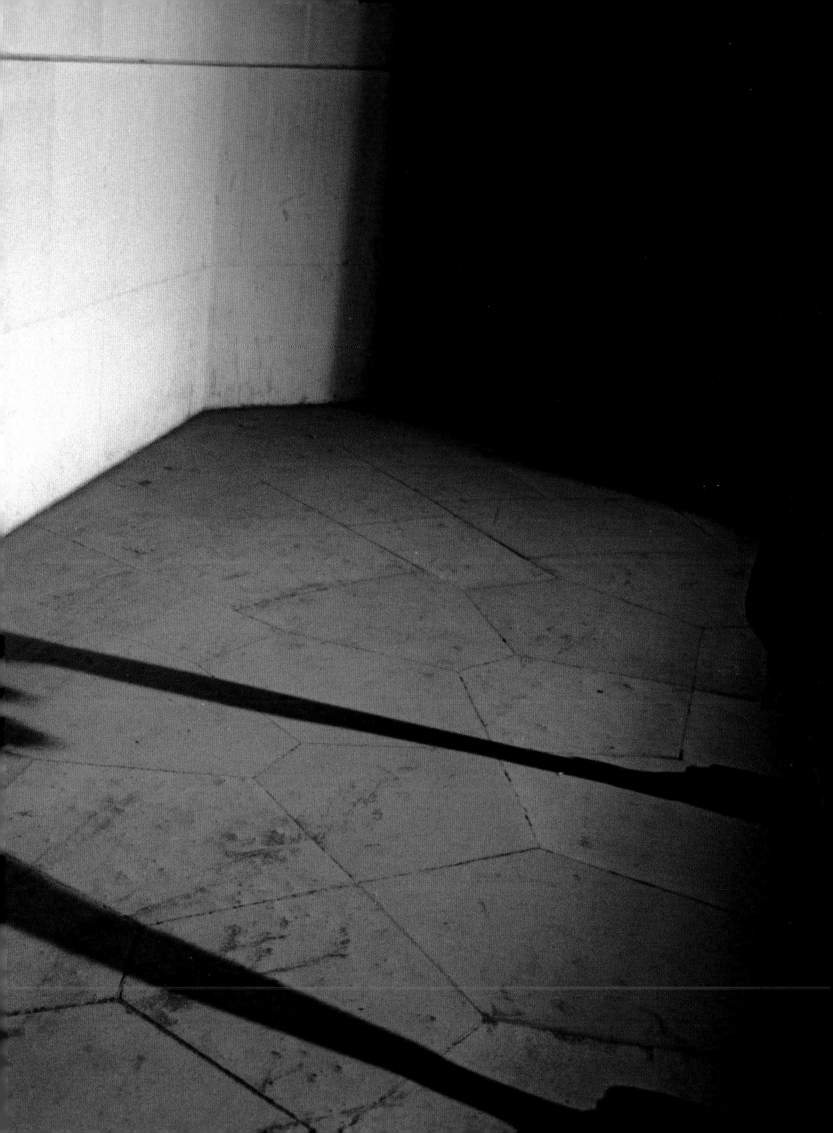

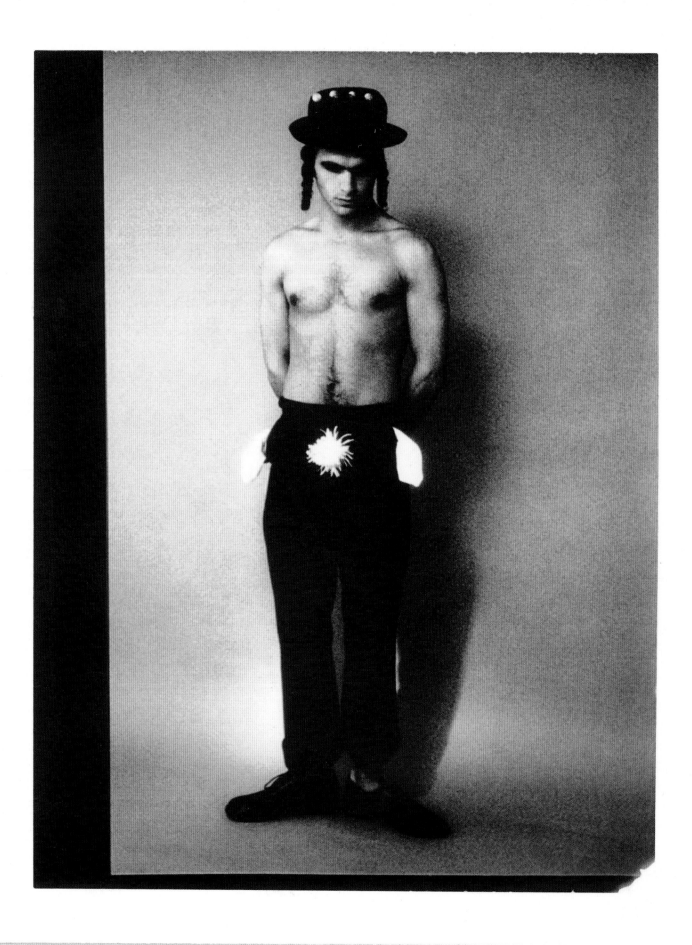

For this shoot I had probably thought about doing a bigger hair look, but in the end it boiled down to just those two locks with everything pulled away. Very simple. I might have got carried away and done what was in fashion on the runway, but what I realised, is that the hair had to be built around the shoot. It was about making the look on the day, on the shoot, rather than having a preconceived idea that I'd want to do, whatever the look.

Mark Lewis, photographer:
Although there were many shoots we did together, the Jewish locks shoot is one of my favourites. I mainly shot with Polaroid film and made prints onto 669 Polaroid, and those 9cm x 7cm prints were used for reproduction. When possible, I shot on an old-fashioned 10" x 8" plate camera, which enabled the magazine to reproduce directly from the 10" x 8" print.

David Holah, designer, Bodymap:
You delved into history for ideas. The way we worked was the way you worked, which wasn't necessarily in a fashion way. The way you styled in the magazine wasn't about trends. We weren't working to trend forecasts. It became trendy. The images are more timeless than sitting in an '80s space. The work transcends time. It was beyond fashion. We weren't out to be fashionable. BLITZ established us as designers.

Rick Haylor, hairdresser:
I loved how you turned up in the studio and altered the old men's jackets. There was one jacket without a pinstripe so you just took out some tailors chalk and drew stripes directly onto it. I went home that night and told my wife Deborah all about it, and she was totally into it. I picked up on the way you worked and it helped me a lot later in my career. You were actually building things on set. On a regular shoot there would be a rail of clothes, and models would try things on, but you were actually working on set. You'd change things about and re-work clothes. You were pushing a lot of different ideas but it was always about the clothes. How you could make them work for the shoot. Being creative was what it was all about, looking different and being different. We shared that same energy on the shoots.

Darryl Black, fashion assistant:
It was never about showing fashion. It was about fantasy and having fun. I always remember this jacket that you stitched like a corset. All my seams are on the outside now.

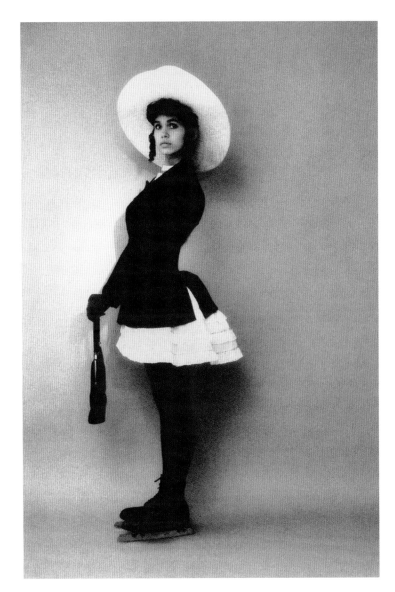

Living along Victorian lines

Photographer: Mark Lewis

Models: David Hume at Z, Elizabeth at Synchro.

Make-up: Stephanie Jenkins

Hair: Rick Haylor for Vidal Sassoon.

Clothes: Help The Aged, Bernstock Speirs, Holts, Oxfam, Past Caring, 20th Century Box, Paul Craig

Yohji Yamamoto showed a collection inspired by upper crust Victoriana, but which of us street urchins could afford a Yamamoto? So, off to the second-hand shops that were a regular starting point, where I bought old men's jackets in brown and navy pin-stripe wool. On the outside, around the waistline, I stitched a row of vertical seams to lend a corset effect, and scissored away the remaining fabric. I wanted to evoke a romantic ideal of dreary Victorian London, and actually these pictures were part of a re-shoot, normally unheard of due to budget restrictions. The original shots, by a New York photographer who will go unnamed, were shamefully glamorous. I was devastated and begged Mark Lewis to re-shoot. Thankfully he agreed, as I count these among my most enduring images. There is a childlike oddness about the styling; the men's trouser pockets pulled out imply poverty, the flower pinned to his crotch – a nod to Victorian prostitution. The Hasidic locks were another look I returned to. The skates were another second-hand find, and reminded me of that painting by Henry Raeburn.

In the style of

Hamish Bowles, a fellow fashion freak at *Harper's & Queen* magazine, attended the *haute couture* shows in Paris. At *BLITZ* we didn't have the budget for the trip and, anyway, *haute couture* was supposedly not on the radar of a trendy style magazine. But I have always loved the glorious glamour of *couture*, so I asked Hamish to review the shows for us. He was delighted, and we ran his story, accompanied by his show notes, as the introduction for a fashion shoot. Because we did not have access to the real gowns, I proposed we make our own versions from denim given by Levi's for the Designer Denim Jacket project. Once again Darryl bravely stitched together approximations of jackets and bodices. Onto these we pinned ball-gown skirts, bustles, bows, and a train stretching the length of the location: the glittering Criterion restaurant in Piccadilly Circus. I remember constructing a giant picture hat *à la* Christian Lacroix, who was reinvigorating the *métier* at Patou.

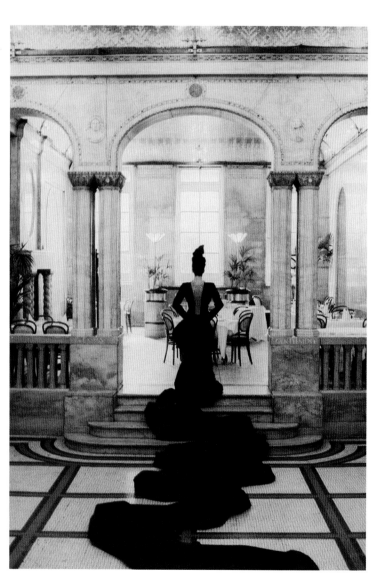

Christian Dinh, photographer:
Brassaï was always a big source of inspiration. I was shooting a lot of night-time stories with available light, as it gave the images a cinematic look and reportage feel. We didn't communicate much before the shoot, and honestly I had no idea what we were going to shoot. My English was very basic, but I was so excited to shoot for *BLITZ* that I didn't want anything to jeopardise it. This was the first time I realised that a fashion photograph was about teamwork, as each element fitted perfectly: the location, the model casting and of course, most importantly, the creations that you built with denim, sometimes at the last minute, directly onto Hilde. I was very impressed by the work you did in the style of the couturiers.

The shoot was on a Thursday. I remember because I never missed a party at the Café de Paris on Wednesday nights. Since we had to be out of the location by 11am so they could serve lunch, and we were meeting at your office around 6am for hair and make-up, I didn't have time to go home and instead went straight to *BLITZ*. I was taking a power nap under a desk when I heard you looking for me. That's when I saw the clothes for the first time and understood your concept. I did panic inside, but was too tired to react.

With so few hours to shoot, there was no time for thinking, and that's when the magic comes – when everything and everybody just clicks. Hilde was not a professional model, the clothes were not commercial garments, and I had only four hours to do it. But when Hilde and three male models came on set all dressed up, and started to interact through my camera, it looked like a scene from a movie. Hilde looked like Greta Garbo with her three *mignons* supporting her. The glamorous fashion and the neo-Byzantine décor of the Criterion transported us back fifty years. Of course, my favourite picture was the last one, when you added the ten-metre-long train. To be able to capture the whole scene, I built a fifteen-foot high pyramid of tables and chairs for me to climb up. It was a pretty rushed affair but to this day it is one of my favourite shoots.

Moose Ali Khan, model:
I used this series of pictures in my book for a long time. I was wearing a tuxedo so I thought this would finally be my entrée to classic work. We just knew we wanted to work as much as we could before it was over. We thought it would be over in a year. There was never an end game to it.

Martine Houghton, model:
What you've done is very inspiring. You just like to make things with whatever materials you can find. You had no rules. It was very art school, really honest. I've been bathed in fashion all my life – modelling, assisting fashion photographers, working with Michael Roberts – but I was never obsessed with it. You just put a look on. I grew up with that as a given. How things have changed. Suddenly fashion houses would say, you have to shoot the whole look. We took it for granted we could do what we liked. It was all very 'make do and mend'.

Louise Constad, make-up artist:
I can't believe how Darryl was so clever.

Photographer: Christian Dinh

Models: Moose at Z, Hilde Smith

Make-up: Louise Constad

Hair: Dean

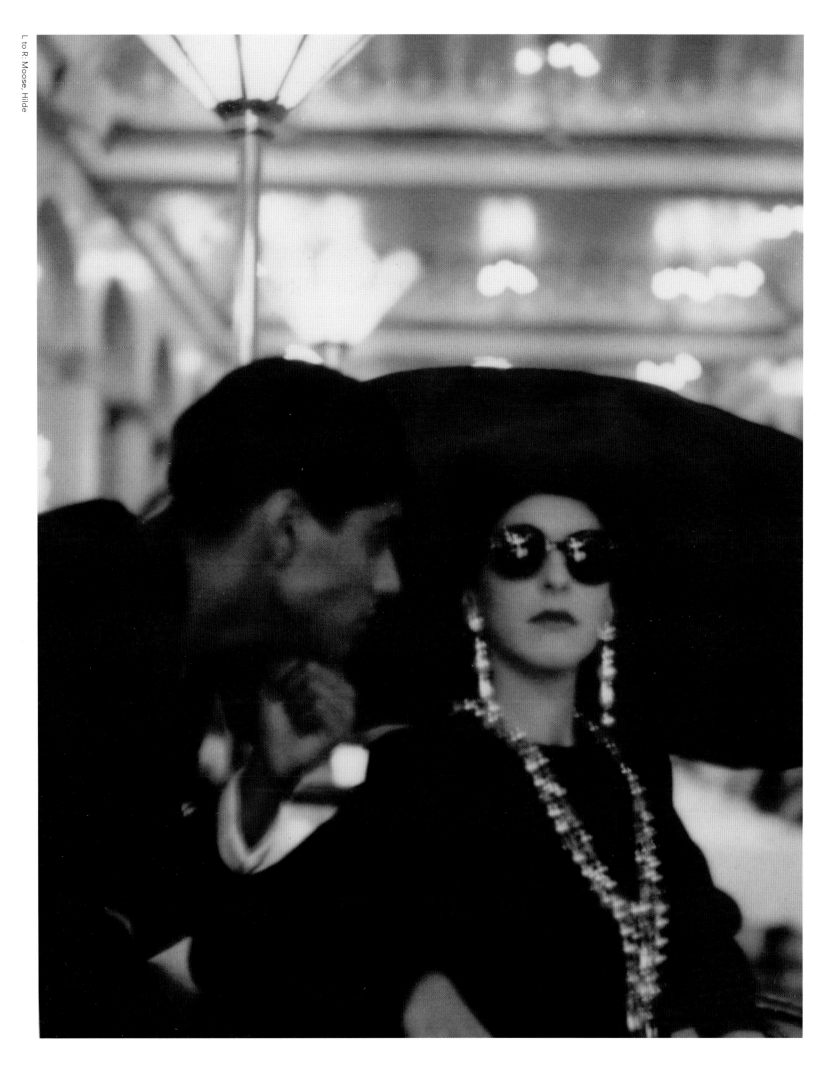

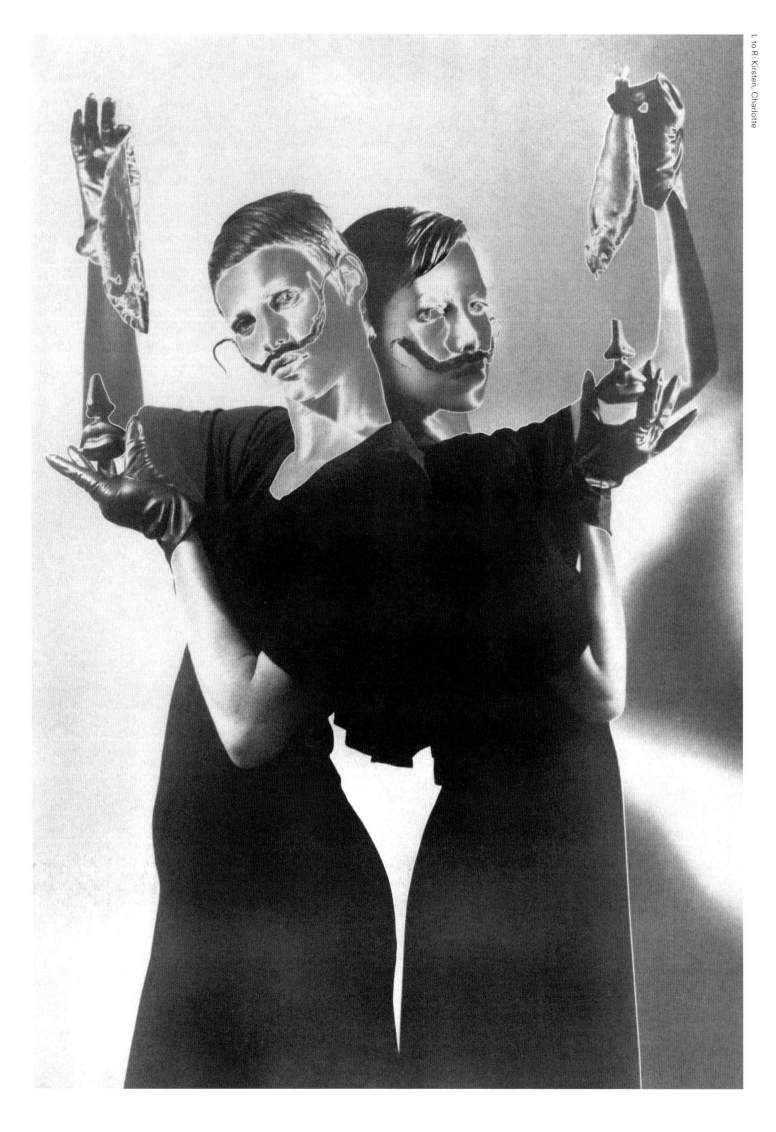

When a new Salvador Dalí fragrance was launched, I thought it a notion as surreal as the artist, yet the bottle was inspired: the flacon was a representation of a pair of lips, the stopper a nose. It came in frosted glass and matt black (the look of the '80s) and was extremely tactile. I seem to remember the perfume being heavy and decadent. The launch offered the opportunity to create images that were even more bizarre than usual. I asked for several bottles to use for the shoot, including the large ones made especially for marketing purposes. Willem had just arrived from the Netherlands and I really liked his romantic, gothic style. We selected two models who looked extremely similar and I briefed make-up artist Jalle that I wanted to reference Dalí. He went about fashioning moustaches from an old hairpiece. He also blocked out the girls eyebrows with wax to enhance their darkened eyes. The effect was spectacularly spooky. I dressed the girls alike, in long black jersey dresses selected from the archive of designer Jean Muir and black Mary Jane tap shoes from Anello & Davide. In one picture they wore black masks with prawns positioned over the eyeholes. In another they held the bottles aloft in one hand, and a fresh mackerel in the other. Willem positioned the girls in equally surreal poses.

Willem Odendaal, photographer:
The picture of the Dalí girl with her moustache sticking her beautiful head through the legs of the other model has always been one of my favourites.

Johnny Rozsa, photographer:
Jalle was such a creative person, so fabulous. I worked with him a lot. What I always tried to do was to create a team. I was really lucky because I had Stevie [Hughes, make-up] and Ray [Allington, hair]. They were my first team, but then Stevie might be in NYC, so I'd work with Jalle. It was everyone working together to be creative. It was about making a picture. That was it. Why? Why not?

Lynne Franks, PR:
The trio of magazines – BLITZ, The Face, i-D – each had their very own identity and fingerprint. When you think of those magazines you associate them with a person. At i-D it was Terry Jones, at The Face it was the graphics (Neville Brody and Robin Derrick), and BLITZ was you. BLITZ was very much about fashion, and you lived it. You were friends with all the people in fashion, the designers, and the photographers. You lived a visual lifestyle. And what came across most was that it was fun. You were highly creative. A lot of the time, what you were doing prompted the question, what came first – the styling or the clothes? What you did was very spontaneous. At that specific time I would say that there was a group of stylists – yourself, Caroline Baker and Ray Petri – who were as creative as the designers, if not more so.

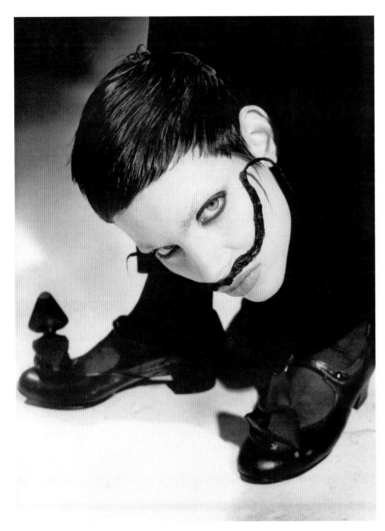

Photographer: Willem Odendaal

Models: Charlotte, Kirsten at Look

Make-up and Hair: Jalle Bakke

Clothes: Jean Muir, Cornelia James, Anello & Davide

The difference between me and a madman is that I am not mad

A menswear story that featured another ensemble cast, each with their own outfit, tailored to their look. The four fashion capitals were used as a stylistic device that enabled me to create characters that embodied each city's stylistic clichés. For London I chose two androgynous models (one male, one female) and dressed them similarly, in layered, hooded raincoats. The boys from Milan were both raven-haired and swarthy. For the USA, the Stars and Stripes was omnipresent, now made over as an *Easy Rider*-style bandana or African-American headwrap. These portraits also featured models of colour, and a Russian (indicated by a red star tattoo in the middle of his forehead). The French youths were the perfect fit for the Gaultier designs — one was blond, hunky and naked (he wore a Gaultier brooch taped to his chest), the other dark and delicate. The editorial spoke of individual style. These pictures were stylish mug shots.

London Paris New York Milan

Photographer: Mark Lewis

Models: Chris King at Laraine Ashton, Christos Tolera

Make-up and Hair: Jalle Bakke

Clothes: Jean Paul Gaultier, Joseph, Nikos, Moschino, Kleins

Christos Tolera, model:
I must say, looking at the Moschino shot reminds me that youth really is wasted on the young. I don't remember being that good-looking, and I grieve for my hair on a daily basis. I do remember though that I was happy to do fashion shoots with you, because even though it may have not been my particular way of dressing, you always managed to make me look masculine – in a 'Gay Icon' kind of way. I don't think I looked queer at all, which is strange considering the ensemble. There has to be an element of trust there, and I had that with you.

Jean Paul Gaultier, designer:
My biggest influence was that I felt rejected as a child. I think that has made me focus on what makes us all different. I hope the people who like my designs enjoy wearing the clothes. That's the best thing. You can express yourself through the clothes. You don't have to put them together in my way. I like when people put them together in a different way that makes it you, and shows that you are unique, because I am frightened by uniformity.

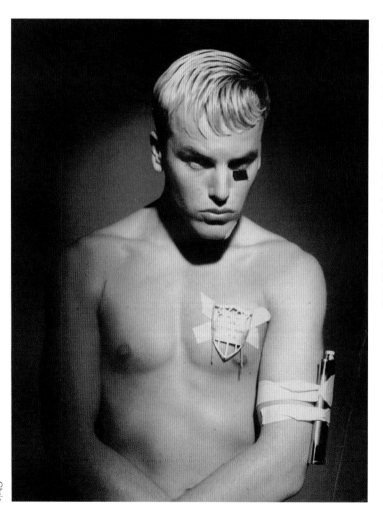

Chris

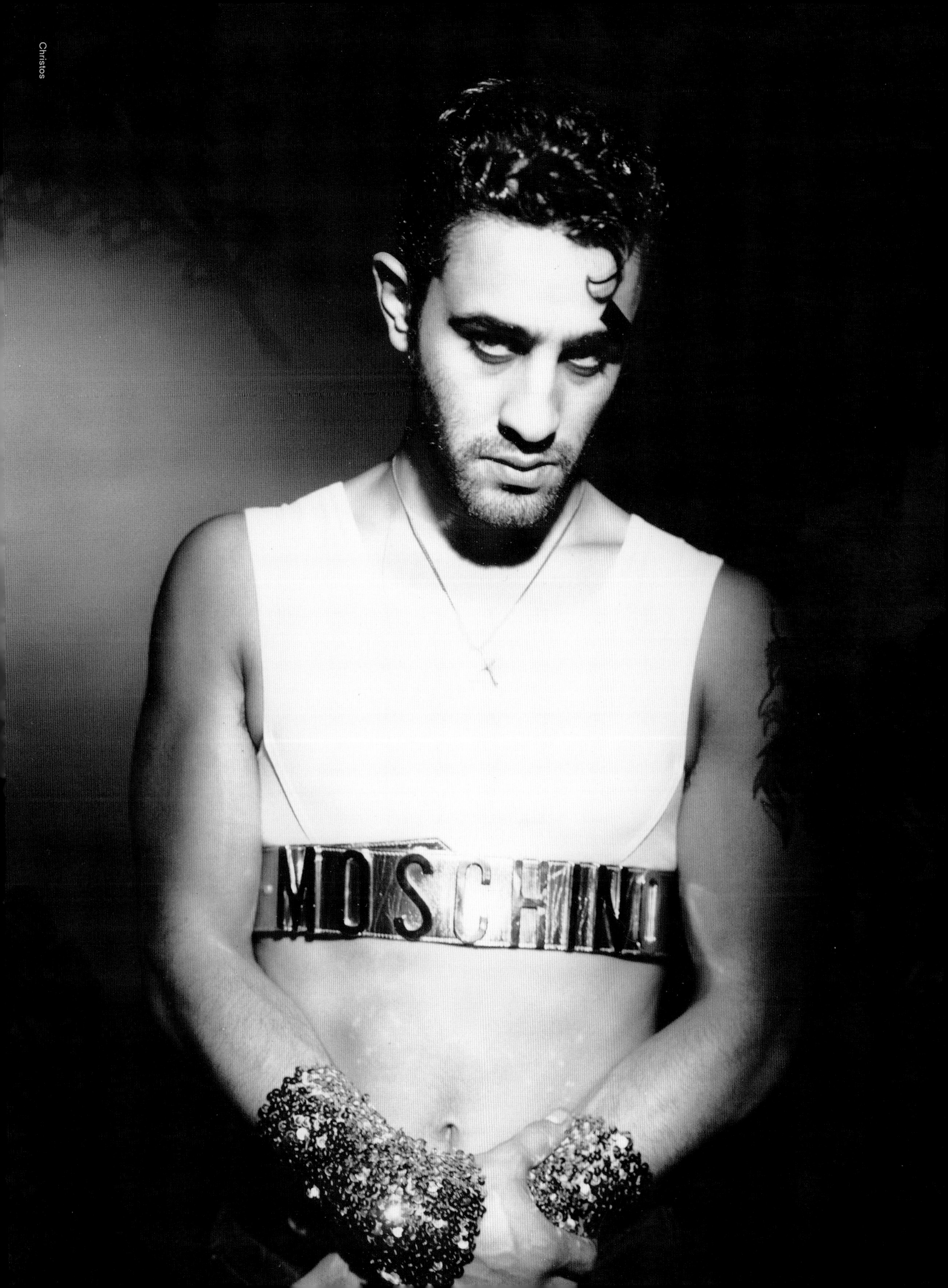

Christos

BLITZ #48
December 1986

Some year, eh?

The idea behind this shoot was simple: a checklist of all the trendy items that you should have worn during 1986. But what if you wore them all at the same time? Martine and David were fantastic sports to participate in this shoot. I particularly like the two-hairstyles-in-one modelled by Martine – a bleached crop (her own) and an Emma Peel brunette flick-up. Surprisingly this made a cover. One for the fashion victims.

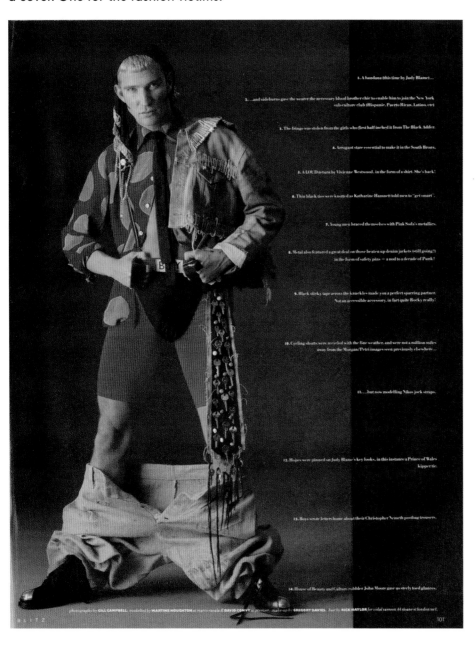

Martine Houghton, model:
I can't say that I looked good but I loved being on the cover. I was in a lot of shows but there's not much documentation of that. I never seem to appear in any footage. I always seem to be on the cutting room floor. The spectacles were cracked. This was before retouching. That look is nuts.

David Convy, model:
That was where I first met Greg. He did the grooming. It doesn't look like me, does it? Did you bleach my hair? A friend of mine still has that issue and they always mention the size of my legs. I'm sure it's just because I was wearing red Lycra cycling shorts, along with everything else. I think I did wear cycling shorts. I've got photos of me in that year in the South of France wearing a pair, and a bum-bag hiding my bits. But it's great, because for that particular year it's like a sort of time capsule, everything we wore in '86. I quite like Martine's look. She got the bloody cover.

Rick Haylor, hairdresser:
She was the total Fashion Victim, wearing everything with no sense of style or taste. She had the blond crop, the headband and the dark flick-up at the back. It was totally mad.

Photographer: Gill Campbell

Models: Martine Houghton at Marco Rasala, David Convy at Premier

Make-up: Gregory Davis

Hair: Rick Haylor for Vidal Sasoon

Clothes: Katharine Hamnett, Azzedeine Alaïa, Vivienne Westwood, Levi's, Johnny Moke, Cutler & Gross, Hermès, Bernstock Speirs, Pink Soda, Judy Blame, Christopher Nemeth, Nikos, John Moore, BOY

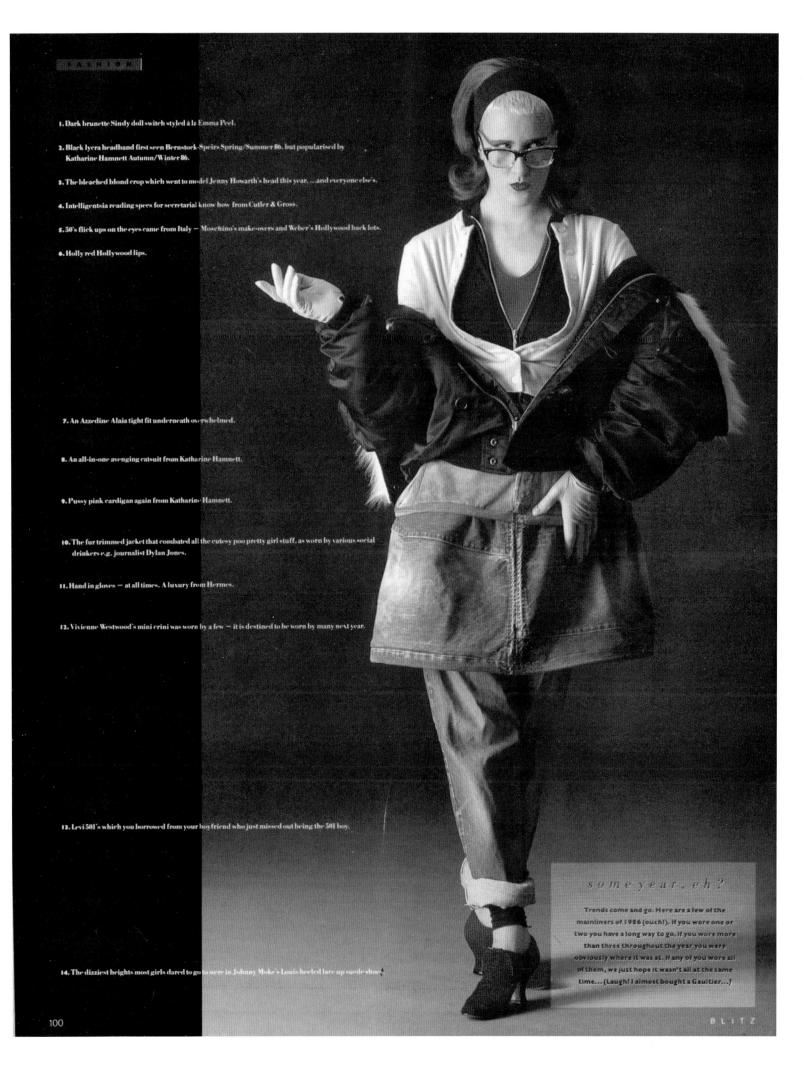

1. Dark brunette Sindy doll switch styled à la Emma Peel.

2. Black lycra headband first seen Bernstock-Speirs Spring/Summer 86, but popularised by Katharine Hamnett Autumn/Winter 86.

3. The bleached blond crop which went to model Jenny Howarth's head this year, ...and everyone else's.

4. Intelligentsia reading specs for secretarial know-how from Cutler & Gross.

5. 50's flick ups on the eyes came from Italy — Moschino's make-overs and Weber's Hollywood back lots.

6. Holly red Hollywood lips.

7. An Azzedine Alaia tight fit underneath overwhelmed.

8. An all-in-one avenging catsuit from Katharine Hamnett.

9. Pussy pink cardigan again from Katharine Hamnett.

10. The fur trimmed jacket that combated all the cutesy poo pretty girl stuff, as worn by various social drinkers e.g. journalist Dylan Jones.

11. Hand in gloves — at all times. A luxury from Hermes.

12. Vivienne Westwood's mini crini was worn by a few — it is destined to be worn by many next year.

13. Levi 501's which you borrowed from your boyfriend who just missed out being the 501 boy.

14. The dizziest heights most girls dared to go to were in Johnny Moke's Louis heeled lace up suede shoes.

some year, eh?

Trends come and go. Here are a few of the mainliners of 1986 (ouch!). If you wore one or two you have a long way to go, if you wore more than three throughout the year you were obviously where it was at. If any of you wore all of them, we just hope it wasn't all at the same time... (Laugh! I almost bought a Gaultier...)

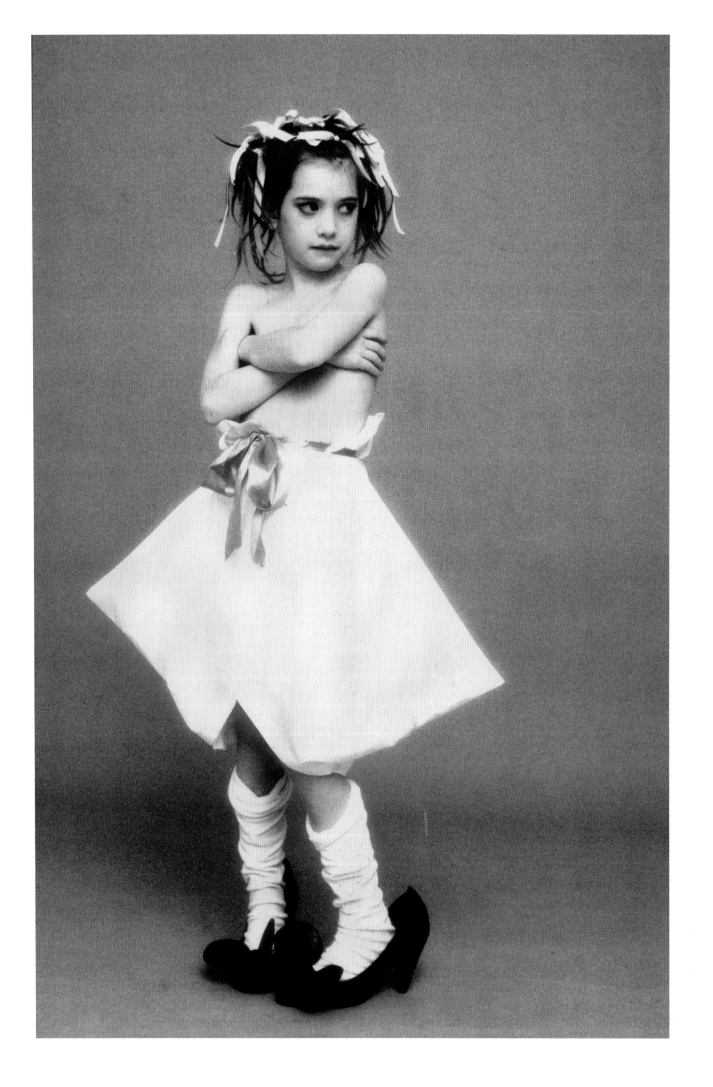

Grandi Scarpe —Westuff

I met Stefano Tonchi and his partner David Maupin during a trip to Florence. They were part of a stylish Italian coterie pursuing a similar alternative ideology. The pair had set up *Westuff* magazine, a large format arts/fashion/music publication. They asked if I would contribute. This story focused on four emerging London-based shoemakers: John Moore, Trevor Hill, Christina Ahrens and Patrick Cox. I wanted to shoot the story on children, as it reminded me of little girls wearing their mother's shoes, so I dressed them up in grown-up clothes. Tamzin had already appeared in *BLITZ*. She was a natural in front of the camera. I loved her *Pretty Baby* style make-up. I think David was the son of one of Mark's friends. Although he was not so sure about some of the looks (a satin Mini Crini by Vivienne Westwood?), ultimately his desire to show off got the better of him.

Stefano Tonchi, journalist:
I have always loved and collected magazines, so I always wanted to have one of my own. We started *Westuff* in a very small way. It was a large format, bi-lingual quarterly magazine of images and personalities. We wanted to be part of the new international independent publishing world, as the established publications were very boring. These alternative magazines were born out of a group of like-minded people who really wanted to make it happen. Florence didn't really have a publishing heritage so that gave us an opportunity for independence, and the space to experiment and do things our own way. Like many other young journalists, you weren't asked to do things for Italian *Vogue* or the other established titles. The fashion world in Italy was centred round Milan and was very boring.

At *Westuff* we commissioned people like you and Mario [Testino]. We had people in New York. We got financial support from Pitti and picked up advertisers.

We always tried to look at things in an original way and gave a lot of freedom to stylists and photographers. All these new things were happening in England and we wanted to put them on our pages. We didn't want to know what was 'in' or 'out' in London, but we wanted interviews with the people that were making London alive. We wanted to let the characters and the images speak for themselves.

This was before the Internet. We would talk on the telephone or communicate by fax, so often I might wait a week or more before a package arrived containing images that I had commissioned. There was always an incredible sense of a surprise, because I didn't really know what was coming until I opened the box. I assigned a project and then waited. Now, a picture can be snapped on an iPhone and delivered instantly.

There was a whole new group of interesting shoe designers doing strange things that were retro or post-modern. You came up with the idea of shooting the new shoes on little children, which I thought was a great idea.

Nowadays we are used to this mix of contemporary art, fashion and music, but at that time it was a big deal. I think it was very much in the same spirit as the style-setters of the 1920s and '30s, or even before, with the Wiener Werkstätte. It was that kind of starting point, having a point of reference and connecting. I think young people still do that. I think it's probably generational. I don't like to look back purely with nostalgia. I guess each era has its style heroes.

Stevie Stewart and David Holah, designers, Bodymap:

SS _ We were definitely anti-establishment. We weren't going to show our clothes in that old-fashioned way. It was a question of resources, or lack of them. We didn't have big financial backing so we'd call on friends in film and dance, the Neo-Naturists, our mums or whoever. Helen Terry wandering down the catwalk singing.

DH _ That sense of rebellion derived from punk times.

SS _ It's in our blood. One of our most exciting pictures is by Peter Lindbergh for Stern. Everyone's in it. The Bodymap family. Lizzie Tear, Barry and Nick [Kamen], my mum, Lesley's mum. It's quite humorous as well. It was fun. Everyone's laughing and happy. And David's four-year old niece, Nico, is there too. When we got a US licence they wouldn't allow those pictures to be shown. We were innocently making art, and they got stopped at US customs. They considered the images to be pornographic.

DH _ Nico was in every one of our shows, so we have a Bodymap mini-collection in miniature sizes. So cute.

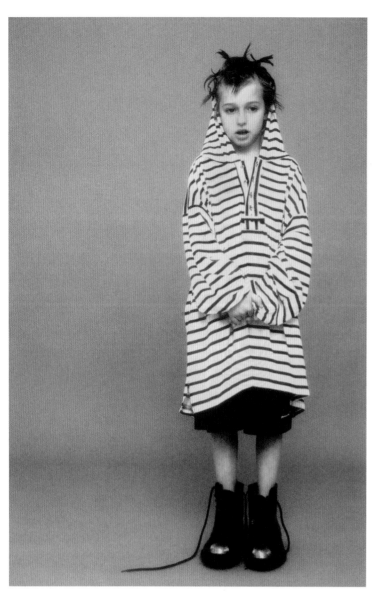
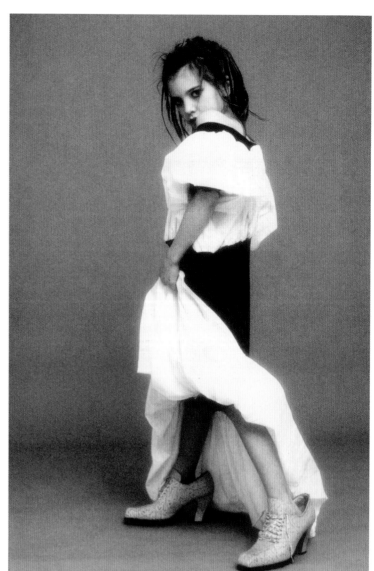

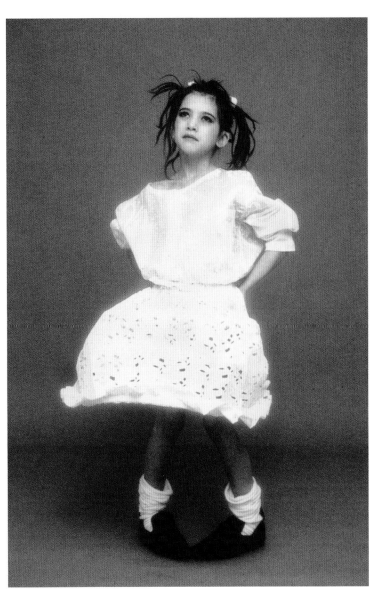

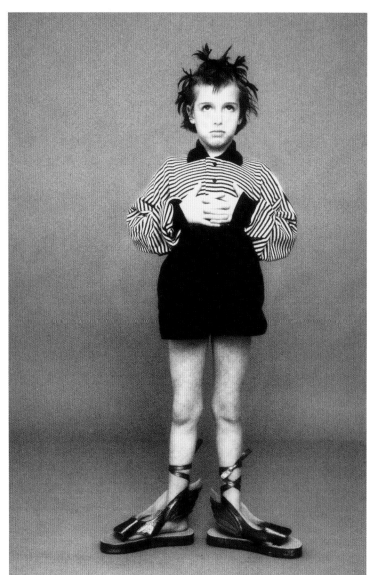

Photographer: Mark Lewis

Models: Tamzin Davis, David

Make-up: Gregory Davis

Hair: Debbie Dannell

Clothes: Bodymap, Richmond Cornejo, Vivienne Westwood, Flex, Pamplemousse, Patrick Cox, Trevor Hill, John Moore

Old favourites

Comme des Garçons were a constant in the magazine.
I chimed with their raw aesthetic, but also with the respect
that they afforded tradition, history and heritage. I wanted
to make a series of pictures that were the antithesis of the
trendy image that had come to surround the label. So,
Robert and I travelled to my family home in a tiny village
in Wiltshire to photograph my mum and dad, along with
my spinster aunts Ethel and Violet. They were posed at the
bottom of our stairs, with fabric pinned up behind them.
We had bought this from the Cloth Shop in Soho, and it was
intended to look like old-fashioned patterned wallpaper; this
was at the height of the vogue for matt black minimalism.
The fur trapper hat was a reference to Ray Petri's Buffalo
styling. My dad became the oldest Buffalo boy in town.

Robert Ogilvie, photographer:
They are great pictures. In the
magazine they never quite looked
the way I had imagined them. I
saw them far more like they are in
the contacts; that's how I'd hoped
they'd look. There is a tremendous
strength of character that comes
across in all of them. If you look at
that picture of your father, if you
showed that to somebody and
said, this is the guy that heads up
Comme des Garçons, even with
it being a Japanese label, they'd
buy it. But actually your dad was a
milkman. That's just priceless. He
could have been a huge model. I
love that we transported them off
into that world, and for them to
actually hold it so brilliantly.

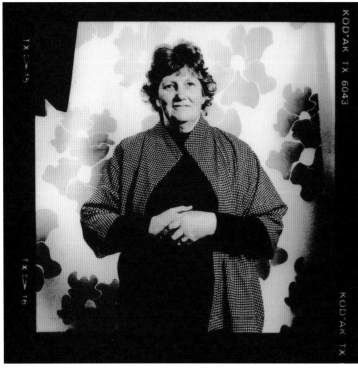

Bet

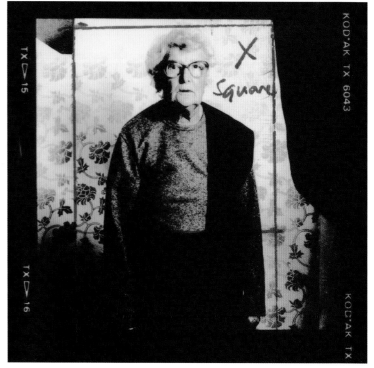

Eff

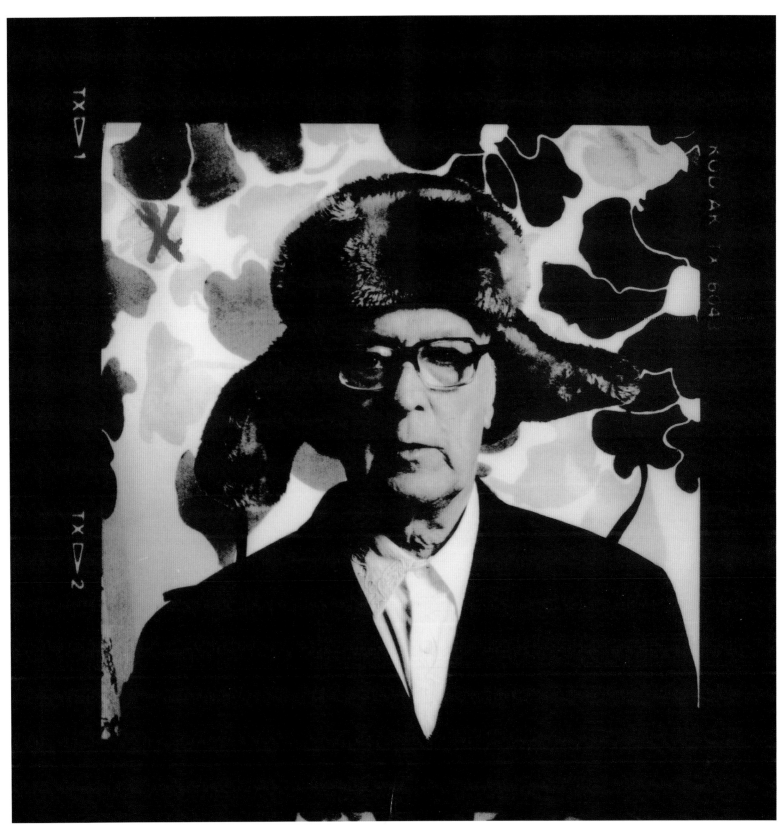

Photographer: Robert Ogilvie

Models: Reg, Bet and Ethel Webb

Clothes: Comme des Garçons,
Comme des Garçons Homme,
Fred Bare

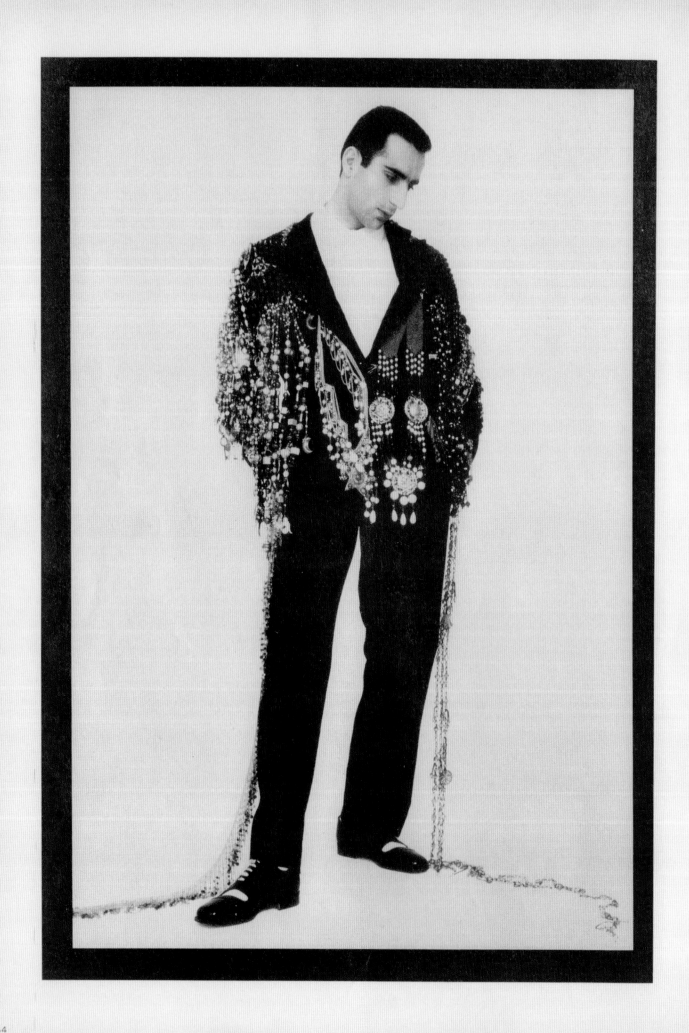

jewellery from a selection by **ERIC BEAMON**, *mary jane men's shoes by* **JOHN MOORE**.

This image was part of a major London S/S 1987 collection story that accompanied my seasonal show review. Chris Hall was a favourite model of designers Mark & Syrie. He was a big man for a model, but had the gentlest soul. The jewellery all came from Erickson Beamon, and I just pinned it directly onto the suit. This took a while, and Chris just posed patiently. He was a truly lovely man. The shoes, by John Moore, were the male equivalent of Mary Janes.

Vicki Sarge, jewellery designer, Erickson Beamon:
I arrived in London somewhere around 1985, from a New York scene that was just beginning to reel from the most traumatic health crisis I hope to ever see in my lifetime. London felt fresh and optimistic and, although not meaning to stay long, I am still here. In New York I was living on the edge, between fashion and the '80s nightclub scene, which was pretty amazing. I was quite a snob about what was cool and London felt like I had arrived home. The scene here was so creative and with a cast of characters that was full of surprises, ensuring that I could never get bored. I loved extremes.

BLITZ magazine, which had its origins in the same DNA I had emerged from, was a highlight to look forward to each month, recording these amazing times. Somehow BLITZ was just that bit more glossy, edgy and glamorous than its competitors. Meeting and working with you was a joy. You were immersed in the scene up to your eyebrows, which shaded those amazing blue eyes. When working on this shoot I recall sending jewellery, however you were not satisfied until we had sent every piece we had in-house. What a thrill for a jewellery designer to have your pieces shot this way. There was nothing like this happening in New York at all, especially the delight of having our pieces shot on menswear. I absolutely loved it. You continued to push the boat out on your shoots, and they really were something exciting to look forward to. I would have done anything you asked.

Darryl Black, fashion assistant:
Boys? We did have our favourites didn't we? Mmmm, Chris Hall.

Growing up in public

Photographer: Mark Lewis

Model: Chris Hall at Z

Make-up: William Casey/ Stephanie Jenkins

Hair: Rick Haylor and Scarlett at Vidal Sassoon

Clothes: Erickson Beamon, John Moore

Pete Moss, photographer:
BLITZ was very good commercially for me, and it opened the door to the fast-expanding advertising and design market of the late '80s. It was a similar time of expansion in London to the sixties, I suppose. Things just got a little more sophisticated and a little more luxurious. Although I wish someone had said, 'Be careful what you wish for', because London lost a lot of its character and openness after that, and became a very commercially driven city with a much harder attitude.

I also shot a few portraits for the magazine of celebrities such as Isabelle Huppert, Neneh Cherry and Marc Almond. I went on to shoot fashion for a number of clients but somehow never worked so successfully with other fashion editors. After that period, everything seemed to take on a much more serious mode of conduct. Magazines and editors became advertising whores, and were just not willing to allow so much pure creativity or take so much risk. That's why these shoots are looked upon as being so special; they were driven by pure creativity, and not the need to feature the right designers who were paying the bills.

Louise Constad, make-up artist:
How ahead of its time. Art follows fashion.

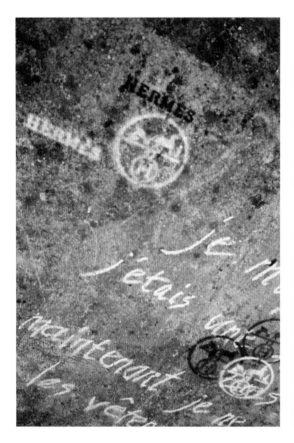
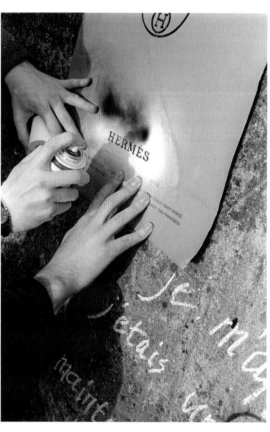

J'ai faim pour le style

Another visual love letter to Hermès. Inspired by the house's heritage, this shoot told an imaginary story of a once-famous Parisian model who was now living on the streets as a down-and-out. There was a touching poignancy in the chalked messages and sad-looking cardboard signs used by the people I had seen living on the streets in Paris to tell their story and ask for help. At a suitably grim location somewhere in the East End, we chalked the model's 'story' on a wall. To this we added spray-canned Hermès logos. We had cut the stencil from an Hermès shopping bag (Banksy? Who?). Hermès prints were notoriously bright, to the point of being garish, so on a piece of torn cardboard I wrote, 'Je ne distingue pas les couleurs. merci.' We did this shoot in two parts, and on the second day we photographed the image of the Hermès shoe pounding the pavement, surrounded by a swirling fringe. I liked the idea that, against all odds, this woman still walked proud and tall on her concrete catwalk.

Photographer: Pete Moss

Models: Valerie at Look, Louise at Unique

Make-up: Louise Constad

Hair: Tim Crispin for Demop

Clothes: Hermès

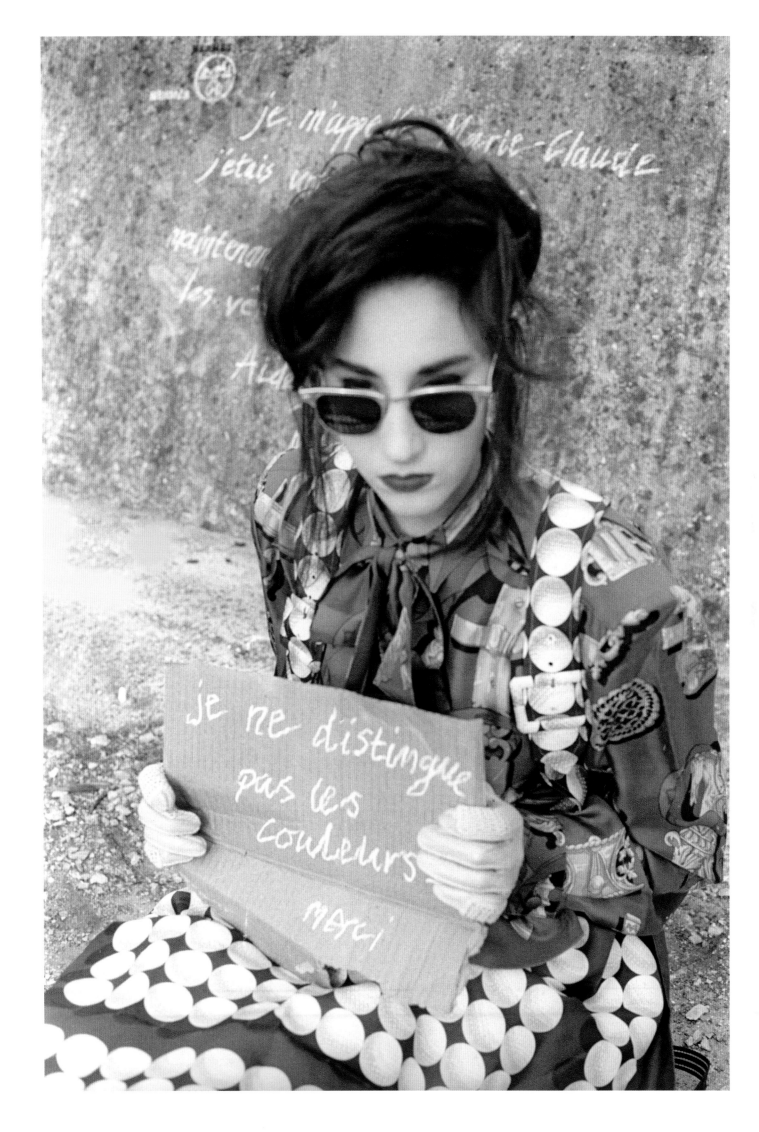

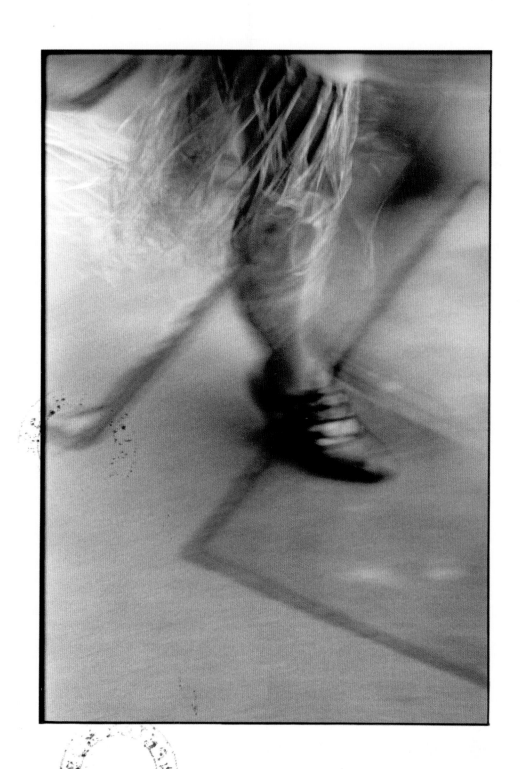

BLITZ #50
February 1987

Photographer: Willem Odendaal
Model: Jaime Travezan at Unique
Make-up: Stephanie Jenkins
Hair: Tony Collins for Pierre Alexandre
Clothes: Dirk Bikkembergs

A contingent of Belgian designers including Dries Van Noten, Ann Demeulemeester, Dirk Bikkembergs, Dirk Van Saene, Marina Yee and Walter Van Beirendonck, who called themselves the Antwerp Six, had been making a big impact on the London scene. 'Anyone who can take orders sitting on a toadstool dressed as a gnome [Beirendonck] has to have something...' one British designer quipped during London Fashion Week. Mainly graduates of Antwerp's Royal Academy of Arts, the designers offered multifaceted visions that at the same time appeared radical and polished. They were an extremely professional bunch.

Foreign affairs — Antwerp

Willem Odendaal, photographer:
It was a big surprise when you offered me my first editorial for *BLITZ* magazine.

I remember we did a story on the Belgian designers from Antwerp who were also just up-and-coming. This was my first job in London. I was stunned. I was a nervous wreck on the day of the shoot, just a week after I had visited you at the magazine's office to show you my portfolio, but you just easily pushed me along on that day, and had me do my thing. I was very inspired with the *BLITZ* interpretation of the Belgians' designs.

When I returned to your office the next day with the resulting photographs, you just sat quietly and looked at them, and said that I gave you exactly what you had expected of me. And right after, you asked me when I could work with you again. I found myself able to breathe again.

Darryl Black, fashion assistant:
This was the first shoot I got to style. It was a long time before you let me do anything. I think I earned my dues. I remember you being on the shoot to oversee things and art-direct, but it was definitely the first shoot I was credited with styling. Oh, I loved Jaime.

Jaime Travezan, model:
When I moved to London from Lima I went to WH Smith and bought *Vogue* to find out what was going on in high fashion. I bought *i-D* and *The Face* as well, but I loved *BLITZ* the most. Imagine how thrilled I was when I met you and then appeared on the pages. I was like a groupie about *BLITZ* and you. You created such a beautiful magazine.

Having been living in Lima where there was really nothing going on, coming to London was like suddenly seeing a rainbow. A friend sent some pictures that Mario [Testino] had taken of me back in Lima and entered them into a model competition. One day I got a phone call from Shola [Akintonwa], who ran the agency Unique, and I didn't understand anything she was saying but I think she said I was a finalist. I lasted about a year as a model. I was the worst model in the world.

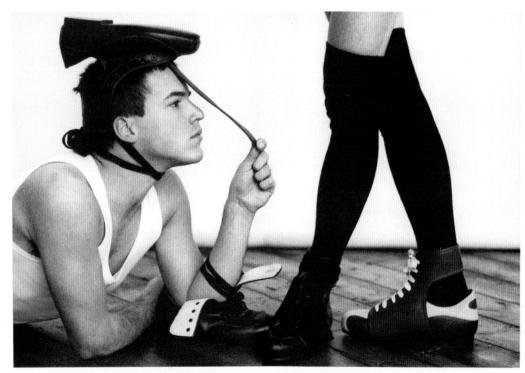

foreign affairs — antwerp

Our introduction to the Belgian contingent began last summer.

The frequent arrival of professionally presented press-packs from graduates of Antwerp's acclaimed Royal Academy of Arts left us much impressed and a further courtship seemed certain. "Anyone who can take orders sitting on a toadstool dressed as a gnome has to have something...", a fellow designer hissed during last October's London Fashion Week, while the corner of Olympia occupied by Walter and his compatriots stole the show. The exhibition was buzzing with talk of their quirky, intricately detailed, superbly made collections and eye-catching stands. The Belgian government gives great encouragement to their young designers and now, under the wing of a top London-based PR and extensive British stockists, a trio of clever clothiers and a crafty cobbler look set to take London by storm.

dirk bikkemberg

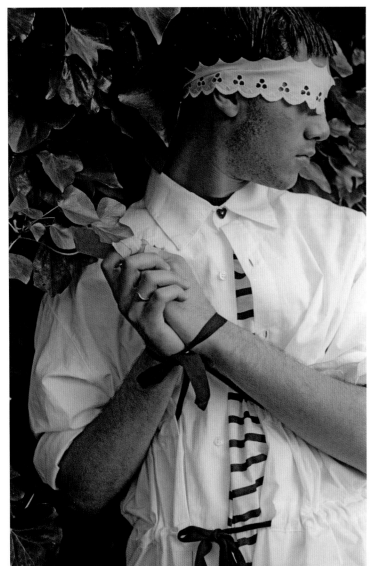

Photographer: Pete Moss

Model: Mark at Z

Clothes: John Flett, Levi's, Workers For Freedom, Pamplemousse

Pete Moss, photographer:
We shot this on Hampstead Heath in the Italianate terraced gardens, which were then beautifully derelict. We would have a meeting to discuss the concept and think about the location, although it was a while before you let me help choose the models. Then we would book a studio if necessary, or think of a location, and ask an assistant along (or a friend who wasn't busy that day) to help carry equipment. The shoots were surprisingly organised with not much fuss, except when some extraordinarily complex make-up and hair was being applied. I think you were very organised clothes-wise, and always seem to cast well – and knew exactly what you wanted. We would shoot according to how much space was allocated, and I was always trying to shoot a killer iconic image to get the cover; but I remember you were very democratic about that, and shared them around with other photographers. On the whole, the shoots were usually interesting social events in their own right.

The newest romantic of all

Tough boys in pretty clothes. I liked the idea of mixing roughed-up denim with lace; *broderie anglaise* worn by a foreign holiday crush. Mark had the look of someone who could happily steal your heart; all soot-black spiky hair and matching eyes. It snowed the day of the shoot, yet not one of the models complained, even though we were asking them to go out in the streets wearing filmy chiffon shirts, ripped jeans, schoolboy shorts and, in one case, a bustle by English Eccentrics, all tied up with lace ribbons.

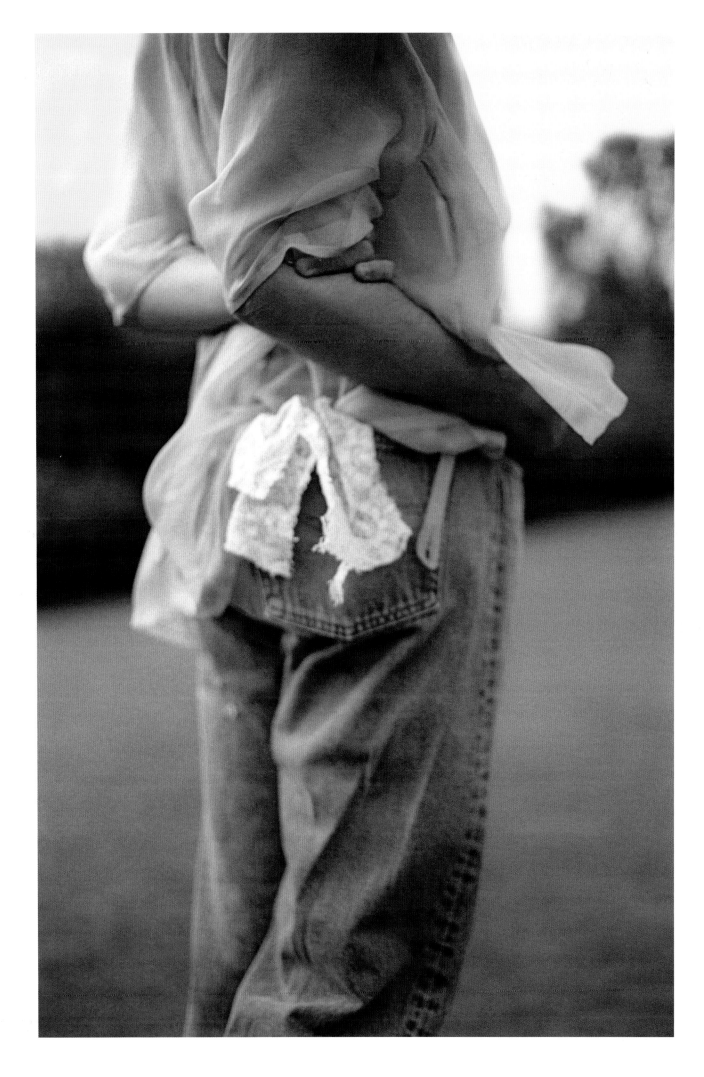

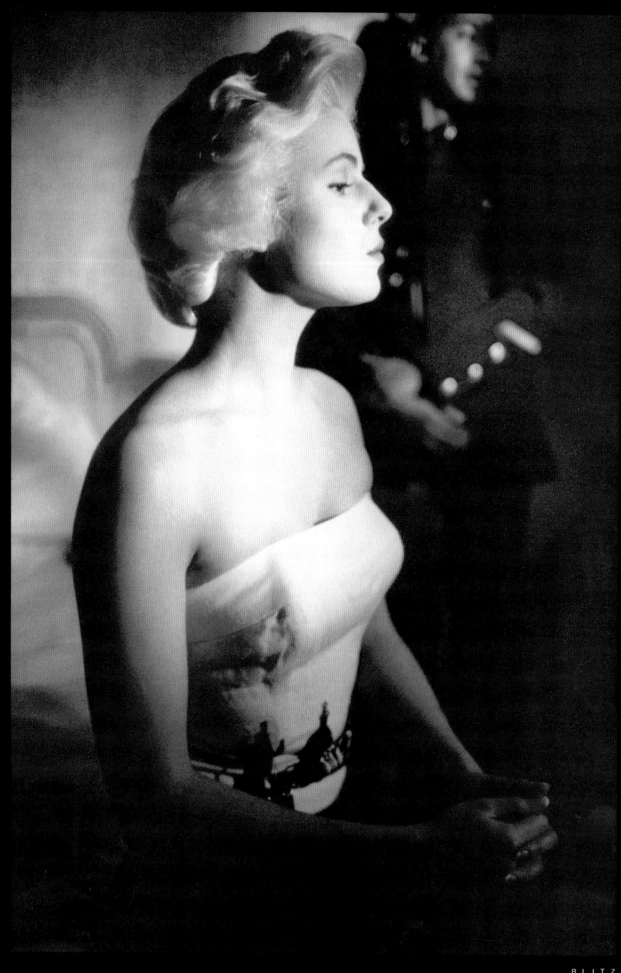

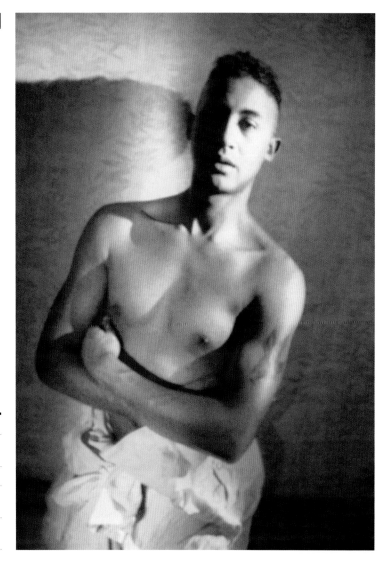

Photographer: Jan Welters

Models: Claudia at Synchro, Anthony (Finn) Kawalski

Make-up: Louise Constad

Hair: Tony Collins for Pierre Alexandre

Clothes: Alistair Blair, Regimentals, Littlewoods

Cruise Wear
Oh what a catastrophe

If I saw a glimpse of something special in a photographer's work, or if they showed an enthusiasm for their craft, then I would often take a chance and set about putting a shoot together with them. Most times, it worked and a new collaboration was formed. I liked Jan when he arrived at the office, and we did a few stories together. This was my favourite. It was very sexy. I think Jan likes to take sexy pictures. AIDS had become a serious problem, yet style-setters were dressing up almost as a parody of sexual stereotypes: mini versions of Monroe in tight pencil skirts and macho, macho men à la Tom Cruise in *Top Gun*. Fly me...

Jan Welters, photographer:
I still have no idea why I was actually shooting for *BLITZ* at the time. It happened quite out of the blue; my book was honestly not that good yet, with maybe only a handful of pictures, and *BLITZ* was a great magazine. But I thought, 'Hey, no problem right, let's try to make the best of it.' I remember being quite proud when the magazine came out.

My assistant and I would travel around on the tube with all the cameras, lights, stands, etc. The evening we did the shoot in the Holiday Inn hotel room, we were quite keen to make the last tube home. At that time home was a squat in King's Cross, so I would sleep with my cameras under my pillow – otherwise they would be gone the next morning.

I was really ignorant about fashion at the time and had, for instance, no idea who Antony Price was. You would tell me about him when we saw each other at the magazine office, which was right in the West End. You were very fashion savvy already then.

And we shot colour transparency slides. Most of them vanished over the years. I'd send the first choice to the magazine and would keep the seconds for my book.

Alistair Blair, fashion designer:
I felt really chuffed that an *über-cool* magazine like *BLITZ* wanted to feature a dress by a (for want of a better word) classic designer like moi. It also, I think, showed the *BLITZ* reader that a simple frock could, with the right styling, look fantastic. Or is the word 'cool'?

I was buying *BLITZ* to read and learn about what was happening in the thriving clubland of London. In the grand scheme of things, that kind of 'out there' representation showed me how to push an idea. If you lift an outfit out of what the designer thinks is its comfort zone – photograph it in a different environment, change the sort of model, add a sharper hairstyle/cut, a certain shadow, heel, angle, etc. – it makes the designer think much more.

Louise Constad, make-up artist:
That shoot became my business card. I think my brief was *Niagara*, the Marilyn film. And I know that was in my mind. The extra white of her skin, and him being so brown. Very, very Marilyn. You absolutely left us to do whatever we wanted, so that was enjoyable. This looks quite calm, but maybe it wasn't. Maybe compared to other make-up around at the time, it wasn't.

Black Power

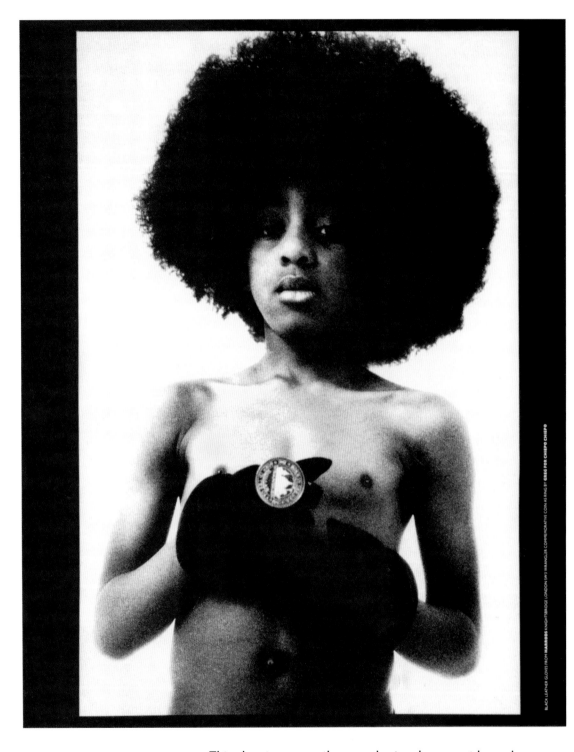

Debbie Dannell, hairdresser:
Adam in that big black Afro wig. He must be 29 now. I still see his mum Jacqueline all the time, and Myrtle. We all lived on the outskirts of society. Every little reject, we all flocked together. How many times did we get abuse for looking how we did? I remember those No Punks signs on pub doors, yet Myrtle never batted an eyelid. All those house parties. It was multi-racial, gay, straight, no bigotry, no abuse. Myrtle wouldn't have tolerated it. I guess it was quite political. Collecting for the miners and going down to Wapping Wall when the printers were on strike.

Photographer: Mark Lewis

Model: Adam

Make-up: Not listed

Hair: Debbie Dannell

Clothes: Harrods, Wrangler, Greg for Chiepo Chiepo

This shoot was another purely visual concept based on the world we were living in. An all black line-up of models, including little Adam, the wonderful Carlos Taylor and Myrtle, a fabulous woman who acted as a surrogate mother to all us waifs and strays. In my own mixed-up, pre-PC way, it provided an opportunity to plunder iconic imagery of black culture, from the Afro of Angela Davis and Marsha Hunt to the black leather gloves of Olympic athletes Tommie Smith and John Carlos. The story sadly went to press without the credits.

When Dylon launched a COLOURFUN range – fabric paints and pens all under £1.50 – and proclaimed in their press release that all you needed was 'imagination', I thought I would challenge four talented textile designers. Brian Bolger, Hilde Smith, Luiven Rivas-Sanchez and Timney Fowler were each given a large cotton sheet, a full set of products and an open brief. The results were fabulously diverse. From Brian's painterly approach to Hilde's minimalist shades of grey, from Timney Fowler's blanket of *BLITZ* covers to Luiven's addition of sequins. "Through this fabric I have seen the eyes of the Virgin Mary," said Luiven, "so I call it Celestial Dreams". But how to present their efforts on the page?

Dye for it?

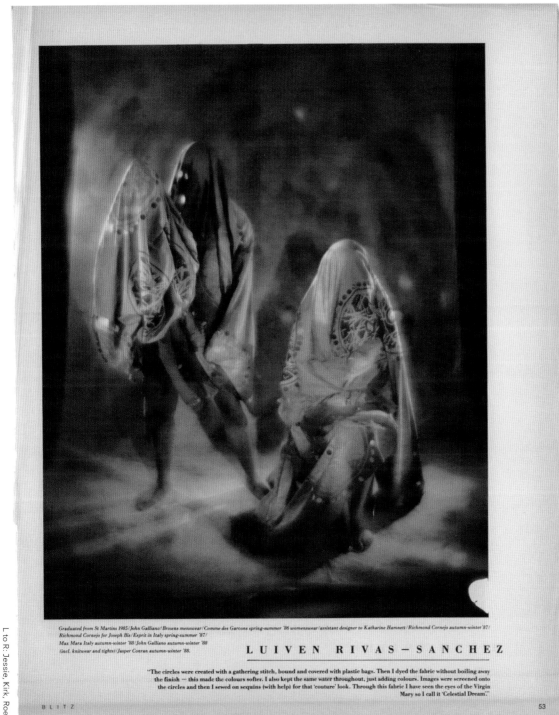

Graduated from St Martins 1985/John Galliano/Browns menswear/Comme des Garcons spring-summer '86 womenswear/assistant designer to Katharine Hamnett/Richmond Cornejo autumn-winter '87/ Richmond Cornejo for Joseph Bis/Esprit in Italy spring-summer '87/ Max Mara Italy autumn-winter '88/John Galliano autumn-winter '88 (incl. knitwear and tights)/Jasper Conran autumn-winter '88.

LUIVEN RIVAS—SANCHEZ

"The circles were created with a gathering stitch, bound and covered with plastic bags. Then I dyed the fabric without boiling away the finish — this made the colours softer. I also kept the same water throughout, just adding colours. Images were screened onto the circles and then I sewed on sequins (with help) for that 'couture' look. Through this fabric I have seen the eyes of the Virgin Mary so I call it 'Celestial Dream'."

L to R: Jessie, Kirk, Roen

Photographer: Mike Owen

Model: Roen, Kirk and Jessie

Mike Owen, photographer:
I had always loved the work of Irving Penn, and in particular his working people portraits. We thought it would be great to recreate a fashion story based on those portraits. I decided to shoot the story on a large format plate camera, as that would have been the same type of kit that Penn would have used. It was an obvious choice. Large format Polaroid gives a wonderful rich and smooth quality to the images that could not be achieved using any other methods.

Each season, we rolled out our version of a collections round-up, usually focused on the London fashion shows. This time around we featured a handful of designers: Stephen Jones, Bodymap, Rifat Ozbek, Richmond Cornejo and John Flett were joined by Belgian newcomer Ann Demeulemeester. The mood was very romantic. We shot the models against a backdrop made from more of the Levi's denim fabric left over from the Denim Jacket project. That fabric had endless uses, and ended up covering sofas, chairs and beds in several homes across London.

Jaime, Kim

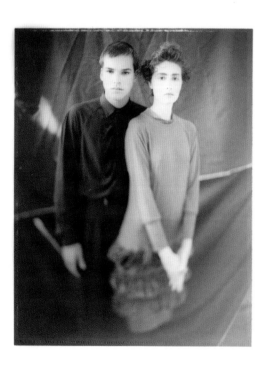

Jaime, Rosalyn

Ronald Diltoer, photographer:
I was still living in Brussels, but running around Europe showing my photographs to as many people as possible. I wasn't officially working as a photographer, but was doing loads of tests and models' composites, making just enough money to pay for the next shoot. I came to London with my then-girlfriend, who was a model, and within the afternoon had an agent. After being rejected in Paris, Milan and Amsterdam, it felt like I was being recognised as a potential talent. London seemed to be the place where it was all happening.

As a young aspiring fashion photographer, I wanted to work for any of the new magazines. The one that looked more likely to give a chance to an unknown young talent was *BLITZ*. I am so glad it happened this way as, with hindsight, *BLITZ* definitely had, in my view, the fashion edge over the others.

We did this shoot in a studio down the King's Road. I actually travelled from Belgium that morning. I remember it as an easy day's work, with me doing pretty much the kind of photographs I always wanted to do. I was working with my favourite format, a 5" x 4" plane camera and Polaroid film. In this instance it was black and white Polaroid with negatives, which I then printed from myself. Working with you was the easiest I have ever worked with anyone. You let me be myself. I really have very fond memories of it all.

Debbie Dannell, hairdresser:
I worked with pop acts so I did *Top Of The Pops* a lot, but because I wasn't part of the union or BBC-trained, I was always stuck in the toilets. Doing the first pop videos was massive. There was nothing like *Karma Chameleon*. Lynne Easton did George's make-up and I ended up doing George's hair for a while after that. It was changing times, working for days at Pinewood Studios making videos. The team there wouldn't let me in the make-up room and I was always put in a room on my own with no mirror. We were out of our comfort zone. It was really, really hard. We weren't accepted at all.

Stephen Jones, milliner:
Suddenly the make-up artist got a credit on the page, the hairdresser got a credit. People saw that they were a valued contributor as much as the fashion designer.

Designer previews

Photographer: Ronald Diltoer

Models: Kim Andreolli and Rosalyn at Premier, Jaime at Unique

Make-up: Lynne Easton

Hair: Tony Collins

Clothes: Stephen Jones, Bodymap, Richmond Cornejo

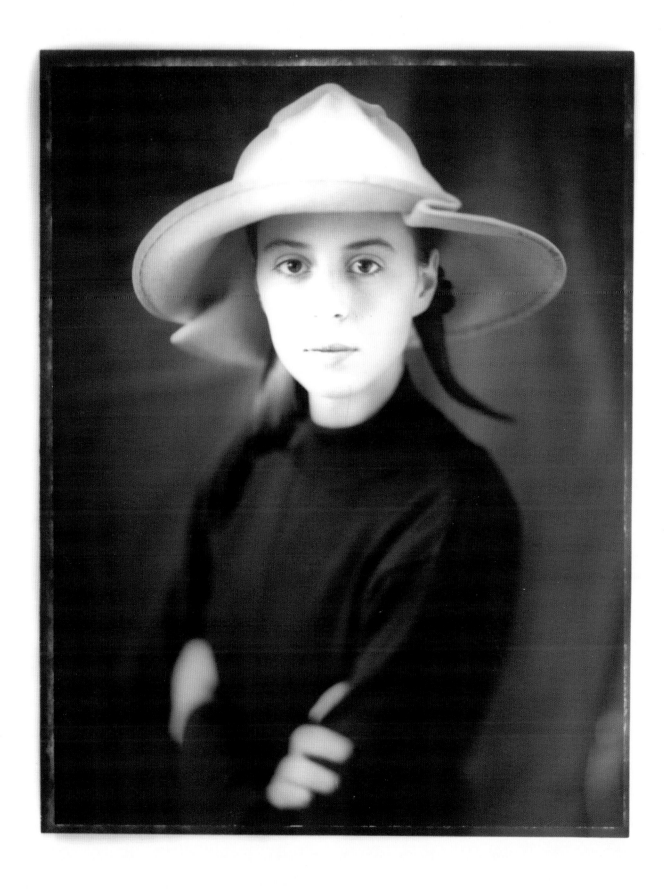

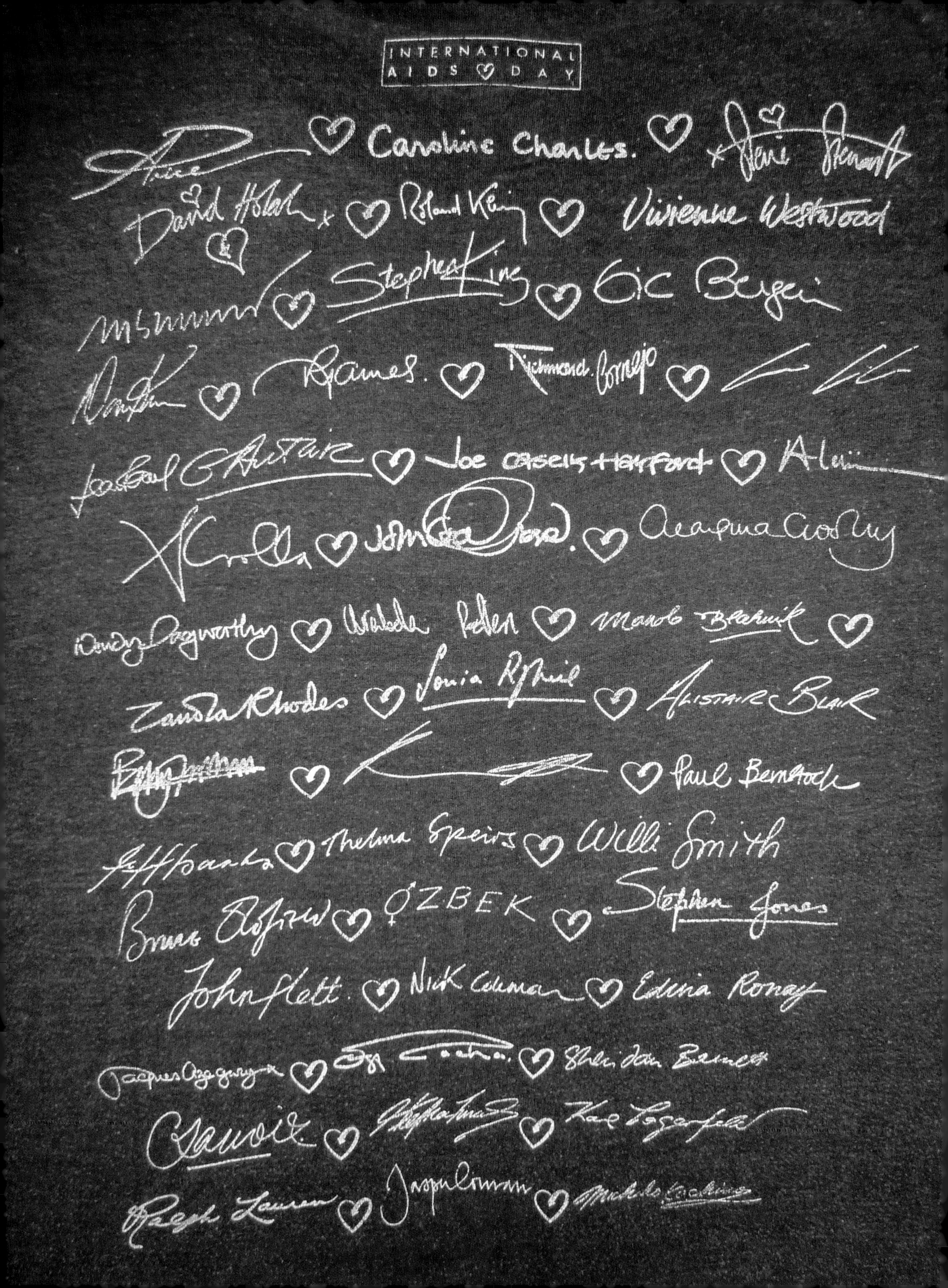
INTERNATIONAL AIDS DAY
Caroline Charles.
Vivienne Westwood
Stephen King
Joe Casely-Hayford
Wendy Dagworthy
Zandra Rhodes
Sonia Rykiel
Alistair Blair
Paul Bernstock
Thelma Speirs
Willi Smith
ÖZBEK
Stephen Jones
John Flett.
Nick Coleman
Edina Ronay
Ralph Lauren

Caryn Franklin, fashion commentator:
Robin Derrick, you and I created the Fashion Cares T-shirt to raise funds for AIDS research. The back was a roll-call of international designers who each gave their support, and signature, to the cause. The shirt was available in both black and white, and became a must-have item. We each photographed it for our respective magazines. Robin used Nick Kamen, model and pop star, for *The Face*; I worked with Nick Knight for *i-D* magazine; and you created this iconic image for *BLITZ*. It's a more subdued photograph than ours was, but is completely indicative of your cerebral approach and has absolutely stood the test of time. I didn't appreciate Jean Muir's contribution in the way I do now that her aesthetic has come full circle. I was surprised even when you revealed you were a big fan; she seemed so 'old school'!

Of course, Muir's brand could have done with your art direction at the time. These days a stylist of your calibre would have been taken into the design house to consult and steer the vision. You could have really influenced the way her brand was perceived by all of us. This has become an important earning stream for fashion visionaries now, but back then we were all pathfinders, working at a time when established fashion houses viewed us as upstarts. They thought street-style had no place to influence catwalk fashion. That would come later.

We all had our own camaraderie though. Despite everyone thinking we were arch rivals, we all went clubbing together and ended up on the floor in a heap at the end of the evening at some warehouse or posh press launch.

Jean Paul Gaultier, fashion designer:
I should say that I love jersey with stitching because of Jean Muir. Yes, she definitely influenced me. I love how her clothes were constructed. She had real style that you can recognise and which is unique. I love her for her individuality. Jean Muir was not about spectacular effects, but the look was strong by itself. It was pure, very simple and disciplined. Very strict and yet feminine. I remember some of the colours. Petrol blue, old pink that was almost mauve and soft brown, colours that were very subtle, and I loved that.

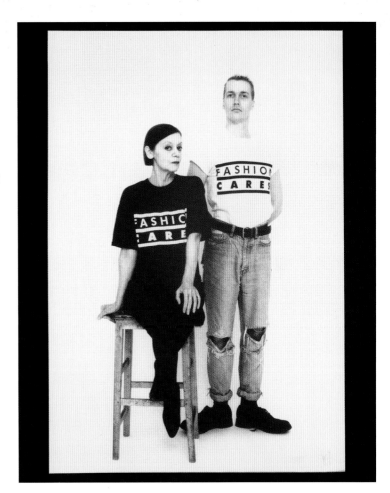

From chic to cheeky
We all care

Photographer: Mark Lewis

Models: Jean Muir, Iain R. Webb

Make-up and Hair: Al Pereira

By the mid-1980s, AIDS had blighted the fashion industry. So although the three new style magazines, *BLITZ*, *The Face* and *i-D*, were competitors, we decided to band together to front a charity, FASHION CARES. Each magazine created an image, which would feature within their pages and could also be used to publicise the product and highlight the problem. I wanted to craft an image that would show that there was no stereotypical AIDS victim. I put in a call to designer Jean Muir, who at first declined the request to pose alongside me. However, within a couple hours, as I was racking my brain to construct Plan B, Miss Muir telephoned back to say that she realised how important this project was and that she would be happy to lend her support. We hastily arranged the shoot with photographer Mark Lewis. And Miss Muir was true to her word, happy to trek to his East End studio for the shoot. I love the juxtaposition of the Lady and the Punk. I loved Miss Muir (even more) for this.

The swot team

Matt was always happy to model, no matter the situation or style. Because he was such a looker, there was an element of opportunistic spontaneity about several shoots. This story was shot on the back of a trip to Paris to film Jean Paul Gaultier for a short movie Matt and I were making together, called *Laugh? I Almost Bought A Gaultier!* Pete Moss also came along to shoot stills and generally support Matt, so it wasn't a leap to get him to take some pictures of Matt modelling Jean Paul's latest menswear collection. The look included short trousers and reminded me of all those well brought up French *Lycée* boys who wore long shorts until the sixth form. I wanted Matt to appear like a cartoon of himself, with slicked hair like Lord Snooty in the *Beano*.

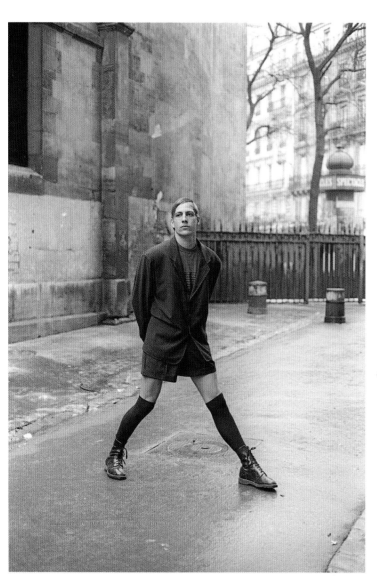

Pete Moss, photographer:
This was such a lot of fun. We were in Paris, all three of us sharing a tiny hotel room. We borrowed some clothes and dressed Matt up and took him out into the street. The light was really good, very grey, and it had just stopped raining so the air was clear. This is a magical type of light for me, and particularly Parisian. Matt was very game.

Matt Lipsey, model:
We intrinsically understood that you had a very different attitude; the magazine had a very different attitude. In the photos there is slush on the ground, but I don't remember being cold, although that might have been because there was fear coursing through my veins. That shoot was an act of sheer faith. I was thinking, 'Iain knows what he's doing.' I remember looking in the mirror and thinking, 'this is the weirdest I've ever felt'. The look was so alien, that's how it felt.

But that whole experience in Paris was alien to me. We went to the Hermès party that was held on the Pont Neuf and there was the most amazing firework display that I'd ever seen. It was incredibly glamorous. Wow! And then I got my first experience of the catwalk shows and realised what a scrum it was. It was a really amazing experience.

Jean Paul Gaultier, designer:
I was always considered the *enfant terrible*, and people would expect me to create a light and funny collection, to make them laugh, and maybe one season I felt a little dramatic but I couldn't do that. Also, you have to sell and maybe you want to change your style and the customer doesn't want to follow. I remember doing big shapes for men, with big shoulders, and I went very quickly to very tight and small and it was too quick and it frightened even the faithful customer and stopped me selling a lot of menswear. You can analyse afterwards but at the time you can't stop to think. When you haven't done a collection before, you can be more spontaneous. Now I arrive at a balance.

In the '80s when I was the flavour of the month, I think I could do either a good collection or a bad one and it had the same result, which is normal because in reality you are more in tune with the essence of the moment. Even if the collection is a big mistake, people are more tolerant because it's like you are surrounded by charisma and means that almost everything you touch becomes flavour of the moment too, even the mistakes. When you are no more flavour of the month that's different because sometimes you can do something similar but people don't see it.

I didn't like it much when my clothes became the uniform of the Yuppie. It wasn't very flattering because all they wanted from me was my name. They weren't buying the clothes for what they were; they wanted my reputation not the clothes I designed. I didn't do this job to be famous. I wanted to make clothes and dress women, and after it brought money and fame. I like it when people love me so I make them love me by my clothes.

Photographer: Pete Moss
Model: Matt Lipsey
Clothes: Jean Paul Gaultier

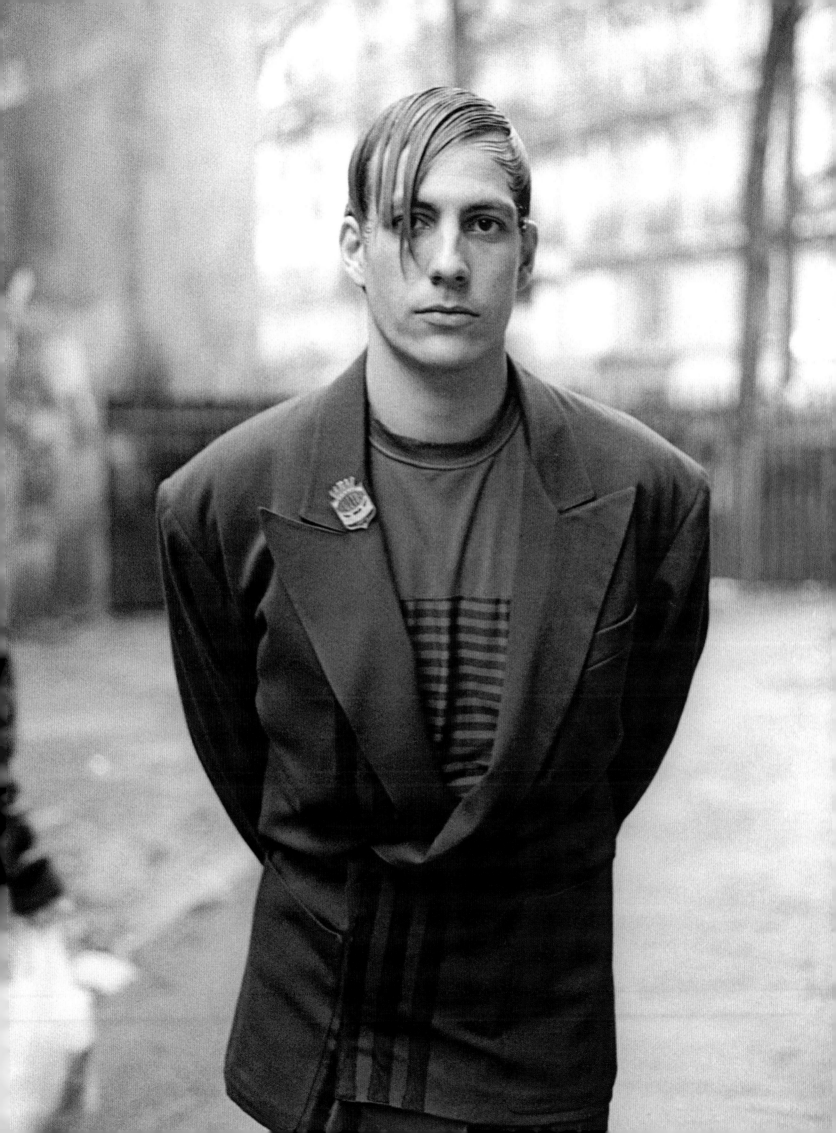

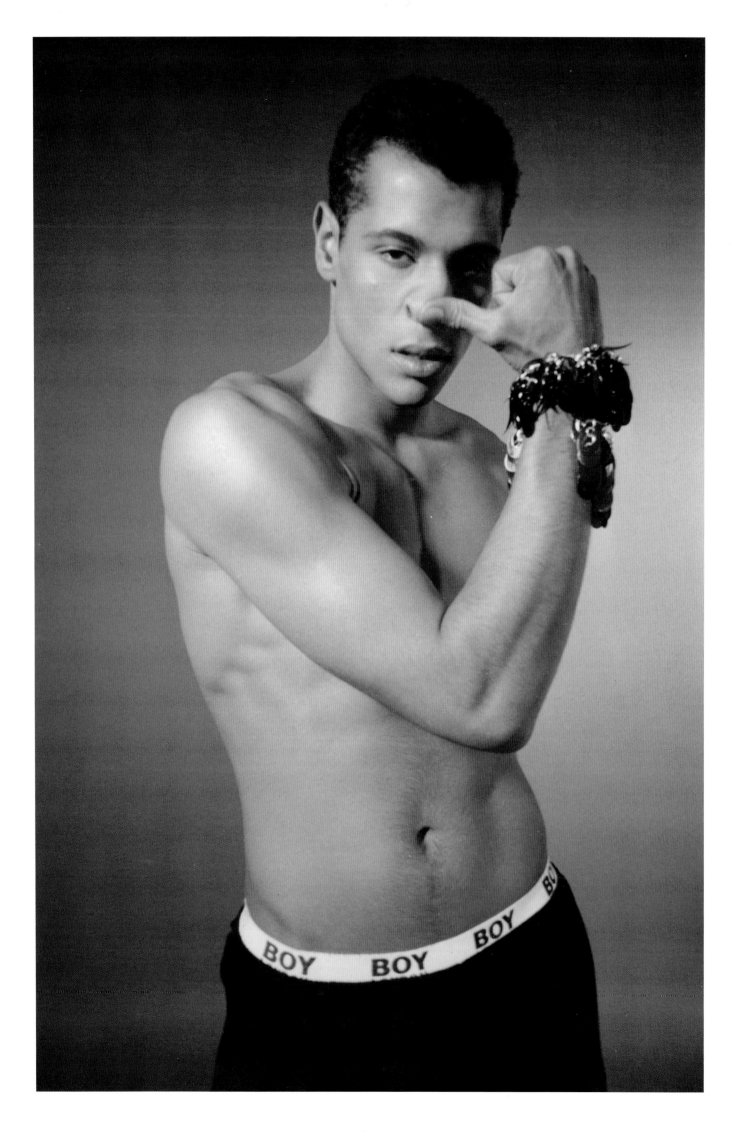

Photographer: Mark Lewis

Models: Isabelle Bondi at Unique, Bruno at Marco Rasala

Make-up: Not listed

Hair: Rick Haylor, Rosie (Bruno) at Vidal Sassoon

Clothes: Katharine Hamnett, BOY, Laura Lee

Rick Haylor, hairdresser:
The thing that struck me more than anything was that, for the first time when working for a magazine, I was doing things that were really part of my life. I had moved to London and was living with my wife, and although we didn't earn much money, we both had great positions at Sassoon's. We were going out at the weekends to Portobello and places like that, and finding something stylish and maybe altering it slightly. I was a straight guy from a working class background. Deciding to be a hairdresser was a big deal for me, and going to London was an even bigger deal.

The process was very much a collaboration. We turned up and were there for each other. It wasn't just me, me, me. It was about the total look. We were given a lot of freedom and had to think on our feet. Working with you, I realised that it was about being part of a team. We all helped one another. I looked forward to those shoots. Working with Mark, we'd work in the front room that he used as a studio. Or we'd go somewhere and set up in someone's kitchen. It was about being together. When we first started working together there was no lunch, no money for anything, but everyone pulled together. Later I remember you booked me and said, "It's only for a couple of hours, hope you don't

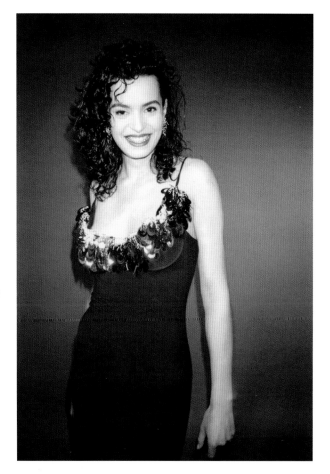

mind? I only need you for one or two pictures." Then when I showed up you said, "I've finally been given the budget for the fashion pages and I'm taking you all for a Chinese lunch." That team thing starts from the top. That Chinese meal has always meant more to me than a lot of fat fees ever did. You never promised us anything but you came good when you could. There were other people I worked for who I stopped working for, even though they were successful. It does have an impact.

David Convy, model:
I hadn't realised that there were so many boys with no tops on. But I was never asked to take my top off.

You Sexy Thing (where you from)

A handful of handsome boys, a couple of beautiful girls and a mattress pulled from the photographer's own bed. The thrust of this story was sex. Isabelle Bondi was another favourite, a wildly sensual woman. Bruno was her male equivalent, one of the new breed of macho Brazilian model boys who had arrived in Britain. They made the perfect couple. I kept the styling relatively underplayed, using body-conscious stretch jersey pieces. Sexy was emerging as the buzzword in fashion. Katharine Hamnett and Azzedeine Alaïa, boxer shorts, stretch jersey, suede and sequins. I used handfuls of oversized sequin earrings and bracelets to decorate a little black dress. I also put a bra over another form-fitting dress worn by another model, although she didn't think it was sexy at all and sulked throughout the session. This only made her look even more alluring.

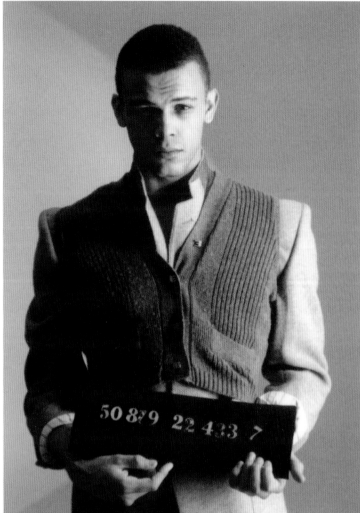

Barry Kamen, model:
Ah, Simon. You did your own version of Yohji. That's lovely. A little War On Want over the top. I love the raggedy holes.

Rick Haylor, hairdresser:
What you were doing at BLITZ was a much bigger representation of what was truly going on. Everyone talked about street fashion and used the words, but the other magazines were still taking so much from the catwalks. What you were doing was more real. It reflected how we would make our own clothes and maybe buy one special piece. Your work wasn't so literal, and I think that's why the imagery looks so much more current now. The styling was more influenced by what you saw around you, on the street, at the movies. I think there was much more variety in the imagery you turned out. There was not a specific BLITZ-type picture. It was more intangible than that. There were a lot more looks because of your approach. *The Face* and *i-D* felt and looked more formulaic and recognisable. The diversity of your pages was definitely stronger. There was also a lot more of a narrative to the pictures. They started off with a storyline and then the make-up artist, hairdresser and even the model could chip in. Everybody felt that there was enough freedom to put forward an idea or to ask, 'What do you think about this?' You were very open-minded even though you were still the person steering the shoot. It wasn't carved in granite. If you felt inspired enough, you would go with it. It really created a culture that was very energising and exciting.

Photographer: Gill Campbell

Model: Simon de Montford at Laraine Ashton

Clothes: Help The Aged, Ally Cappelino, Jennifer Corker, Demob, Duffer of Saint George, Calvin Klein, Damart, Culture Shock, Oxfam

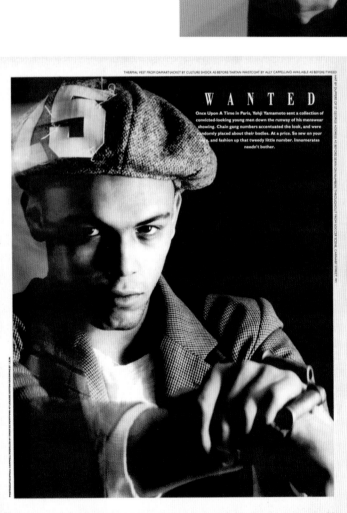

Wanted

I have always loved the movie *Once Upon A Time In America*, so when Yohji Yamamoto presented a menswear collection full of turn-of-the-century tykes, I was excited to make my own chain-gang look. I got some sew-on numbers from a sporting store and tacked them onto tweed and tartan jackets and caps. Knitted waistcoats and sweaters, sourced from the local Oxfam shops, were mostly too small for model Simon, splitting at the seams. Some were layered over bulkier jackets lending the look a hand-me-down, poor-boy vibe. I was happy to be working with Simon, who was one of Ray Petri's inner circle. With a black eye and bruises (courtesy of Leichner make-up) he was perfectly cast. To emphasise the numerical styling, I added tiny children's buttons to a waistcoat and had Simon hold a police booking ID board, which I created with metal number brooches by Bodymap jeweller Jennifer Corker. The pictures and layout evoked mug shot files.

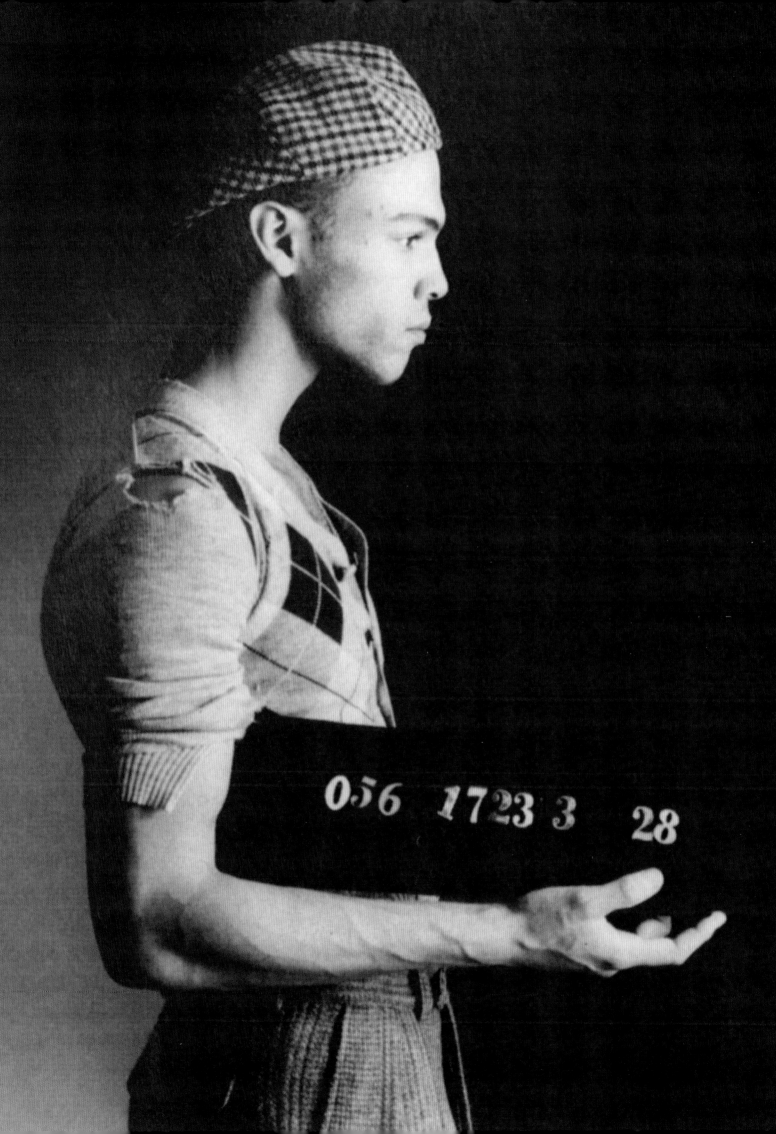

BLITZ #53
May 1987

Skinny models in skinny knits. This was predominantly a colour story. Layers of monochrome jersey pieces and sweaters offset with soft buff, creams and shades of grey. The models all looked suitably gangly. Like teenagers who had grown too fast. I emphasised the length of their limbs with shorts and over-the-knee socks, worn with boots by Dirk Bikkembergs. There is something wonderfully tender about these pictures, even though the models were some of the most wild I had worked with, especially the bleached blond Andre.

Skin and bone and everything in between

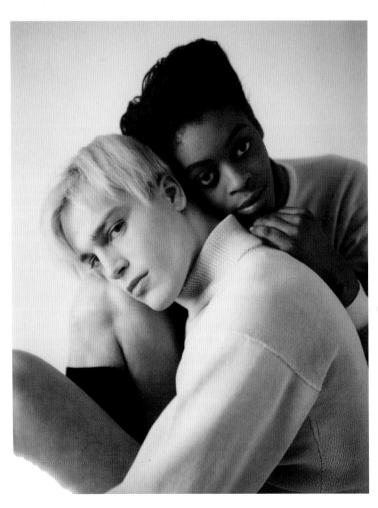

David Woolley, photographer:
When I was first commissioned for *BLITZ*, I was still an assistant and worked with one photographer full-time, and was rushing from shoot to shoot, national and international, which was a real adrenalin buzz. I was beginning to shoot my own work, calling in favours, begging for free studio space, desperate to create my own photographic vision. In my downtime I was living life, hanging out with friends in Chelsea and having as much fun as possible.

I loved the magazine from afar and just decided to go for it. I pulled together the best portfolio I could and called you. Luckily you found time to see me, loved my work and asked me to do a shoot. This was shot at London Studio, lent to me by my boss at the time. This was my biggest break.

The day of the first shoot I was hit by a double whammy of fear and excitement. Your styling was on song, and we worked together to create a vision we both loved. There are pros and cons of shooting single models versus group shots. On this job I encompassed both, but the models' interaction was fantastic, so my job was made easy. A technique I had been experimenting with worked perfectly for the first shoot: slide film, Ektachrome, under-exposed and then pushed two or three stops, making the colour thin and creating an overall vibrant picture.

Andre Van Noord, model:
I came to London in 1985–86. I had just become a model in Holland, working for Mexx. A guy in the pop venue Paradiso asked me. I said yes. Shortly after, I stopped my studies to live in London with my American rockabilly girlfriend, Diana, whom I met on a previous trip.

The modelling did not really hit off. I was a punk with white bleached hair and a lot of eyeliner and it was difficult for me to find an agency. I just wasn't presentable, so I had all kind of jobs. I sold cookies on Elephant & Castle. I was a very bad double-glazed window salesman. I never sold one. I worked for the Rough Trade label as a record puller, organising orders for shops across the UK. The good thing was that everyone was allowed to put records on – Grauzone and The Birthday Party.

Young and restless, my girl and me moved from place to place. Paddington to Shepherd's Bush, just living, fucking and getting the rent together. Something had to change. We started squatting. A guy showed us how to just go in and change the lock. We tried it in Westbourne Park. The door was already open. We changed the lock. We were set. Then a guy came, he started yelling that he'd beat the shit out of me for stealing the house – he had squatted it. Turned out that he broke in, forgot the lock, went to pick it up, and in the meantime we had come by. We found another place.

An agency took me on. Unique was owned by the dear Shola Akintonwa, a beautiful Nigerian businesswoman and artist. She said, "Come back here tomorrow looking like a normal person and I'll take you on." I came back. I had to borrow clothes from people and looked like an office clerk with a hangover, but I passed the test. And then things went fast, doing editorials for *BLITZ* and *i-D*, and shows for Gaultier. In the morning I'd wake up in London in a squat with no heating, in the afternoon I'd open Jean Paul's show in Cirque d'Hiver in Paris. Yeah.

Photographer: David Woolley

Models: Andre at Unique, Roen

Make-up: Anne Marie Lepretre

Hair: James 'Cuts' Lebon

Clothes: Comme des Garçons, Scotch House, Dirk Bikkembergs, Emilio Cavallini

BLITZ #54
June 1987

Photographer: Pete Moss

Models: Jean Luc at Premier, Andre van Noord at Unique

Clothes: Johnsons, Porselli, Reldan, Pineapple

Pete Moss, photographer:
We shot these Bowie/Rocker looks at the Forum in Kentish Town. What used to be the legendary Town and Country Club. It's a classic look now, but was being rediscovered by you back then.

Jean Paul Gaultier, designer:
In 1978 I was very inspired by John Travolta in *Grease*, so I did teddy boy hair and big skirts and T-shirts with no sleeves. It was when Frédérique [Lorca], who was a punk, came into my life, and from that day it all changed. Suddenly all the young ones came to see the show and all the odd girls came to work for me. I didn't like stereotypical models because they had stereotypical attitude. I have always been more attracted by bad boys and bad girls than the good ones.

Princess Julia, model:
Obviously Bowie gave us permission to experiment with various looks. Circa 1972–73, Bowie showed how you could transform yourself, image-wise and musically as well. But it was not only Bowie. I drew a lot of inspiration for role-playing from old movies. Bette Davis playing a different character in each movie; *Whatever Happened to Baby Jane* or *All About Eve*. A film like *Mr. Skeffington*, where the actress goes from really young to really old.

Who cares about a broken arm when you've just touched David Bowie

The title and inspiration for this story came from a concert review in the *NME*. Writer Nick Kent penned this treasure having witnessed the mayhem and madness that ensued during David Bowie's *Diamond Dogs* US tour in 1974. I had noted down his wonderful words way back when, in the knowledge that someday it would prove useful. When Jean Paul Gaultier sent burly blokes out onto his catwalk wearing spray-on Lycra, leopardskin and high-heel boots, I was reminded of Kent's observation. Jean Luc and Andre were the kind of models who could take on any role asked of them. They both had a lovely, laid-back, louche approach to modelling. The blackened eyebrows and liner were purposefully heavy-handed, as if applied night after night on a never-ending tour. I think we even replicated Gaultier's heavy metal high heels with some glued-on kitchen foil.

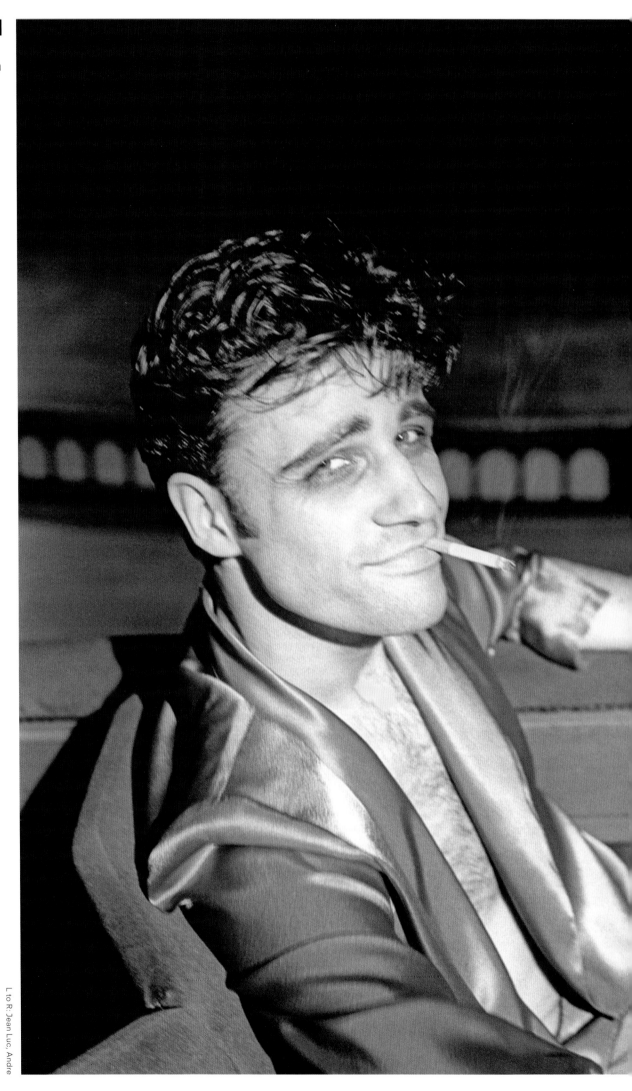

L to R: Jean Luc, Andre

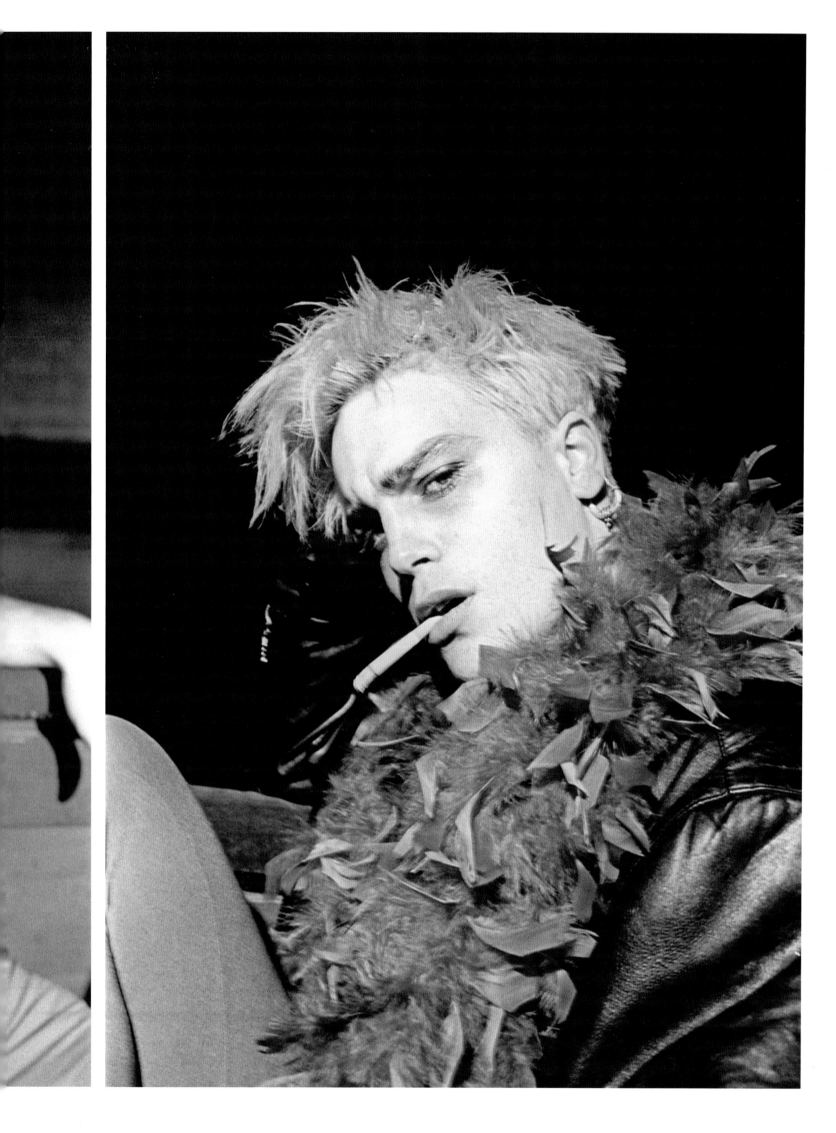

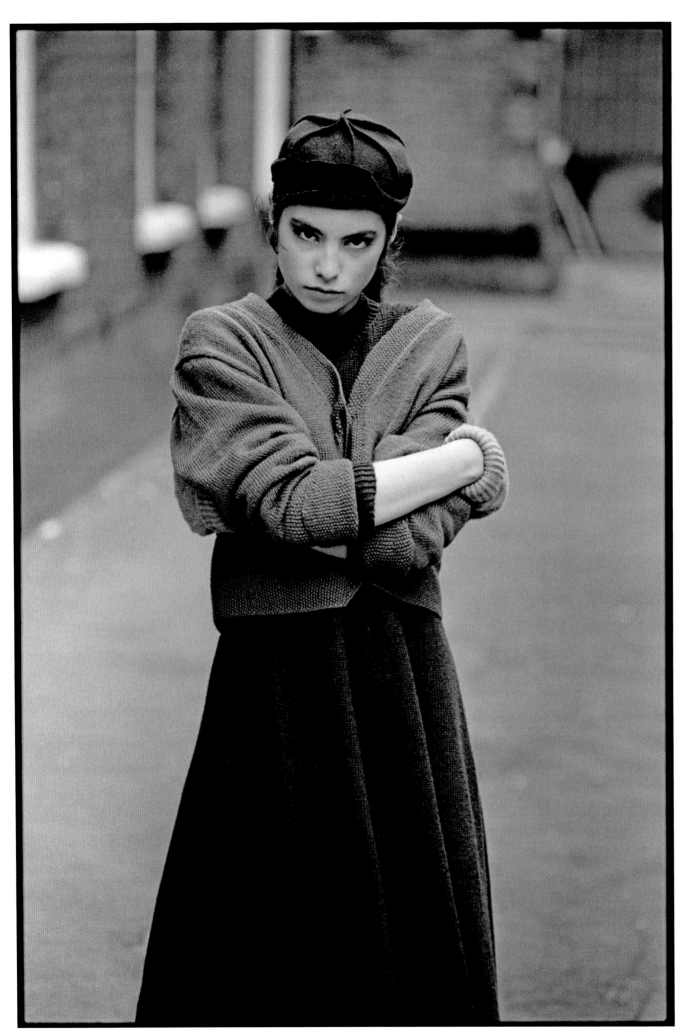

Photographer: David McIntyre

Models: Apple, Chris Hall at Z, Robert Abernethy, Tony Felix at Select, the Roeber Triplets at Laraine Ashton

Make-up/Hair: Wakamatsu at Z

Clothes: Marion Foale, Comme des Garçons, Bernstock Speirs, Ghost, Romeo Gigli, Go Silk, Matsuda, Vivienne Westwood, John Moore, Laurence Corner, Help The Aged

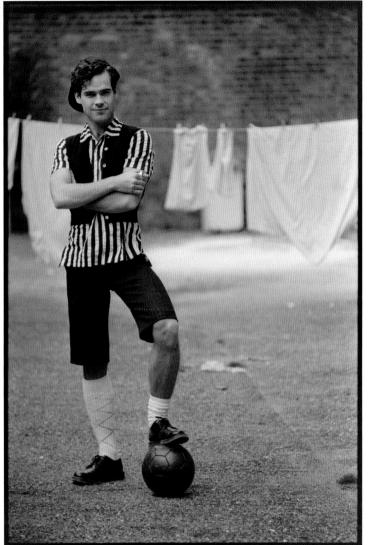

Robert

David McIntyre, photographer:
Every new generation of young photographers, fashion designers, models, make-up artists and hairdressers needs a magazine like *BLITZ* and a stylist like you. My career was just beginning in the mid-80s. I'd been living in Milan for a few months trying to get a break, and upon my return to London I visited you to show you the new work I'd been doing, and pitch some ideas. You were great in this way, because you always made time to talk and listened to ideas.

I'd just moved into this tiny studio apartment in Miles Buildings, off the Edgware Road. They were originally built for factory workers at the turn of the last century and had a wonderful North of England 'Hovis' feel about them. I suggested shooting in the area, perhaps using a lot of models, like a gang. I could tell the vagueness of the idea wasn't exciting you, and I had to put some meat on the bones. I can't remember if it was there and then or at a later date that I had the idea of a gang playing football in the street, but now the idea caught your attention, and I could see you were spinning through present and future fashions, bringing it all together.

For the shoot we based ourselves in my apartment, which seemed even smaller with a huge crew. Plus a ton of clothes – as you can imagine, with so many models and each having four or five looks.

The day was a blur, there was no rest. As long as I had the energy to shoot, you had new looks ready, always calm, always willing to try something new. It was a great shoot, and this story and others published in *BLITZ* were very instrumental in launching my career.

Can I have my ball back please?

I have always loved cartoony clothes that are too big or too small, and children wearing hand-me-downs when nothing quite fits. Transpose the whole thing to grown-ups, and the look becomes more exaggerated. The shorts suit for men was something being proffered and worn by trendy designers. These images have a nostalgic quality that David captured beautifully. The models played their roles with such tremendous gusto, they soon became lost in the game of football. This was always a story I saw in black and white. The clothes were mostly monochromatic or shades of grey. Marion Foale was a knitwear designer I came across at Olympia Fashion Fair. I liked that she wasn't a trendy young thing (she had been part of the Youthquake explosion in London in the Swinging Sixties), and loved her plain, unfussy knits. They looked like something your gran might have knitted for you, or more likely for an older sibling – and then handed down.

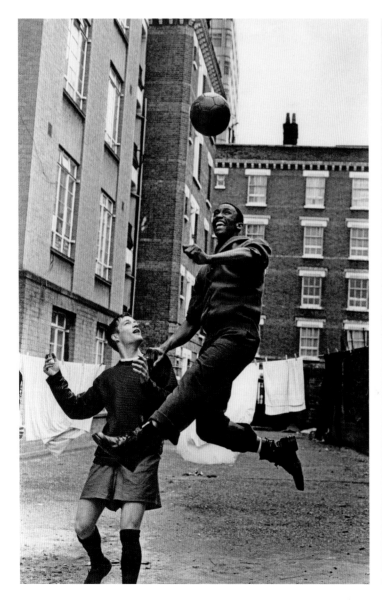

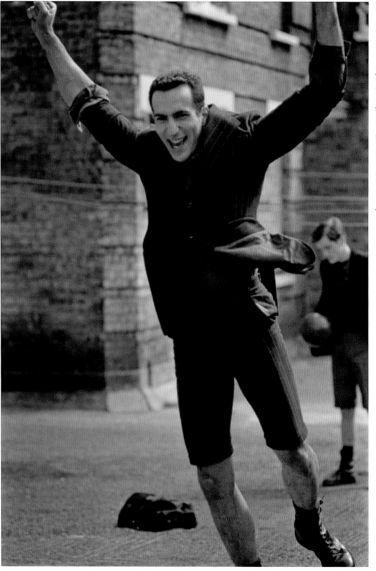

L to R: A Roeber triplet, Tony, Chris, another Roeber triplet

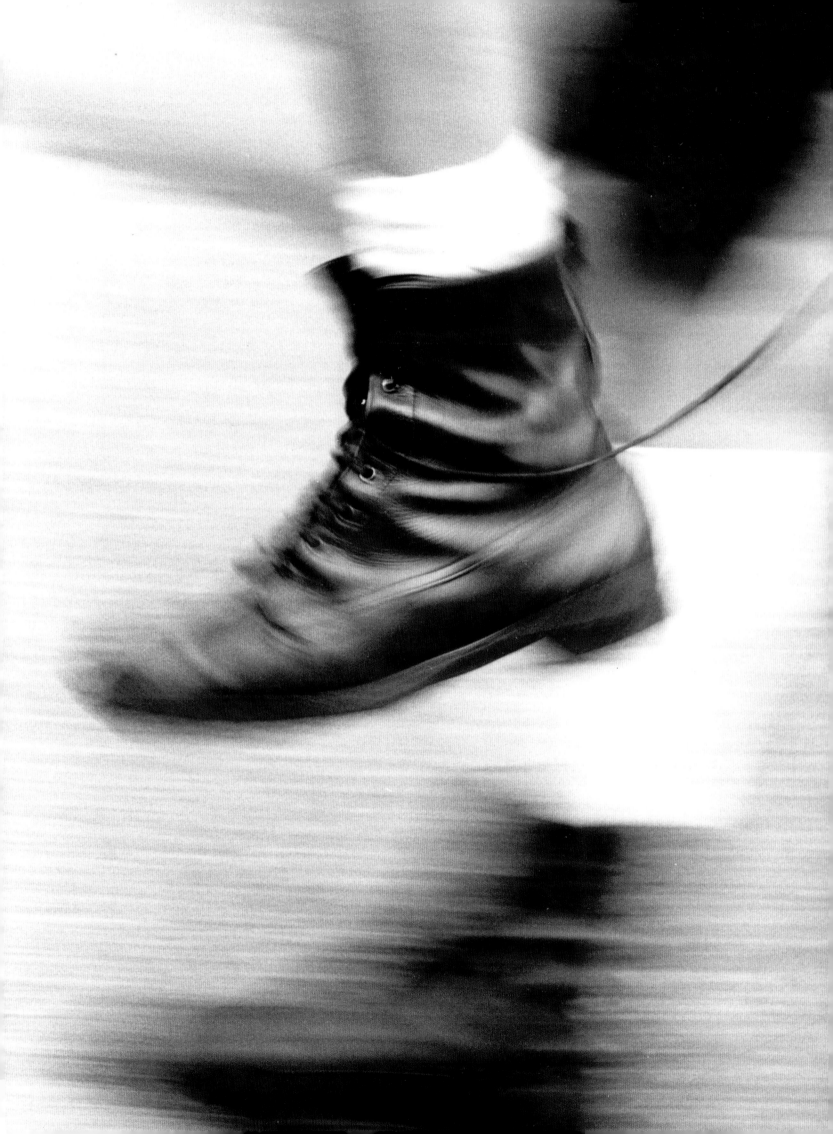

While bridalwear was not particularly the concern of style magazines, it provided another opportunity to play with an establishment uniform; and it was June, so why not? Brides tend to conform. Although fashions may change (at this time Princess Di had prompted a meringue moment), the look rarely deviates from a romantic ideal. I wanted to present wedding looks that were more individual and fun. If you liked wearing bondage pants, then wear a gleaming white sateen pair under your dress! I am still surprised how willingly people collaborated; for this shoot Jane Packer created bouquets, one of which ended up on Lori's head, along with a floral display that read 'MONOGAMY'. This was photographed on Louise's bed with a wedding picture of her parents, Judy and Mervin.

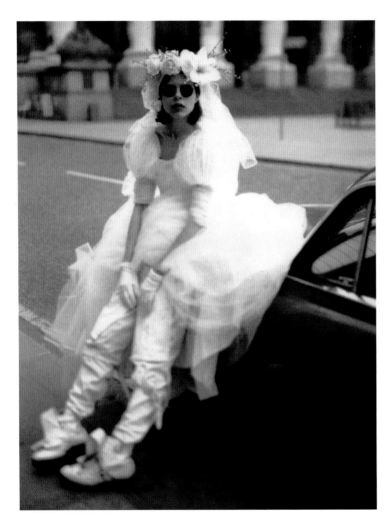

Ronald Diltoer, photographer:
The shoots we did together have stood the trial of time. I recently photographed a friend's wedding, and the bride was dressed in a similar style. The model was very beautiful and I probably fell in love with her, but then I did with all the models I worked with. We drove to the Stock Exchange to do the shot against the car, and another by a bandstand, where she smoked a long hand-rolled cigarette held in a Slim Barrett knuckle-duster ring. At the time I thought this was the best way to smoke. We also shot inside a flat (was it yours?) with flower arrangements laid across the bed.

This fashion story was simple, stylish, tasteful and timeless, which is always what I have been about in my work. When something has style it lasts and becomes inspirational.

I don't remember casting models. I think you did it, or we may have faxed each other suggestions. At the time in London there was a definite change in the perception of what models should look like, with new agencies like Z (who were my agent) and others trying to establish a new type of beauty. They didn't promote bimbos or pretty stupid things, but girls with balls and brains, and boys without the chiselled American faces. It pretty much changed the fashion world's idea of what is beautiful forever; and I was all for those changes.

I was delighted with the way the stories came out. I was so proud of those images, and they kick-started my career. From that moment, I was going to make a living out of photography, so BLITZ will always be very special to me. These stories have opened many doors for me. Suddenly people would listen to me or ask for my advice, which was new for me. In a way the reason why I eventually moved to the UK is all down to BLITZ. I just wish I had done more stories with you.

On these shoots David Sims was my assistant. What a lovely guy he was. I met him when I was doing a test. He was the studio assistant. We got on and I ended up sleeping on his floor for a few weeks. He assisted me until a more famous photographer wanted him. That was pretty much the last I saw of him until one time in London when I heard he was working in the next-door studio, so I popped in to say 'hi'. When I entered the studio I saw David and went up behind him and tapped his shoulder. The other people in the studio were looking at me like, 'How dare you?' but David turned around and gave me the biggest hug ever. We chatted and were sure to meet up again, which never happened. That was ten years ago.

Louise Constad, make-up artist:
I didn't think putting frou-frou dresses with bondage pants or bouquets on her head looked weird. I thought it was normal fashionable bridalwear. I believed that I would wear the same if I got married, the same way I cut up my own jean jacket and remade it after that denim jacket shoot. I would have gone to Pronuptia and got an ordinary dress like you did and just trendied it up, because I couldn't possibly have worn it as it was. I love that I had tidied up for the shoot.

Photographer: Ronald Diltoer

Model: Lori Vincent

Make-up and Hair:
Louise Constad

Clothes: Pronuptia, Seditionaries, BOY, Cutler & Gross, Stephen Jones, Jane Packer

The bride wore on

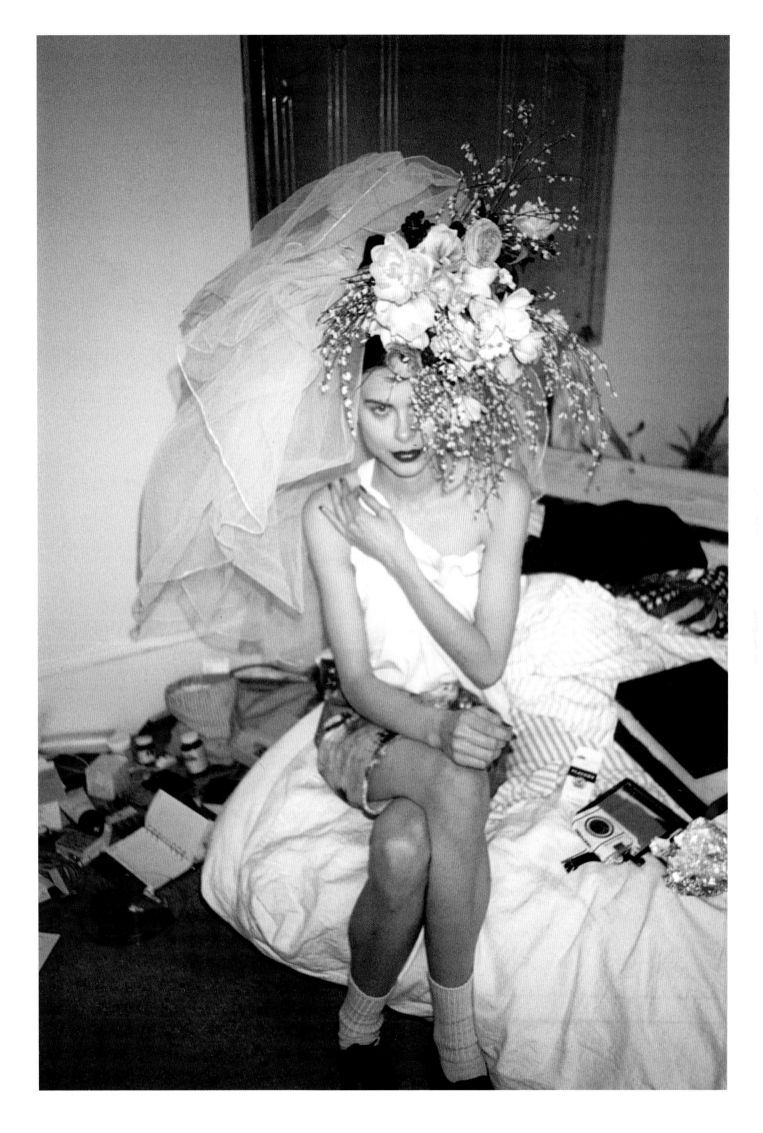

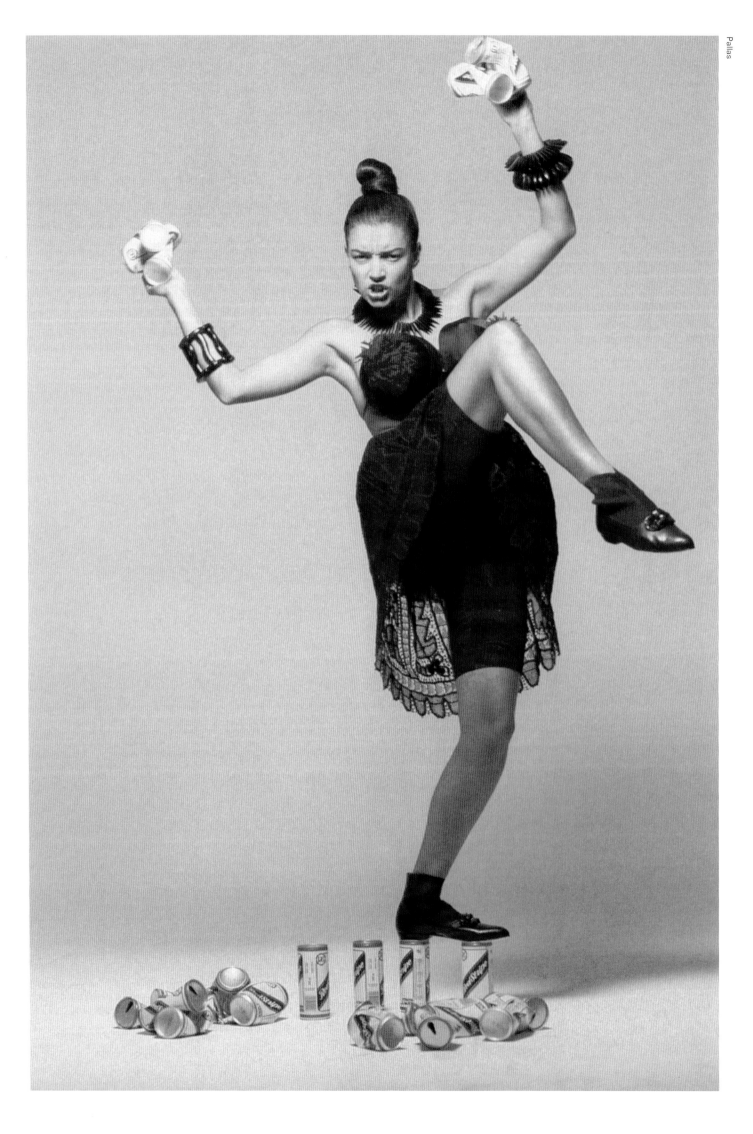

The shoot featured pretty much the entire stock of World, a tiny store owned by Michael and Gerlinde Costiff, who were two of London's style-setters; they also ran the nightclub Kinky Gerlinky. The merchandise was a mix of ethnic souvenirs they brought back from their travels and urban club kid sportswear. The shoot focused on the lust for labels and the omnipresence of giant companies. I guess this was the start of global branding.

Gerlinde and I were often referred to as pioneers. World was before coffee shops and mobile phones, so it was as much a social centre. People would meet there and leave messages with us for their mates. Soho has had it now. It's so corporate. And everything has moved over to the East End. I call it downwardly mobile. You don't have to bother to shave over there.

We were always quite wary of stylists when they came to borrow things but we liked *BLITZ* the most. We'd say, 'Take whatever you like. That way you have a bit of choice.' Those two boys wearing the sarongs. We never sold any of them. I've still got some in a box somewhere, and I've got one of the Brazil football shirts left that was mine.

Wear in the world

Photographer: David Woolley

Models: Chazz, Moose, Pallas Citroen at Z, Tai-Shan at Marco Rasala

Make-up: Melvone Farrell at Z

Hair: Gordon Pindar for Toni & Guy

Clothes: World, Martine Sitbon, Bernstock Speirs, Budweiser, Marlboro, Obsession Calvin Klein body glistener

David Woolley, photographer:
It was the most exciting experience of my life. A new world was opening for me. *BLITZ* had a much rawer energy than magazines today. Productions now tend to be much slicker. *BLITZ* had an inspirational creativity, a vitality and authenticity that inspired my generation.

Michael Costiff, designer:
BLITZ was good to us. You always used lots of things. One thrilling moment was when we went to London Fashion Week and on every seat was a copy of *BLITZ* with about twelve pages of World. That was when Kim Bowen became fashion editor.

Gerlinde had a stall in Antiquarius market on the King's Road but we wanted our own store, so we opened World in Litchfield Street on the Covent Garden/Soho crossover. We had a ball.

Our trips abroad were all about the shopping. We never went to the beach. I still love a good airport gift shop. We bought things we never saw elsewhere. Now everything is on the internet, everything is everywhere. It's difficult to find things that are different. We had exotic taste. World was a very eclectic mix. We lived in a world of our own. I still avoid real life now. It's just too ghastly.

We'd travel and bring back whatever took our fancy. Sometimes we got it right, sometimes we didn't. I remember when Lycra cycling gear was coming in, so we bought a lot of it in Brazil, by the time we got back it was all Acid House. If we bought stuff when travelling and something sold out, there was never any chance to replace the stock.

Chazz Khan, model:
I remember the hairdresser putting egg yolk in our hair. You couldn't follow that as fashion. It wasn't that direct. It was the feel or the mood. It's got to be more blatant and obvious now. Your shoots were so brilliant. I thought, I'm never going to be doing this ever again.

Moose Ali Khan, model:
We just wanted to part of anything happening – a show, an editorial or an event. If we were in Paris or Milan there was always the same British contingent of models, then a few years later there would be a different group from a different country – the Brazilians, then the Eastern Europeans. But at that time everyone wanted a bit of London energy, the mixed-race models and the edginess.

L to R: Moose, Chazz

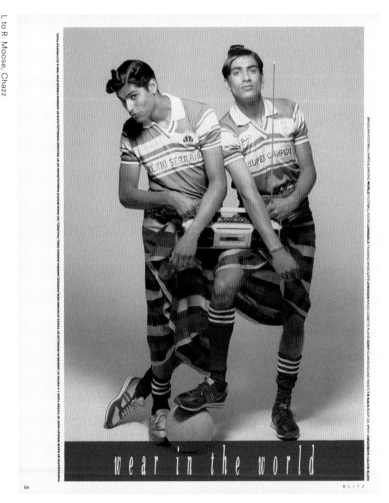

wear in the world

Pallas Citroen, model:
I didn't do catalogue. I did editorial in Italy and Paris so I didn't make lots of money. My colour was an issue. I wasn't one thing or the other. Naomi was black. I wasn't even exotic-looking. I was brown with English features.

You were doing jobs with your friends. Everyone was treated as an equal. We'd have a laugh. It wasn't like working with the toffee-nosed women on the more establishment fashion magazines. I often felt intimidated by them and the whole process. Working for *BLITZ* was fun. It felt like a jolly day out.

At this time everything was emblazoned with logos, which was horrible. We used to wear mental things. I remember wearing tutus and big woolly jumpers. As models we'd pick things up on our travels, so you could call my personal style eclectic if you were being nice, but really it was a bit of a mess. You'd just put stuff together. Do your own look. You'd never buy top-to-tail looks.

This shoot was great fun with Chazz and Moose mucking around. We were very unprofessional in one sense, but we were also very politically aware. What we were doing was the opposite of the 1980s ethos about making lots of money. This shoot pre-empted the Acid House look that was very tribal and about embracing all cultures. This was very counter-culture. It said, 'We are not interested in capitalism'. That was too restrictive. In the mainstream the 1980s were actually quite boring, very grown-up. It was wine bars and Sade.

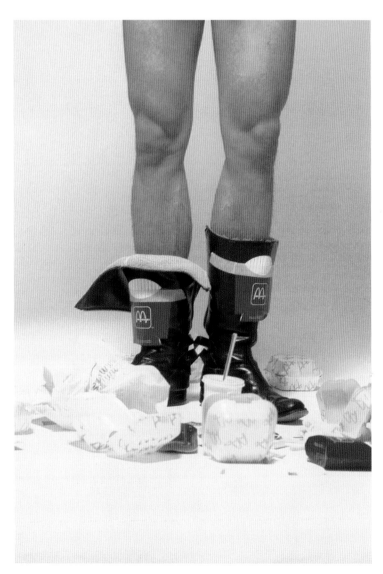

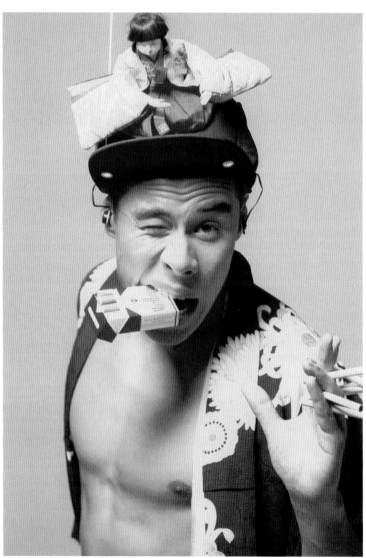

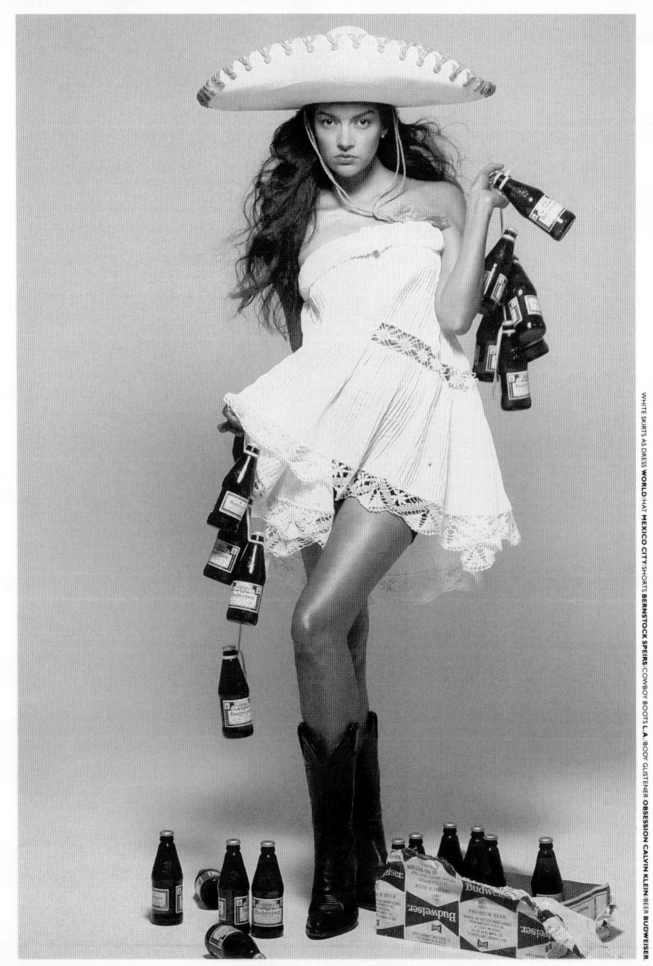

WHITE SKIRTS AS DRESS **WORLD** HAT **MEXICO CITY** SHORTS **BERNSTOCK SPEIRS** COWBOY BOOTS **L.A.** BODY GLISTENER **OBSESSION CALVIN KLEIN** BEER **BUDWEISER**

BLITZ

This was one of the last shoots I did for *BLITZ* magazine, and the wide open-brief was starting to unravel at the edges. I don't think there was any major storyline for this shoot. I pulled together some clothes and, as usual, did a bit of customisation (random red felt flowers stitched on a shirt collar). Denim pieces were jumbled in. It was a strange day, with most of the team strung out on a bottle of Southern Comfort. Ricardo was one of the new breed of Brazilian boys. He was a golden Adonis who (after a few shots) seemed game for anything. Although his English was limited, Marcus persuaded him to make leaps of faith on the chalk mountaintop. In contrast we photographed a female model in formal close-up portrait mode.

Sky Blue Pink Denim

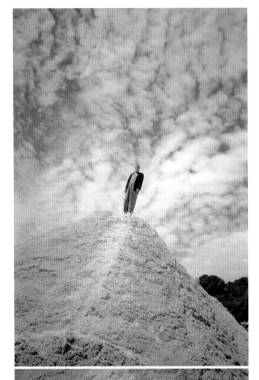

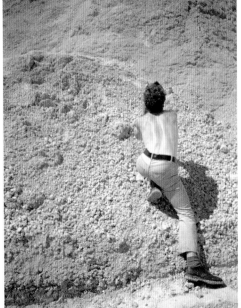

T to B: Ricardo, Marcus

Photographer: Marcus Tomlinson

Model: Ricardo Herriot at Marco Rasala

Make-up: Louise Constad

Hair: Not Listed

Clothes: Momento Due, Wrangler, Bernstock Speirs

Marcus Tomlinson, photographer:
It was always so much fun to work on *BLITZ*. As a newcomer to London I fell into a world of remarkable, strange and beautiful people that I often tried to look like, but somehow I could never manage to pull it off. I felt the only thing to do was to transport you and the rest of the *BLITZ* team to my neck of the woods. So, packed into somebody's car (maybe the make-up artist's?), we drove to a disused quarry in Dorking. I seem to remember that we actually had to break in to the quarry as there was no access; everything was fenced off. The day was the hottest I can remember for a long time; this was probably due to the fact that we were essentially working in a giant reflector that intensified the light and heat, and felt like a furnace. I don't know how the models were able to do their stuff but, styled as if they had just fallen from another planet, they made a day of it and revelled in the madness. One to treasure...

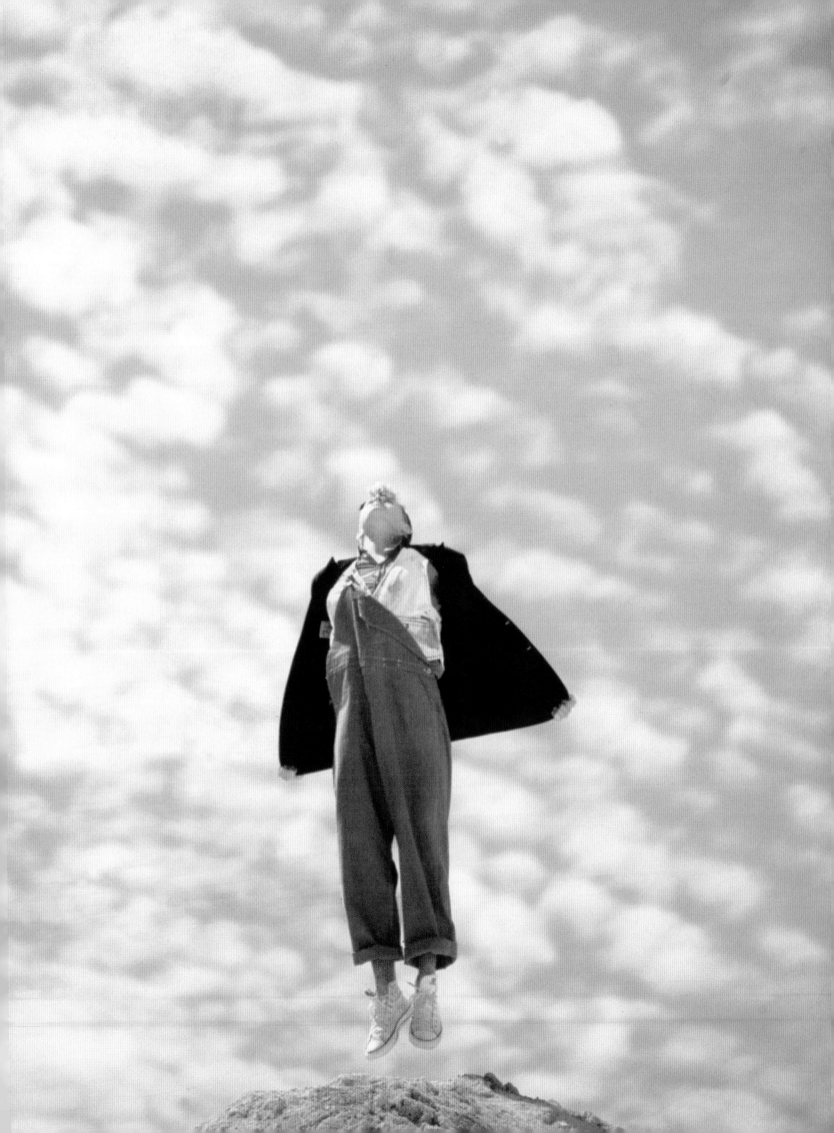

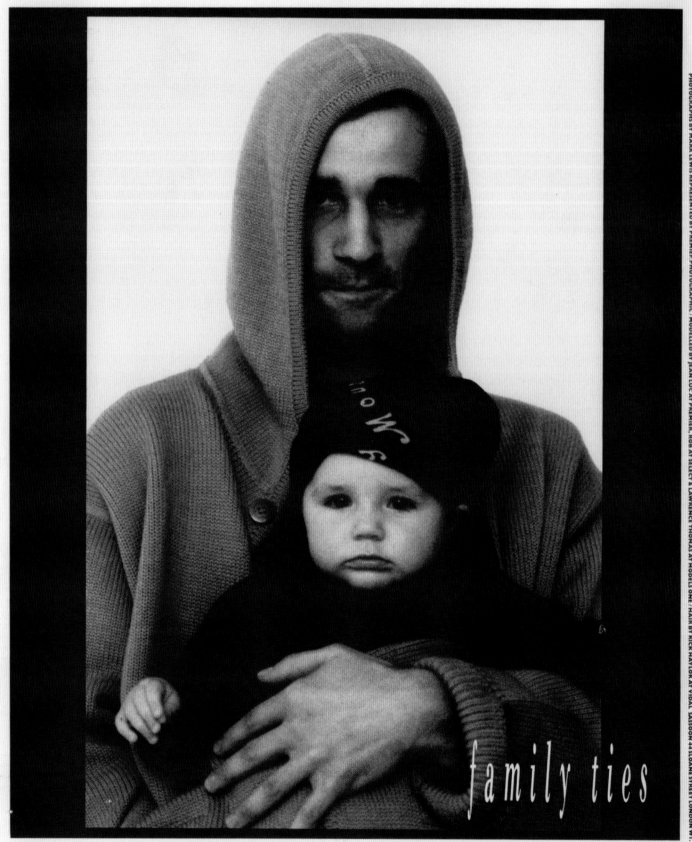

PHOTOGRAPHS BY MARK LEWIS REPRESENTED BY PREMIER PHOTOGRAPHIC / MODELLED BY JEAN LUC AT PREMIER, ROB AT SELECT & LAWRENCE THOMAS AT MODELS ONE / HAIR BY RICK HAYLOR AT VIDAL SASSOON 44 SLOANE STREET LONDON W1.

family ties

KNITTED HOODED CARDIGAN **DIRK BIKKEMBERGS** / MICKEY MOUSE BANDANA **DISNEYLAND**

BLITZ #57
September 1987

Photographer: Mark Lewis

Models: Jean Luc at Premier,
Laurence James Thomas at Z

Make-up: Not Listed

Hair: Rick Haylor at
Vidal Sassoon

Clothes: Dirk Bikkembergs, Dries
Van Noten, Wendy Dagworthy,
Disneyland

Fashion was becoming more conservative, as designers such as Dries Van Noten, Katharine Hamnett and Nicole Farhi were appropriating classic menswear mainstays. This presented a problem: how to shoot these trad items in a modern way? Perhaps the most obvious solution was to use a classic portraiture style, so Mark photographed the boys in a very formal way. The styling was relatively simple, a shirt and tie(s) or a sweater or two. I did have a bit of fun with how I tied them up in knots, and introducing a bow that came from Disneyland. This childish element also crept in with the addition of a baby (I am not sure where he or she came from?) whom I wrapped in a Dirk Bikkembergs sweater and positioned among a group of Jean Paul Gaultier shoes. I dressed the baby in a bandana (another Mickey Mouse reference) that I found in the street outside the office.

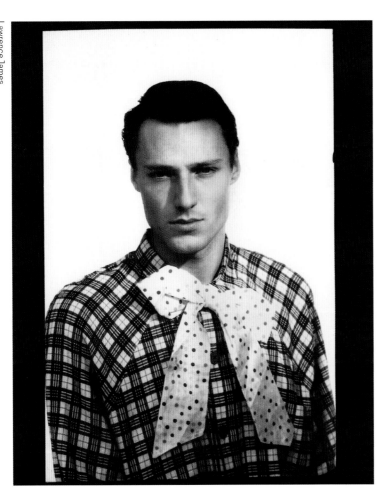

Lawrence James

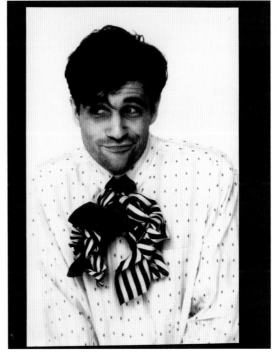

Jean Luc

Rick Haylor, hairdresser:
As a hairdresser, you tend to think about what style you want to do before the shoot; you want to make a bit of a statement. Working with *BLITZ* stopped me from doing that. I wanted to wait until I got to the studio to see what the shoot was about. Looking at the Polaroid after each shot, I'd want to change the hair to make it stronger or to calm it down. It taught me to look at the overall picture of everything.

Family ties

BLITZ #57
September 1987

Martine Houghton, model:
I don't know how Jean Paul Gaultier knew about me but I guess he saw pictures in BLITZ, so when I went to see him he said, "You're so Jean Paul, you're booked!" He really embraced me. I did Martine Sitbon as well as Wendy Dagworthy. I was so shy so I wouldn't naturally put myself on a catwalk, but I saw it as a challenge. But when you come off the catwalk you want to get straight back on.

I was very attracted to the hideousness of it. It's translated through time. Back then I thought, 'Oh, my God!' but actually this image is very pretty. I had a brief spell taking fashion pictures and I didn't really like it. Everyone had an agenda, unless you stomped in and made demands.

For the seventh anniversary issue we asked Jean Paul Gaultier to make us something special to celebrate. We certainly did not expect him to cook up a fabulous birthday cake outfit, featuring a fishbowl helmet fitted with candles. Of course, nobody but Martine could model this outfit, even though she wasn't too keen on the head-to-toe second-skin Lycra ensemble. She also wore a swimming cap that we piped with real pink and white icing (intended as an approximation of a 1930s sugared finger-wave hairstyle). Under the hot lights the icing refused to set and slid down her face throughout the session.

Jean Paul Gaultier, designer:
For me, girls like Martine, Amanda, Missy, Laurence Treil and Eugenie Vincent are the supermodels, because of their personality. They have more character. When I make a show I am very specific for the hair but the make-up not so much, you know why? I often let the make-up artist do their own thing most of the time, first because I respect their work, but also because I think that make-up can change a lot the face of the girl, and I don't want them to look uniform. If I choose Amanda and Martine for my show, I want them to be Amanda and Martine. You can have an extreme look but I still want to see the personality of the girl. I don't want the make-up to hide their beauty and make everything disappear so you will not see her beautiful nose or lips. I like those girls so much that in reality, even if they had no make-up, I should love it. I like them like that.

To be honest, the choice of model is super-important for me. For example, when I am doing fitting for ready-to-wear, mixing the clothes, sometimes I don't find how to mix, and it comes from the model.

I think I am drawn to strong women, from Jeanne d'Arc to Madonna, because I have been educated by women – at school, of course, but also by my grandmother and my mother. They gave me love and they were strong women. They were maybe even stronger than men.

Robert Ogilvie, photographer:
That's so Angus McBean. The colours are stunning. It reminds me of the photo of Carmen Dell'Orefice underwater with Norman Parkinson, putting her hand in his helmet.

Gregory Davis, make-up artist:
This is Bourjois make-up again. I loved their pearly pink lipstick. I remember the icing sugar kept slipping off the swim cap. Quick, retouch the make-up. Eyebrows! I had that shot in my book for ages.

Carol Brown, make-up artist:
There was a very different London/European vs. American look: American models were usually tall, tanned and commercial, whereas our lot were pale and interesting, and took risks with bold statement haircuts. I loved the freedom of working on shoots for BLITZ and I think the models did too, because they knew that their individuality would be celebrated instead of homogenised. Yes, BLITZ took risks with the weird and wonderful.

Photographer: Mark Lewis

Model: Martine Houghton
at Marco Rasala

Make-up: Gregory Davis
for Bourjois

Hair: Iain R. Webb

Clothes: Jean Paul Gaultier

Bon anniversaire

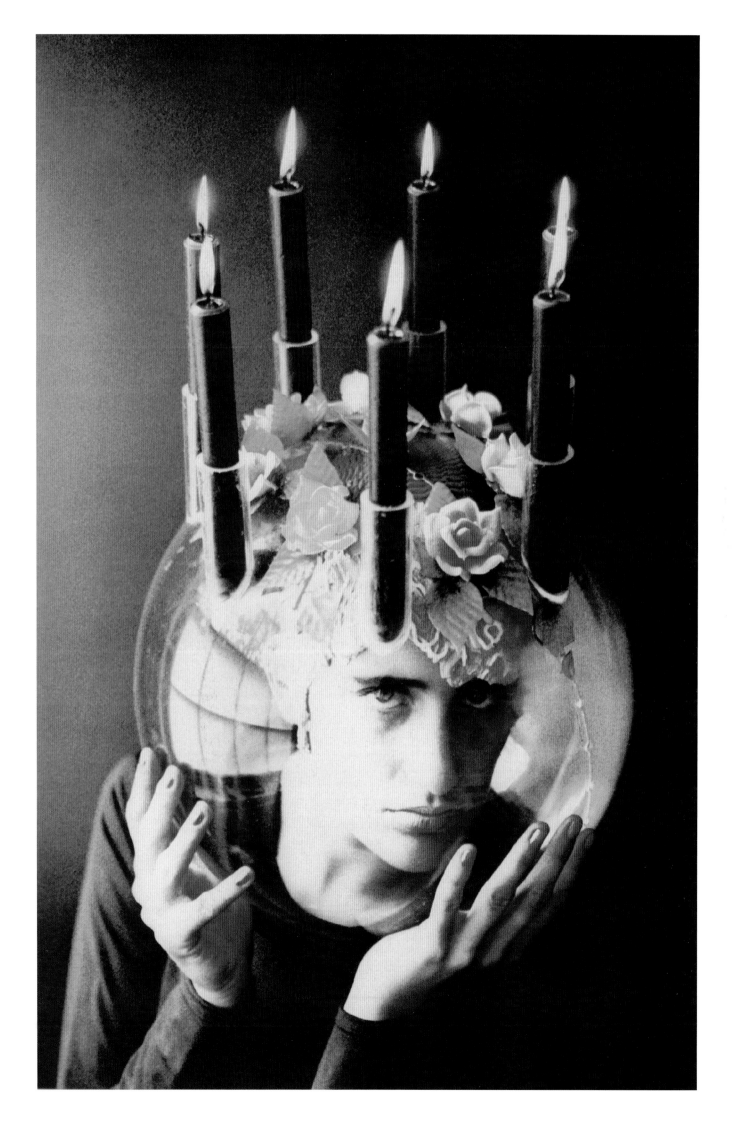

BLITZ #58
October 1987

Photographer: Pierre Rutschi

Model: Lucy Goldman at Unique

Make-up and Hair:
Louise Constad

Clothes: Ann Demeulemeester,
Marina Yee

Girls do it better

The emerging Belgian design school was predominantly male, but I always admired the work of two of the original Antwerp Six: Marina Yee and Ann Demeulemeester. This story showcased their uncluttered, understated and somewhat innocent aesthetic, something that would later be billed as deconstruction. I met photographer Pierre Rutschi through Jean Paul Gaultier. He was a handsome ex-model who burned the candle at both ends at the Bains Douches and Le Palace. With his greased quiff, white T-shirt, washed-out jeans and winklepickers, he looked like a latter-day fifties bad-boy. I was immediately smitten. I loved his work too, which had a surprising stillness, especially as he had a peculiar way of shooting, jumping around in the studio.

Pierre Rutschi, photographer:
Even though I'm not nostalgic this was a really lucky period, when being friends with Jean Paul Gaultier opened some doors, and generally speaking, work seemed easy. I travelled to Milan and London, most likely for partying and having the best time ever. The London scene was all about fashion, music and clubbing and *BLITZ* was part of that creative era.

After studying film and art history, I started as an assistant, mainly with Barry Dunne, a rather trendy and commercial fashion photographer. Coming to Paris in 1977, I met Thierry Mugler at a party and, to my surprise, he asked me to model. I also got to know Jean Paul Gaultier and did many of his shows. I was never with an agency. What I liked most was the opportunity to see the whole creative process from sketch to runway, and to learn about fashion by observing backstage or at the studio.

This shoot was very relaxed; a sunny afternoon with beautiful light coming into the studio. London had a flavour of alternative fashion, the fetish scene, the goths, the skins and the teds. Youth culture was more alive and creative than in Paris, always related to music and a way of life. I used to love Vivienne Westwood, and saw the first shows John Galliano did, thanks to Marie Sophie, who modelled for him. I was mainly interested in Comme des Garçons and my friends Jean Paul and Thierry. I was very happy when the story was printed in *BLITZ* as, along with *i-D* and *The Face*, it had a certain prestige in Paris. The whole era offered opportunities. Exposure helped me work on campaigns in Italy for Fuzzi, who produced Gaultier's knitwear, and whose own collection was designed by Martin Margiela.

I loved London for its club scene, and used to go out a lot rather than thinking too much about work. Through the years there have been so many parties. Taboo, of course, on Thursdays, Total Fashion Victims at the Wag on Tuesdays, Café de Paris on Wednesdays. I was around for the first Torture Garden parties held in Shepherds Bush. Well, I could go on and on.

Ann Demeulemeester, designer:
I will never forget the warm welcome I received in London. The air was full of positive energy when I showed my first little collection. Thank you with all my heart for all the encouragement on my first steps in fashion.

I felt more comfortable coming to London, as it seemed younger, more open, more easy than to go to Paris, which was a bit scary to me at that time. Also, London was a city that was attached to music that I liked, to all this kind of energy. Back then what was happening in the music scene was so fantastic. It was a city that young people were dreaming of. It was exciting to go to London but I wasn't very much aware of our impact as a group. I didn't even feel part of a group; we just wanted to come together because we didn't have the money to go separately. I built my little stand at the British Designer Show and I put out my rack of clothes, and I was open for business. I didn't really know what would happen, but the first day, the first hour, I had important clients sitting down and actually writing an order. This was really a surprise for me. It was a bit *Alice In Wonderland*, you know. I thought, 'This is actually happening.' Also, the reaction of the press was very positive. I think because the press couldn't pronounce these difficult Belgian names they thought, ah, there are six of them – so they made the Antwerp Six, and this has become the thing, like folklore.

It was a combination of people who are at the same place, the Antwerp Academy, at the same moment, who are all ambitious and hard workers. We all wanted to do our own thing. There was this kind of energy in the school back then, because we were all very individual and very hard workers, so when one person did something, another did more. Out of school it just continued, because all these individual people had really big ambition and were very serious about the job. It was a love and hate relationship between us. There were big discussions but we never agreed on anything. We disliked the work of each other, but that was good because it made everybody get stronger defending his or her own thing, and this was the strength, the individuality. I never liked the word deconstruction; it's like you are breaking down something, while I was trying to construct something, to start from zero. For me it was about breaking rules and a reaction against the conservative, that's how it started. It was also an act of freedom.

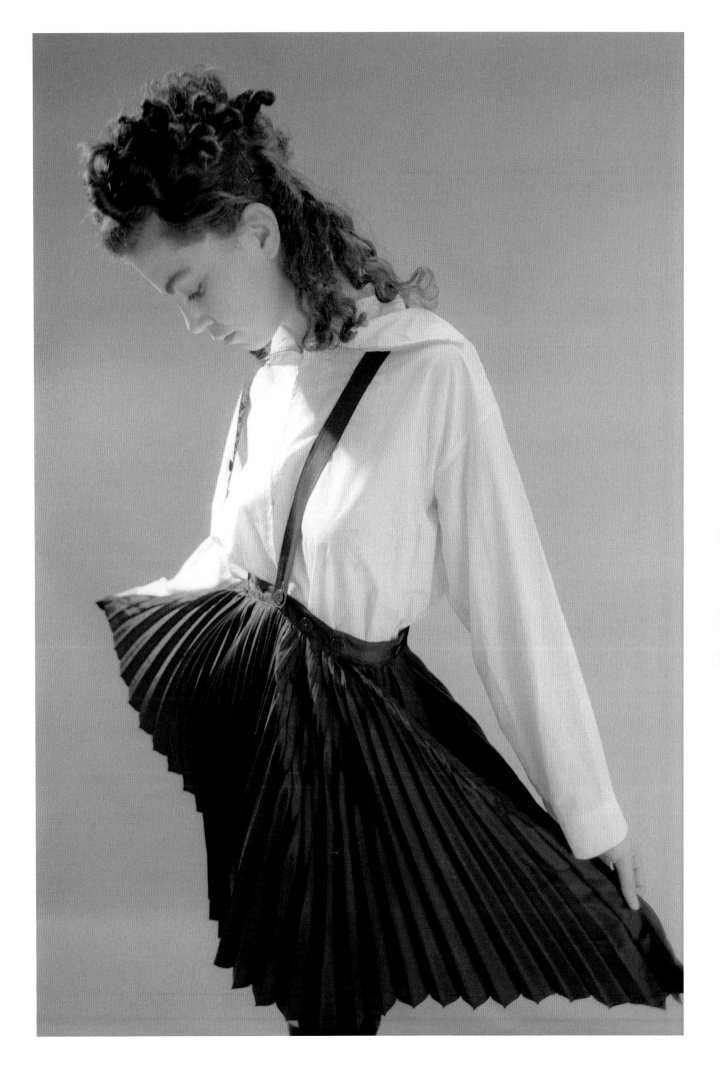

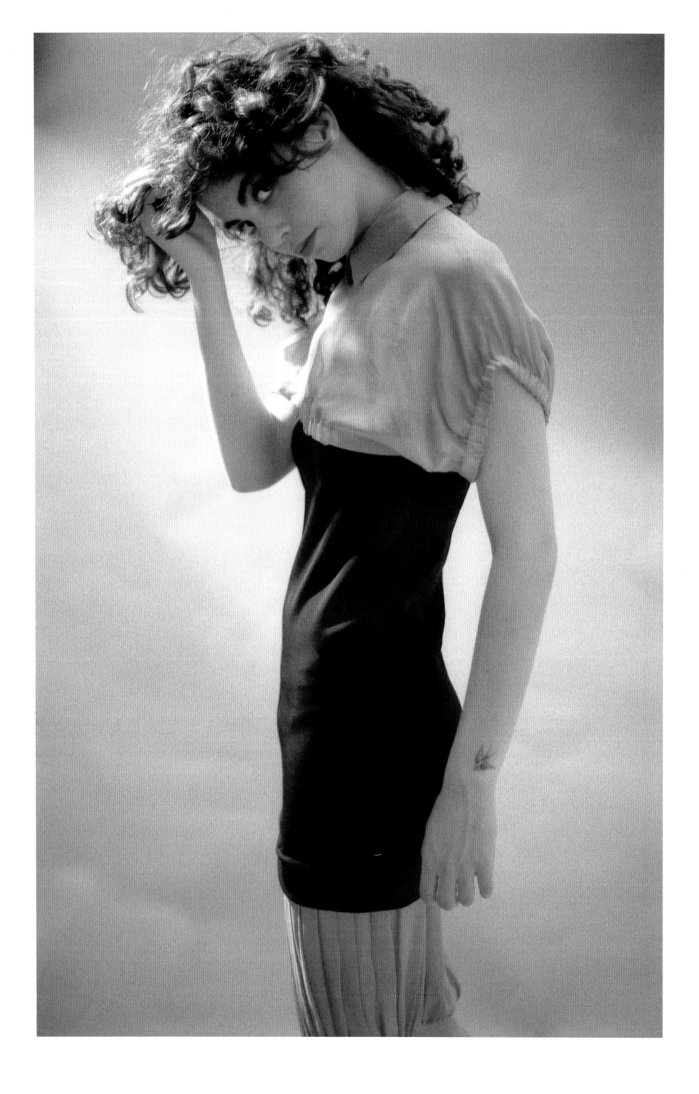

THE LONDON EVENING STANDARD
11 August 1987

IAIN R. WEBB

Peter Brown, photographer:
We worked together for many years. I always enjoyed working with you, and you were the most inspiring. Kim was inspiring too, but in different ways. Your wings were definitely clipped being in Fleet Street. We all were, whereas on *BLITZ* you had the opportunity to do whatever you liked. Kim and you were very different in your approaches, but what an opportunity *BLITZ* gave us. It gave me a portfolio of tear sheets that I could take around and get advertising and other editorial. I took my *BLITZ* tear sheet book to Milan and phoned, cold calling Italian *Vogue* from a payphone and ending up going to see Alberto Nodolini, who was then the art director, the next day. Imagine today, some twenty-five-year- old kid on a pay phone, calling whoever on a major magazine and them saying, 'Oh yeah, come in tomorrow!'

The main thing about this whole time was we had so much fun doing it. I remember laughing, laughing until we cried on some of these shoots. Hilarious, hilarious stuff. It's become so corporate now, and I don't think you could go on a fashion shoot and have that level of hilarity and that kind of spontaneity, because now everything is so driven by money and has become so serious. The money didn't matter to us because there wasn't any.

Mark Lewis, photographer:
So when you left *BLITZ* for the newspapers on Fleet Street, and later for *Elle* magazine, it kind of spelt the end of fashion for me. Firstly because I loved the social document aspect of the fashion that you were doing – that it wasn't only about beautiful clothes and bodies, but about society, politics and economics – and secondly because there wasn't another you, and the thought of working with hysterical, insecure fashion editors was rather daunting.

Photographer: Mark Lewis

In 1987 I left the *BLITZ* magazine family, and with it the creative security and sartorial safety net. My Jean Paul Gaultier pour Stephane Kelian shoes were filled by Kim Bowen, yet another ex-St Martin's fashion graduate and fellow Blitz club kid. Enticed by Features Editor Maggie Alderson, I took a job as fashion editor of the *London Evening Standard*, located on Fleet Street. It was a big deal, as a career move and, indeed, financially. On my first day I received a bouquet from my new comrades on the features desk. The card read: 'Welcome to the Street of Shame'. The transition to Fleet Street was a shock, but naïvely I tried to continue to approach the job with the same mindset and dress sense. I think wearing a shorts suit to the office caused cardiac arrest for some of the old boy staff. But editor John Leese had employed me knowing my pedigree, and Maggie was incredibly supportive and encouraging, so I tried to continue to create fashion pages with an inspiring narrative. This did not always go down well, especially with the printers, who lived in the basement and took delight in brandishing prints that I produced around the office as they barked, 'What the fuck is this? Well, it's not fucking fashion that's for sure!' This portrait was used in the newspaper to announce my arrival. I was as lost on Fleet Street as I looked in this Gaultier jacket. Welcome to the real world.

... our new Fashion Editor

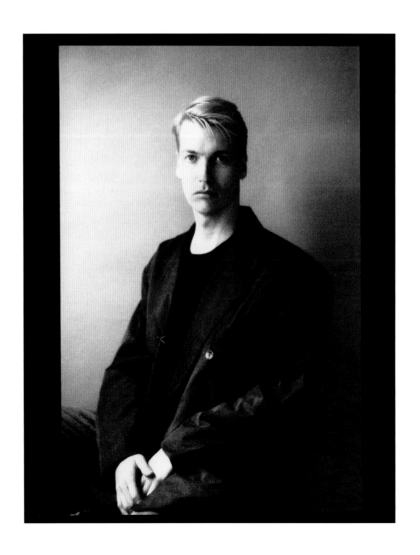

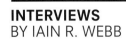

In conversation...

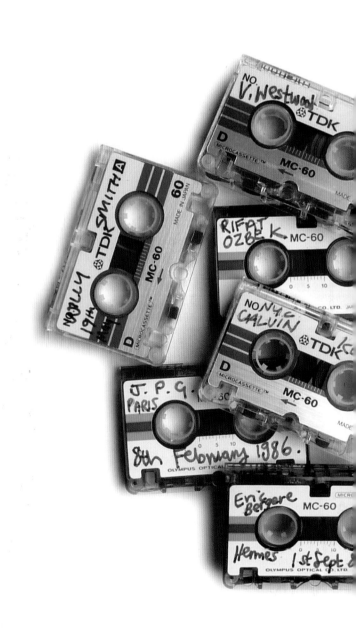

JUDY BLAME
TAKE THE BLAME!

Judy Blame... Judy Blame. That's all you ever hear in our house. Judy this, Judy that. It's one thing sharing your life with another person but something else again sharing your home with a fan of Judy Blame's over-sized jewellery.

"Bought another necklace today."

"Where are you going to put it?"

"Around my neck, dummy!"

"And then?"

"It can live in the spare bedroom."

Judy Blame's jewellery is BIG, but then so is its creator. Larger than life as they say...

———

How did you become Judy Blame? When I worked as a coat check boy in a nightclub I met Antony Price, and he nicknamed me Judy ... then I thought of Blame, and it just sounded like some trashy B-movie actress ... so it stuck ... I'm using it as a brand name. ——— **So it's a product?** Yeah. But it does get a bit confusing at times... ——— **So what should people call you? Chris or Judy?** Most people call me Judy Blame... both together... Antony still calls me Judy or Miss Blame. ——— **Do you call yourself a jewellery designer?** That's how I pinpoint what I do but there are lots of spin-offs from it... ——— **Are there any restrictions on what you would deem a piece of jewellery?** The more I've done it, the more the things have become garments as opposed to being just pieces of jewellery ... I'm just pushing jewellery design a bit further than most people do. ——— **Are people overpowered by it?** Yeah, most people; but it is different. ——— **How did you begin to use 'found objects' in your pieces?** Money! I stole the takings from 'Cha-Cha' (a nightclub he ran with model, Scarlett) and never went back. I thought, 'What the hell am I going to do?... so I showed Antony my ideas in a tiny little book of Polaroids I always carried... He was really pissing himself laughing between every picture, and I was getting more and more wound up, and then he closed the book and said, 'One day when I do a show, Judy you can do the jewellery' ... but it didn't happen for twelve months... ——— **Shall we look at your press cuttings?** (Opens book) Oh... *Tatler*. ——— **How did that happen?** I'm a very social person... I like to meet people. You know the phone goes and they just ask if I've got anything ... it's always worth following up leads because you never know what will happen ... I'm a great believer in fate! I wish I'd had one of those Hollywood mothers who PUSH their children... (turns page) Oooh, look! Antony Price... He's someone whose work I've followed ... people like Roxy Music... On the first show we did I just turned up and looked at the frocks and he told me which spaces I had to fill ... it wasn't fashion, it was show time! (turns page) Oh, this is my first bit of publicity, Judy's Jewels... God, look at those prices! ——— **How often is your jewellery presented the way you see it? Say if the *Sunday Times* does it?** I actually liked the pictures they did ... normally they don't use enough ... I know some pieces

are heavy and cumbersome, but you should just pile it on... ——— **How did New York react to Judy Blame?** They really looked after me ... it was ridiculous, I was staying there and staying there ... it's so fast you can get so much more done. ——— **Is it different to the reaction you get in London?** I believe the reaction I get in London... if someone doesn't like it they'll tell you...in America turning yourself into your image is part of their lifestyle, so every time I went out it went with me...They are all party people, so you never really meet anyone, it's all done on a kissing-on-the-cheek level. I can do that till the cows come home... (turns page) This is Judy Blame in his rubbish dump... my studio... Good haircut! That was really fun because this Japanese magazine asked me to pose with my head shaved, so someone did this huge prick and balls across my head... I arrived at the session wearing a hat, and when I took it off they were just like (fakes mouth agog) ... I mean, they shouldn't have asked me in the first place... ——— **Did they do the portrait?** They said it was 'too strong'... The times I've heard those two words strung together by the media. ——— **Is that a problem?** I think it's worked to my advantage ... I never went to college so I've built up through experimentation ... struggling away at it was my way of working it out, like going to college ... no grant, mind you! Now I'm ready to do whatever people want ... on my own terms. You know people think I'm pissy and stand off-ish... I'm not at all, but because my stuff was not readily available people had to come to me... (turns page) Oh look, Boy George at the Grammys. He just said, 'send over all your gold stuff' and I thought 'Oh, he'll choose a necklace', and he just put it all on... I thought I was over the top... Standing next to Joan Rivers it works really well... Next to Joan Rivers it just looks fabulous. ——— **On the subject of George, do you believe that those who hang on in there will come through so long as they believe in themselves enough?** Yeah, you have to believe in what you do. I did... I was on my own believing in it for a l-o-n-g time... It's very much about me. I do care what people think, but I don't let my ideas be dominated by anyone... ——— **So what's next for Judy Blame?** I'm doing New York with Susanne Bartsch and it's the first time I'm really attacking summer... Japan has been a great ambition of mine because I love what they do ... so to go to Tokyo will be a great treat... ——— **And personally?** I'm doing a lot of Rock'n'Roll work and obviously you're talking to a different business there so you clash with them a lot of the time ... but I'd like to do something like TV ... like *Doctor Who* ... ——— **Do you still get elated when you see someone wearing your jewellery?** I'm always surprised when someone does! ——— **What's you ultimate ambition Judy?** To have a Judy Blame ice cream company. 402 flavours. That's my ultimate passion in life, and that's why I have to go around the world – to investigate all the ice creams...

KATHARINE HAMNETT
HAMNETT

I can remember a T-shirt my older brother bought – at about the same time he decided to stick a psychedelic 'Mr Tambourine Man' poster on his bedroom wall. The T-shirt bore the slogan,'WHAT IF THEY HAD A WAR... AND NOBODY CAME?' As far as I can be sure, the design is not hers, but the dream is one most definitely shared by Katharine Hamnett. Over the last year nobody, but nobody, has been copied like KATHARINE has. Her sloganeering T-shirts have been worn by anyone who wants to wear their conscience on their chest...

———

Are you described in your passport as a designer? Is that how you see yourself? Yes I do... I don't see myself as a company director... I try to be a designer who is just surviving, and therefore has to run a company. ——— **Do you think you need just one label for yourself?** No. I think people are enormous, they're infinite ... they have everything. ——— **Then how do you relate to fashion? How do you perceive it?** It's a lot of things. It's very hard to talk about because it comes from an area of the mind which we are not educated to use in a way which we can see or touch, and yet we use it the whole time. It's unexplored like the New World. Jung talked about the collective unconscious and that's about the nearest we can get to it. It's a level we communicate at without words and without even being aware that we are speaking to each other ... it's like a subliminal level because we form our opinions of people absolutely on how they look ... we judge by looking at their clothes ... the relationship between the colour of their clothes and socks, even the fibre their socks are made of gives you enormous information about somebody... ——— **Do you think that to be able to read such signs comes naturally to everyone?** Yes, I think we all do it. Unfortunately European fashion has taken over the world, but people do it a lot more in Africa, Australia, all the Central American tribes. In these places people have their own personal message systems which are more sophisticated than ours... ——— **So do you think that it is not as specialised and elitist as people would have us believe?** I think it's universal... I think everybody has the same taste, and all the good people have good taste. I think there is only one good taste, but you don't have to be rich to have it. Poor English kids at sixteen have got more taste than anybody else in the whole of the West ... they express themselves in their clothes better than anyone ... they have tremendous fluency in the language ... the only trouble is we don't know how to commercialise on it ... at that level we're ignorant. ——— **What professional training have you had?** I went to college, but worked freelance as I didn't have enough grant to live on ... to answer your question, I learnt a hell of a lot of professional experience by kicking around in the industry. ——— **I understand that you did not receive the attention you deserved from the press because of the statements your T-shirts make?** Yes... ——— **Do you think that they were**

scared of the political statements you make? Shit scared... In this country they are shit scared... —— **Does it bother you?** Not at all. I sell them like shit... I can't make enough, and I've got people copying me all over the world. —— **Why did you put messages on your garments?** Because I'm so furious at what's going on ... not only in this country, but the whole world. Another reason is because I've been so copied, so I thought it would be nice to do a collection which would be wonderful to be copied. At the same time I was seething at things which were going wrong, things people were accepting through ignorance that are damaging the planet irrevocably... Nuclear radioactive water being dumped into the sea is horrific, and people say, 'Oh what can I do?', and I'm fed up... So I wanted to demonstrate what one person can do, although I realise I am in a very powerful situation. —— **So do you think that one person can change the world?** Yes, people have got to start using democracy and if they think something is wrong they should form pressure groups. I'm totally opposed to violence, and marching is stupid because they cordon off the marches and the media don't cover them because they think it's boring. You should contact your MP. If everyone did that we'd have some effect...The Parents Teachers Association [PTA] is wonderful because all they care about is their children, and this is when you get concerned... When you're young you tend to think, 'oh shit, if it goes up now I've had a good time', but once you have kids you think 'What about them?' I've got two boys ... this is when I've changed. When you become a mother to your own kids, you become a mother to them all... Anyway the PTAs are fab because they are spread across the world. If putting pressure on your MP doesn't work you ought to form rotor systems for telephoning organisations who you feel are contravening public safety, and just block their telephone lines. All you do is get people to dial the number, ring it, and when they pick up, disconnect... Right? And then you ring again ... and that way, POW! —— **Do you think people perceive that there is more to Katharine Hamnett than simply slogans on shirts?** Yeah sure. I'm a combination of a threat and a Fortnum's hamper. They think I'm mad ... don't understand me at all, but they understand that my clothes sell better than anybody else's... —— **I read a piece a while ago in one of the Sunday supplements which said that you had the trendiest accessory of the season, which was a Rastafarian boyfriend... How do you feel being in a business with such clueless and tactless people?** I laughed because it was totally wrong, but I also thought it was a disgusting thing to say about a human being, and I thought the girl who wrote it was really stupid to use such a phrase, and not to check her facts ... but you get used to it ... the whole of the West is stupid ... what worries me is that we've got our values all wrong, and we're being conditioned from infancy to believe in things which are worthless and not respect things which are of enormous value ... that scares the shit out of me...
—— **Were the T-shirts your way of proving your responsibility to the world?** Well, I don't really want to get involved, but I don't see any alternative...—— **You've got the chance to do it?** Yeah, to have a chance like that and not take it... I just couldn't respect myself ... and the Downing Street thing was a good laugh, and let's have some more... It's a bit like streaking, but it's not as silly. —— **Do you think your designs have a relevance to today's youth?**

Yes. One of the basic things I put into them is quality fabric ... they're made well, good cut, flattering to most people's figures. There is real utility in them... they're functional. They're easy to look after, and last a long time. —— **Do you hope they are timeless?** I aim to design things which are fairly classic... I look at it emotionally, but also very clinically ... it's got to work on several different levels. —— **Do you like the idea of people buying your clothes and putting them with somebody else's?** Oh God yes, it's ingredients you're offering... I think it's essential that the public do that... —— **Describe your lifestyle now.** It's not what people imagine … it's certainly different from anybody else's. —— **Because you have a family?** Having a family I try to be as unobtrusive as possible when I'm not working... I think that's good because as soon as you become successful, people think you are useful to them ... either frightening or desirable. The first thing they try and do is prove you are a wanker, and you have to put up with this completely unnecessary shit. I travel a lot, and I've got a house. —— **What are your loves?** My loves? My kids. My family. Life, laughter ... everything ... I love learning, pleasure, nature, artefacts. Everything apart from things that are horrible. —— **What is your ultimate aim?** Professionally, I'd like the company to become more creative. In my own life I'd like to have more time to do things which I wouldn't have to sell... I think that's a horrible problem for creative people, because you love everything you do for fun, but in the end you hate the thing you started doing because you're not earning enough money from it... —— **Do you think as your company grows you'll be able to remain in total control?** The only way that it works is because it's planned well. I'm interested in the autonomous control system ... it's really quite easy to sit down and write a concept, and then you can leave it to itself. My ambition as a kid was to have a machine that you put designs down one chute, and have money coming out of the other ... closer and closer.

BLITZ #32
June 1985

STEPHEN LINARD
THE RELUCTANT EMIGRÉ

In 1981 Stephen Linard was St Martin's School of Art's most celebrated graduate, the first established 'New Romantic' fashion designer, whose Reluctant Emigré collection and graduation show made his name in both London and New York.

A year and a half later, in February 1983, he was previewing a large and very adventurous new collection, Angels With Dirty Faces, based on three different themes – Gangsters and Molls, male and female convicts, Cowboys and Tomboys. In the end the collection was never produced. Linard's company went out of business, and despite his reputation he couldn't get it started again.

His new collection, Beyond Stephen Linard, is his first in this country for two years. In the meantime he has been working as a designer for the Japanese Jun Company, designing women's thirties-style eveningwear as 'Stephen Linard for George Sand'.

Stephen Linard is timid when it comes to talking about the past. He says he wants to be represented by what he will do, not by what he's already done.

It must be remembered nevertheless that it was Linard who was responsible for grown men wearing Nancy's shirts, for pinstripe prima donnas, and for that religious look that has hung round our necks like so many crucifixes for the last four years. Linard has long since confessed, accepted and swallowed his penance of two half lagers and three Bloody Marys...

Although he's been quiet of late, he's now fronting the appropriately titled club Total Fashion Victim at the Wag, and there are few who do not expect to hear plenty of ranting and much raving soon...

——

When you left St Martin's you were surrounded by publicity. How beneficial was that to your career? At the time it was good fun, and it was a good thing ... it's kept me going over the past four years ... people have still heard of my name. Six months after the show it was quite bad because I was a very well known designer but I didn't have anything to show for it. I had no money but loads of press cuttings... —— **Why do you think you've been ignored recently?** For the past two years there was just nothing available. While I worked in Japan I wasn't working here at all ... until Bazaar suggested that I do a freelance collection for them... —— **Your designs tend toward the classic lines. Is it your intention to create timeless clothes?** The clothes I design – even those from four years ago – can still be worn today... I don't want to design fads or fashions. It's very stylistic – there is a certain lifestyle behind it... —— **Do you think that, because the clothes are so refined, it makes it easier for the press to overlook them in favour of more quirky and off-beat numbers?** Probably, especially at the moment when London's got the reputation for wild, craazzeee things, but I think that the discerning eye does realise that my clothes exist above the street fashion level... —— **Does it worry you whether you're particularly 'In' or 'Out', or top of the pops in the fashion world?** Well it's nice to be 'In' ... it's nice to be 'In' all the time. It just worries me when I don't get invited to parties and things, and when I don't get invited to 10 Downing Street with everyone else... —— **You've had problems with companies and contracts. Does that business side of fashion depress you?** The business side of fashion is a little shady, and there are some nasty people involved, but once you understand that, you have to accept it and live with it. You can't really change it. —— **There were rumours that you earned vast amounts of money in Japan, and then squandered it on Lagerfeld's 'tap' and 'spanner' jewellery. Is that true?** It was large amounts, I suppose compared to what I was earning ... and yeah, I did squander it, but that's because I hadn't had any money for years and when I got this wad of money in an envelope I just decided to go to Paris and blow it all ... which I did. —— **Do you regret that now?** Yeah, of course ... but money's there for spending ... I don't really use it as a cushion... —— **It seems strange that you can be treated like a star in another country yet can't pay the phone bill at home...** Well that was mostly irresponsibility on my part... I don't do it as badly now as I did. —— **What was it like in Tokyo? How were you treated?** It was brilliant, I was treated to a limousine, and a driver, and five star hotels with expense accounts. It was all quite glamorous, like a designer on a catwalk and a bunch of flowers at the end of it kind of thing... —— **Whose work do you admire yourself?** At the moment I think Eric Bergère, who designs for Hermès, is good because he's very witty and expensive, and totally unobtainable, and Andre Walker ... Leigh Bowery because he's got so much front, and gets away with it... I like Bodymap because they've come through all the press and are actually making money, and they've got a good company going... —— **Who influences you?** Lots of Edwardian pattern-cutting books, and films. At the moment I'm trying not to be influenced by Andy Warhol and Edie Sedgwick... —— **Who are you aiming your clothes at?** I think the discerning 20 to 30 year old with a bit of money to spend. I mean, my clothes aren't expensive, no more than Yohji or Gaultier ... they're just good time clothes. Not street clothes, but more restaurant, brasserie, disco clothes! —— **Worn by anybody?** It surprises me the kind of people who do buy them. From Rockabilly boys who buy a shirt, to pop stars who wear the whole outfits ... people like Peter Stringfellow buying a whole outfit. I was quite surprised. —— **A lot of your work, particularly the early designs, has been quasi-religious, seemingly influenced by Judaism and religious imagery. What is your fascination with religion?** Because it's so elaborate and over the top. It was very tongue-in-cheek. At the time I was living in that big Victorian squat, surrounded by candlesticks and religious paraphernalia. I got given a big black coat and the whole look revolved around that, and then a homburg... —— **The St Martin's show had the models wearing halos and carrying crucifixes...** Yeah, it was just... I don't know really what possessed me to design it really ... probably because I started dressing as a Catholic-Rabbi-Greek-Orthodox-priest, and the collection sort of grew around that. Then that club called Hell started and everyone began wearing religious things...

—— **What is the most essential quality in a designer?** To be aware of what people want and not to be impose your own personality on them. For instance, I wouldn't dream of designing a collection based around the more wild outfits I wear ... oh yeah, and not fiddling people. Giving them good quality, good material, good value for money, good cut, and something that will last... —— **Tell me about the show you had in photographer Perry Ogden's studio.** That was the collection that received the most press – it was the floral bias cut dresses, and floral shirts for men ... lots of bag suits... —— **Was there a theme?** *Badlands* with Sissy Spacek. The dresses were meant as Parisian rip-offs that the department stores in the mid-west sold; and there was the convict collection. The whole thing had a thirties feeling, but that never got produced because the company fell apart straight after that ... the worst six months of my life... —— **Is that double-think important? Do you like the clothes to be intelligent?** You can start off like that, but I don't think you can really expect the people to whom you are selling the clothes ever to worry about the idea behind them so long as they look nice. They're not going to think, 'Oh yeah, this is like Sissy Spacek in *Badlands*', or 'It's meant to be like a rip-off of a Paris original' ... it's a bit naïve to think that people are interested in that. Maybe the real fashion aficionados are interested, but I don't think the people who buy clothes are... —— **What do you design most successfully?** I think the most successful thing I've designed was the organza man's evening shirt from my degree collection in 1981, which is kind of quite popular at the moment. The ubiquitous organza shirt. —— **What do you feel is your contribution to fashion?** I think I did make people look at menswear in a different light ... and I think I was the first to use organza for making men's shirts ... in the Eighties... —— **Tell me about your up and coming show. What will the collection be like?** Summer '86. It's my comeback collection, and is going to be the biggest thing I've ever done ... very expensive men's and ladies' wear, because Bazaar are opening a ladies shop in London ... and also the sequinned and beaded collection. It will be a continuation of everything that I've done previously... —— **You always dress in very complete looks. Do you see yourself as a complete person?** The looks I put together are more my sense of humour than anything. I'm quite happy to go out in jeans and a T-shirt, or full Theda Bara drag. It's what I feel like that day, or whatever happens to be clean... I like to wear something completely different all the time because its funny if people don't recognise you because you've got a wig on, or put different make-up on ... it's just amusing for oneself... —— **So finally, are you a total fashion victim, Stephen?** I'd say most definitely yes! I can't help it. The only thing which Lydia Kemeny (Head of Fashion at St Martin's School of Art) ever said to me which I thought had any significance was that if you're going to be a designer you've got to live, breathe and eat fashion... I think that was the only thing I learned at St Martin's really... —— **And that's what you're doing now?** Yes... breathing and eating it.

BLITZ #36
November 1985

RIFAT OZBEK
IN CONVERSATION

Rifat Ozbek is an arbiter of style, and has the lucky fortune to be blessed with EXQUISITE taste. In an incomplete design studio, he lolled playfully on an overlarge settee, hidden from view by dust covers made of deepest red velvet, as we talked of things he cared about, and of others he could not care less for ... He is witty; charming company to be with; and is the possessor of an apparently unconcerned attitude which allows him the appearance of being 'all style and no content'. The content IS there ... and here for you to read.

——

Your background. You attended St Martin's... Yeah I went to St Martin's to study fashion, but originally came from Turkey ... Istanbul ... to study architecture, but realised it wasn't for me because I couldn't do all the technical part of it. I mean, I could do a fabulous building, but it wouldn't stand up. I met some friends who were into fashion, so I thought, 'I'll get into fashion'. I showed Muriel Pemberton (Head of St Martin's at the time) about fourteen sketches and she immediately accepted me. —— **Did you enjoy it there?** Loved it. The best years of my life. —— **Why do you think its so successful?** I think because it was so free. We were there just to design clothes, you just did whatever your fantasies were. —— **Is that what you're still doing now?** Yes, but they have to be more wearable now. Yeah, I think clothes have to be or there's no point. —— **Were you always into clothes?** Oh yeah. I was the dressiest architect student in school. All the other guys wore corduroy pants and big sloppy sweaters. —— **What did you wear?** What did I wear? That was the time of Glam Rock – all that Bowie, Aladdin Sane, Ziggy Stardust stuff. —— **Tinsel?** Tinsel stuff. Beyond! Glitter, tinsel, maquillage for days (laughs). —— **Who do you admire?** Designer wise... I don't like many of the living ones (laughs). I like Azzedine Alaïa. I like Saint Laurent. I like Karl Lagerfeld. —— **Are there no British designers you actually like?** Mmmmmm... not really. —— **Even though your designs are crisp and curt, you yourself are very eccentric. Why don't your clothes echo that?** I don't think just because I'm eccentric in my own lifestyle it has to reflect into my clothes. I like dressing things up, but I also love to be able to dress down into nothing as well. I can design a very simple dress but then put really eccentric fabric or jewels on it, and make it look eccentric. —— **So you have the choice...** Yeah, exactly, rather that giving them something they can't get rid of. —— **How did it feel when you dressed up as Diana Vreeland for *The Tatler*?** It felt great, I loved every minute of it. I was paranoid in case it didn't come off, but it did. It took Barbara Daley about four hours to put the make-up on. David Bailey couldn't believe it when I came down the stairs, he was screaming, 'Diana! Diana! She's here, she's arrived!' —— **What about the poses? Did they come naturally to you?** Very naturally (laughs). —— **Do you live in luxury?** Luxury? No not at all. I live in a friend's house in a little room, but I'm going to get my own flat soon.

—— Do you think the women who buy your clothes live in luxury? I guess so. You have to be rich to be able to afford them, and when you're rich you live in luxurious surroundings ... yeah. **Were you immediately successful when you left college?** Yeah, people wrote about me. I really don't know what success is. It must be different from the outside than how one sees oneself. It doesn't really mean anything. —— **But you enjoy the attention?** No. I don't like getting too much attention, and I'm very shy actually. I realise to further my career I have to do interviews and have my photograph taken, but if I could, I'd do without it, because I'm not very relaxed in this kind of situation. —— **Would you be worried if somebody suddenly picked you as the Next Big Thing?** I don't think I'd let people do that to me. I don't think that sort of thing happens here anyway like it does in America. I wouldn't want to be a commodity. My collections are very small, they're very personal. My first under my own label had eighteen styles. Last season I had twenty three, and this season I'm going to have about thirty. It's growing gradually. —— **You're not going to have a show this time?** No. Unless I could have a catwalk as long as a runway at Heathrow and two thousand models on it I'm not interested. —— **Not even a showroom show?** No. I have two girls I think are right for the look each season, so they come and prance around the room showing the collection to buyers and press. That's it really. I don't have a big numero. —— **Do your friends wear your clothes?** My friends can't afford to buy them. —— **Don't you sell them to them cheap, or give them away?** I wish I could. Yeah, I've given a few as presents, and of course I do give them wholesale prices. —— **Are you affected by criticism?** Yeah, it's natural that bad things in the press upset you. —— **Would you let it affect your work?** No, I know what I like doing, and there are people who like it. —— **Do you think that the inner being of Rifat Ozbek is represented successfully exteriorally?** What does that mean? —— **Do you think others see you as you see yourself? Do you get the reaction you want?** Oh dear ... but how would I know that ... yes, yes, I do. Actually I'm a bit of an open book ... how difficult is this question by the way? —— **Your future. What do you hope for?** Immediately what do I want? Happiness. —— **And for the next few years?** I don't think of things like that. I live from day to day. I don't plan the future, I don't say this is my aim in ten years' time. At the end I'd like a nice place by the seaside. —— **A suitable ending...** Yeah, How fab. Thanks, readers!

BLITZ #37
Dec/Jan 1985/1986

·····························

ERIC BERGÈRE
FRENCH DRESSING

Designer labels come dear, but none more so than those which bear the HERMÉS label. It is a combination of rare quality, superb fabrics and luxurious opulence that keep the prices high. Way high, but if your credit rating holds up, you too may share some golden moments wrapped up in a python's skin, or the minkiest of sweatshirts. The man responsible for putting you in them is Frenchman Eric Bergère. Eric smiles coyly, while his designs wear permanent grins. They are both, at present, being worn out by insatiable fashion editors and inscrutable fans. At twenty-four years old Eric Bergère is Le Chien Surtout (TOP DOG) in Trend City...

——

Has your success, especially with the trendy young crowd, been a surprise to you? Oh yes, of course. I was very proud, but I do not understand very well why it has happened. In Paris nobody thinks the same. —— **How do they react in Paris to what you're doing?** I get compliments from Jean Paul Gaultier when I see him, but that's the only one I know about. The other people don't speak to me about my work... —— **What do the fashion press make of you?** The fashion press in Paris don't notice me at all at Hermès ... ever. —— **When I was in Florence recently all the young people had Hermès headscarves around their necks. Does that please you?** Oh yes, it's wonderful ... I think that Hermès is now a fashion, is in fashion. I think it's easier now to work for Hermès than it was five years ago when I began. —— **Was your aim when you went there to make Hermès fashionable?** To make fashion not too boring for the Hermès customer. When I arrived it was a little bit... old. Old customers and too serious, too conventional. —— **So how have you tried to change this?** Not a lot, but just by putting a little bit of humour into the designs, and using bright colours... —— **Will you continue to take it further and further from the traditional image?** Yes. It takes a long time, nine or ten collections. But it couldn't be another way because Hermès has a lot of customers, and they must not be shocked or provoked too much. They must understand little by little. —— **Do the clothes still have to sell to the original customer – more traditional women – or are you trying to find a new, younger market?** We try to have different lines in the collection which sell to different women. We try to have things for young girls, but the prices are rather ... expensive. It's possible to buy one thing to wear, but to be dressed in it all is very expensive. We do sweatshirts in cotton, ties with the Hermès print on it, which are not very expensive. —— **Would you like to do more things that could be bought by younger people?** Of course, because when you go to Japan and other countries you see Hermès prints on other cheaper synthetic materials. It's a problem. We try to do Hermès for the young on natural fabric but at a low price. —— **You apprenticed to Thierry Mugler. How was that?** It was only for a short time, but great experience. I suppose he's the only one who has such

enthusiasm, and the best philosophy in fashion. —— **How does working for someone like him differ from working at Hermès?** It's two worlds ... I was lucky to get the job with Hermès with my style, because it is difficult to get the chance to do anything different with them. —— **Is it a challenge?** Yes, I think so. Thierry Mugler, not enough for me... —— **Because you could do what you wanted?** He knows what he wants and all he wants is done because he has a lot of people around him, and he has one idea every minute. He does it all. For me, he is a real creator. —— **Which other designers do you admire?** In Paris not so many... —— **Where?** I like the work of Americans, like Anne Klein. Very simple clothes, very elegant. When you go to New York you see women who are elegant and it's wonderful to present shows and make clothes which are so wearable ... in the road ... out; maybe because American women are often very tall, and wear just big gold jewellery, flat shoes, a little sportif ... a little bit Katharine Hepburn... —— **What do you think of London fashion?** I suppose all the world copies London for fashion. I go to Tokyo, and all the little Japanese are like people in London. It's incredible, even the States copy. I suppose it's the same for music and art. I feel that it all begins in London and after that the world commercialises on it. But London doesn't make a profit – with all your ideas you could have a lot of money. My feeling is that the others – Italians, Japanese – make money from London. —— **Anyone specific whose clothes you like?** I like Jasper Conran because it's a little bit similar to what I do at Hermès, maybe. But I always like the new ones. Bodymap are a very important influence in the world now. —— **Would you like to design things as extreme?** Oh, it's difficult for me to do it. Maybe it's possible in another life. In another place. In Paris it's very difficult. You don't have the desire to do it because in Paris you have no places where you can dress in extreme ... just for evening, maybe. —— **Is there not a great chance for young people in Paris who want to design?** I suppose that if you want something so badly, you can have it. You are willing to do what you must do to get it. It's not a problem, I suppose, because if you truly want to work in fashion you don't suddenly decide that you want it at eighteen, but when you are five years old... —— **So you always have it inside you?** Yes ... and you design all your life. When I went to art school everyone around me had waited eighteen years to draw their first sketch. It's natural that I have something more because I had designed for years before. —— **Tell me about your home. Do you live in Paris?** Yes, it's not very stylish. I have no furniture. All is very yellow, and I play a little piano, so I have a piano, a bed. Not so much furniture. I live out of my home a big part of the day. I am looking for a place with a garden, but it's very difficult. That is the only thing I would like to have ... or a terrace. —— **Are you always working?** No, not always. In fact I can't design in my studio now, because you have people who come to ask you questions, you have phone calls, and you can only design at the weekend. —— **Are you always seeing things which inspire you?** I see a lot of TV. I have a TV in my apartment and it is very important for everything, because you can't design now without the world, I think. It is important to feel the world, and what people desire. TV is a great instrument for that. —— **How else do you relax?** I go to the cinema. I walk across gardens, and I like very much to go to the sea. I love the sound of the sea to design to after the week in Paris – it's very noisy, it's dreadful. I don't go out nightclubbing too much, not too much, just a little bit ... but in Paris I don't think it's very important for fashion to go nightclubbing. —— **Would you like your clothes to be timeless?** Oh yes, but I know it's not possible, because you have to change your designs every six months and if you change just a little bit it's not enough for customers. You must change colour. It's the women's taste, I suppose. Women like to change a lot, and like to have different silhouettes. Even if everybody says fashion doesn't move, it's not the truth. Customers want you to change things always. —— **Is making those changes difficult for you?** No. It was difficult five years ago, because when I arrived at Hermès I said, 'I do one coat, I do one blouse, one pair of pants, and no more. In grey, in navy blue, in black, ok? Everyone looked at me and said 'He's crazy, you can't sell it, it's not Hermès', but I said 'It's Hermès to have the best quality in fabric.' It's not enough. You must give more. You must give colours, luxury, something more feminine, more seductive. —— **Would you like to live anywhere else in the world?** Oh, I'd like to live in London. I regret the fact that, seven years ago, I had the choice to go to St Martin's college for a year. But I had the proposition of Hermès at the same time, so I had to choose. St Martin's or Hermès? —— **I think you chose wisely.** I don't know. —— **Have you always been very stylish, and considered the way you look?** Not too much, because, I suppose, for the people who work in fashion, fashion must not be of too much importance for their life. Today I wear a suit and tie, but my preferred clothes are the clothes of the church. Mono colour. Very simple. Like someone who wants to be a pastor. Very straight. —— **Anyone who you'd like to wear your clothes?** I suppose today it's very important for a singer to wear them, because video is the best advertisement for designers. It travels all around the world, even to people who don't know who Thierry Mugler or Jean Paul Gaultier is. It's very important. —— **You** mentioned that Jean Paul Gaultier liked your clothes... I suppose he likes them. I don't know exactly, but when I see him he's very happy to speak about the collection. —— **What do you think of what he's designing?** It's very elegant. Before, it was a bit too much, but this last season it was very elegant and very rich. I went to see the ballet he designed the costumes for, at the Pavillion, and all the people there, even thirty- or forty-year-olds, looked very elegant. It's very important, I think, to see customers wear and wear well. —— **Are you happy when you see people wearing your clothes?** Yes, I am very happy because in Paris, even if customers are very old, they are always elegant. I never get a bad surprise. I don't see someone every day (laughs) but when I do, I never get a bad surprise, no. —— **Do you think you'll always be a designer?** I don't know. I hope so, because it's very interesting and it's a wonderful life, more than a lot of other kinds of work. I hope so. —— **Is there anything else you would like to do?** No ... I don't know what!

BLITZ #39
March 1986

MARK & SYRIE
IN CONVERSATION

For once Iain R. Webb is speechless, as Mark Lascelles (one half of Carnaby Street couturiers Mark and Syrie) talks and talks and talks and...

——

Mark and Syrie. We've become established, which is good, but the majority of the press don't know what we're about at all. They think of us as tea towels and carpet and gimmickry and that's it... —— **The beginning.** The very first dress we made was eighteen months ago. The old floral curtain. The Sanderson print – before Crolla. We were selling in the street and Ursula Hudson of *Predictions* magazine bought a pair of our trousers. We were selling outside Covent Garden tube and kept getting moved on by the police. Browns bought that very first dress. —— **Workmen and Cats.** I did very figure-hugging lurex dresses with wet-suit zips up the back. We saw Sarah Jane Hoare (Fashion Editor at *The Observer*) even though we didn't know who she was. She said, 'How do you know about these things? How are you getting it right? Do you know about Stephen Sprouse?' and I said ' No.' She tried endlessly to get it into her newspaper. —— **The Fashion Business.** I thought this would be the business where you could come from anywhere, but I found it so established. So serious and so straight and heavy about everything! —— **Fabrics.** Materials are terrible. You're talking about £40 a metre. I went to a place and said I wanted to do a print of London and they said it would cost at least £28 a metre. Now if I made that up, I mean, who could afford it? I've always tried to do fashion which is affordable. On the rail at £15. I used the tea towel because it was a serious way of using another good quality fabric. It was the same way I used the carpet. But all the press saw it as sixties. I mean, Elizabeth Smith (Fashion Editor of *The Standard*) came in and just put the whole thing down. 'You're a skinhead aren't you," she says to me. 'I smell skinhead.' —— **Selling souvenirs.** The souvenir thing was when people found out about us – and I found out about the Individual Clothes Show. I phoned Joanne Davis (the organiser of Olympia Fashion Week), and asked for a square metre of space as I wanted to build Nelson's Column and put a girl on top of it... She told me to phone Lesley Goring, who was brilliant, and put us in the show. We just got together a few pieces. A long black velvet thing which was the policeman; a carpet Crombie; the donkey jacket; houndstooth leggings, a whole outfit out of headscarves; a gold sari; little beefeater punk skirts; and the Union Jack outfit. We got applause, and Vivienne Westwood said we were the best. The very first time, we took £35,000 worth of orders. —— **Baby Blues.** Then we did the 'BABA' collection, the frilly baby look. Then Gaultier does the same, so did Vivienne Westwood, who also did the Union Jack look. —— **Showing at the swimming pool.** I wanted to do the show near water. We didn't want a massive show. Unlike someone like Gaultier who will show 150 outfits, and only one is available in the shops, I'd rather do a smaller collection and sell it all.

—— **The beer towel jacket.** People hated it. They thought it was tacky. But if you look at beer towels, the fabric is woven, not printed. It's really good towelling. If you try and join beer mats together, as with tea towels, or carpet, it's harder than just using a length of fabric. It's the punk side of my personality, and it's taking these things and making them really good, well made and wearable. It's telling others you can make this too... —— **Mark and Syrie (again).** The conception and the philosophy behind it is me, and all the immaculate conception is me and her. —— **What' stylish.** What kind of things do I find stylish? I think anything in life has a pure version. —— **Mark.** I don't see myself as a designer, I see myself as someone who makes clothes. We've had our stuff in Country Life, we've had it in *BLITZ* and *i-D*. We've got skinhead girls and boys wearing the stuff to Oi! parties, and I've got young royals wearing the same things. That's a real achievement. There are people who HATE it, and people who love it. That's good. —— **Fashion.** It's sad when people get too into the fashion, because it's just clothes, and you can buy them and wear them and look good in them. —— **Gimmicks.** We're not gimmick designers. We're serious. Across the media the sad thing is that very few people are actually doing what they want. People aren't really allowed to do what they want, so you can't really say we're being represented. I think Bodymap aren't even accepted by some people. I'll be doing a magazine soon with no restrictions and I don't think it has to be militant. Also a shop somewhere like Regent Street, for everybody. If a person comes along and they're good, they'll go in and they'll go in the window. —— **The business.** It's getting to the point where it really kills you, and you might as well forget it, but I want to see a bigger support for people. I was unemployed and I got up and did something, and I want to show other people they can too. I mean, I wrote to Mrs Thatcher and she wrote back telling me to speak to some other bloke, so I said, 'if I write to the Gas Board, I don't expect the Electricity Board to answer.' I go lecturing at college and the first thing I say is GET OUT! The students do all these looks. They do my look. Galliano's look (which is Vivienne's anyway). I set them a project and I said, 'Go and design something you would want to wear, make something you like.' And they make these really good clothes. So I said, 'Why don't you take that around some places and sell a few?'

JEAN PAUL GAULTIER
JPG

In an early 'definitive' article about Jean Paul Gaultier it was claimed that 1983 was definitely his year. Since then though, 1984, 1985, and possibly even already 1986 have also been under his control, full to brimming with Gaultier-isms. Even the laced contoured constrictions of the new 'Prince of Paris', Azzedine Alaïa, hark back to the severe lacing that Gaultier forced down the backs of women who wore his original elongated corset dress.

Gaultier is influential. His images are that tiny bit sacrilegious, his cut that little bit better, his visions always quite literally breath-taking – enough to wind any fashion editor who has braved the scrum to get to into one of his shows, as his fantasies wing their way down the runways. Backless t-shirts; cutaway jackets with less pattern pieces than space between, riots of print; the pointiest tits in Paris; curlicue cigarette holders; burlesque brassieres; insanely be-skirted men's pants; beautifully besuited women ... and so much more.

Gaultier is hard to tackle. Physically and aesthetically. Over a weekend in Paris I met with the man who is for some the Prince, while making others paupers (his clothes cost a fortune...).

Accessible, hugely likeable, very funny, he is all the things that I had not expected, and one that I had: brilliant. That I had suspected already.

——

Tell me about working with Patou. I was a lot younger then. It was 1974. But it wasn't as much fun as working for Pierre Cardin, and I was a little disappointed. At Cardin, everything was possible. Almost. At Patou it was much more conservative, and the big boss was a very old, strict man. He used to tell me things like 'Don't use negro models in your shows, because the American buyers don't like it.' That kind of thing. I was very shocked. They used old models and old stereotypes, and it could sometimes be funny. But there was conflict, they were narrow-minded. I would be wearing cavalier boots, and they'd say, 'Why are you wearing those? Do you ride horses?' Always like that. Confrontation. I stayed for two years, and then left. I couldn't work at a place where nothing was possible, where I couldn't make what I wanted to. —— **Did you set up your own label as soon as you left?** No, I went to the Philippines and worked for Cardin again for a lower price collection aimed at the States. I had a heart attack, it was so difficult. Then I came back to Paris. —— **How young were you when you began to design?** Since I was twelve. My grandmother was a faith healer and I would sketch her customers, dressing them like stars, like Marilyn Monroe. And then I made my first collection at fourteen, telling everyone that it was a very Parisian collection. Very beautiful, very successful, you know? I used to tell people that there was a marvellous new perfume as well – I'd look at the newspapers and that's what they said about the designers, and so I did the same. Before my eighteenth birthday I'd sent all sketches of my collections – I was making 350 sketches for each – to all the couturiers, and then had the first answer on my birthday, April 24th 1970. Monsieur Cardin told me to come to his house and work with him. —— **Were you a stylish child?** You mean in what I wore? No. From when I was a small child the only thing I liked was my anorak – blue with white fur around the hood. Oh, and also short trousers. I thought I had nice legs and I liked showing them off! I also loved my first communion. I had to wear like a priest's robe, all in white. I loved that. It was my first dress! Afterwards it wasn't so important how I looked. I preferred worrying about my work, so I would buy from the flea market and places like that. —— **Have your designs always been off-beat?** When I was with Cardin I was influenced by Cardin, Saint Laurent, Courrèges. After that, when I started on my own, it was in the same mood as Castelbajac. Then these people began to influence me less and less, and my ideas came more from the street. —— **When were you first taken seriously as a designer?** Not quickly. My first collection was in 1976, and people thought it was too jokey. Not until 1980 or 1981, I think, about five years. —— **Is it difficult to break through Paris?** Well, what I like about London is that the young sell their designs in the markets, but it's not so in Paris. Always in Paris the young want to try and prove how professional they are, they want to start with a big showroom and everything. When I began, I certainly didn't tell anyone that I had no money. Quite the contrary – otherwise I would have not been taken seriously. It's perhaps better in London with places like the Great Gear Market in the King's Road, where the designers are mixed with things from India. I think that's great. —— **I saw you getting your haircut when you were over here last.** In the Gear Market? Yes, always. Unfortunately I'm not in London enough, so I'm obliged to get my hair cut in Paris. You can see that it's not as good. In London the colour and the cut is perfect. There is only one place that is good in Paris, Rock Hair in Les Halles. It is good, but not as good as in London. —— **I spoke to a French photographer recently who said you were treated like the Pope here. How do you take this kind of deification from the Parisian press?** The Pope? Can you imagine how old that makes me sound? That's horrible. They don't really treat me like a Pope. —— **How are you treated then?** It depends. Le Figaro and newspapers and magazines like that don't like me, others have liked me from the very beginning. —— **In London you're adored by both the trendy magazines and the likes of *Vogue* and *Harper's*.** I'm very glad. I'm pleased that it's both sorts. In England the magazines have a wider mixture of the extreme and extravagant with the classical. In France, magazines are either one way or the other, much more restrictive. —— **Did Punk affect you?** Of course. But it was very funny here. It was fashionable not sociological. We did not have real punk. But it influenced me a lot and changed my thinking, not just superficially like with black and safety-pins. —— **What do you think of Vivienne Westwood?** I love her, I have great admiration for her. She has been very influential. I admire a lot of British designers. I love Jean Muir. I like also Galliano, Bodymap... In France I like Mugler and Alaïa. Also Yohji Yamamoto and Comme des Carçons. —— **You said that the street inspired you when you began. Is that still the case?** Yes, but not the same way as before. It's also the way people behave, movies, music, everything. I am very visual, I take in all these images and mix them up and then the ideas come out. —— **You've cut away your outfits to reveal most parts of the body – armpits, stomachs, bottoms... Which bit do you find most appealing?** To be honest, I should say the face. After that, I don't know, it depends. If someone has nice legs, it's nice to show them; the same with the stomach. But I don't prefer. You can have a nice face with a very ugly ass, you know... Or vice versa. —— **French *Elle* described your designs as futuristic.** Not at all. I can't tell you what will happen in the future, I just care about now. I am obliged to work six months in advance on my collection, and in the meantime I might meet someone or go somewhere that will change my ideas, so that the final result is only part of the original. How can I tell what will happen in ten or twenty years? I think futuristic is wrong. —— **Are you very business-like?** Definitely, I have to be, or I die. Sometimes I make advance cuts of ideas because I think that they might be too much. But then I come to London and see people wearing what they want, and I realise that I must do what I want as well... But then I'm not always in London. I also sometimes work with Italians, and they are so chic. They say 'But your fabrics aren't silk...' and I say 'Yes, yes, but there are other fabrics.' It makes me depressed sometimes. But then from depression you can get energy. —— **Your shows have been described as over-indulgent.** Not exactly. People find them extreme, but they are not as much as they used to be. For example, four years ago I had a coffin at the end of the catwalk, and a vampire climbed out of it. She had scarlet nails, and smeared the colour onto the models. People were frightened because it was about death, but I think that they would love it in London. I did it because I thought it was funny, and because I love horror films. —— **What's the purpose of your shows?** It's very important. The clothes are made to worn, I don't design them to be in a museum as if dead. The show can demonstrate a way of moving. For example, the boys and girls of today don't walk the same as they used to twenty years ago, so it has to be shown. They have different attitudes, and music reflects an ambience. I like the idea of the show in general – the day I stop doing shows is the day I stop designing. —— **Do you have any particular favourite out of all the things you've designed?** No. Well maybe the corset dress because it comes from my young days. I opened my grandmother's wardrobe and found this corset, all pink, with lacing, and thought of making a long dress for evening out of it. Maybe that, but otherwise I love them all, or hate them all, equally. —— **Does it make it difficult to know that everyone is waiting to see what you'll do next?** To tell the truth, it was easier at the beginning. Because I was not successful I was more spontaneous, I did whatever I felt like. I remember a collection I did in 1978, I think, just before ska, when I didn't have any money for accessories, but I wanted black and white glasses. I went to London, but all the markets only had fifties, not sixties glasses, so in the end I made them out of linoleum ... in that position you find more ideas because you have to think more to get what you want. Now I try to make every show different, not just the designs but also the presentation. Sometimes I have a singer, or some strip-tease artists, and then another show might be very straightforward. I never think, 'Oh, yes, people like me for this, so I'll do more of it'. —— **How do you react to people who say you've lost your**

crown to Azzedine Alaïa? I don't care, because I never felt that I had a crown. I love what he is doing. It is very different, nice and interesting. So very different from me as well. It is nice that he is recognised, there's no problem for me at all. —— How does it feel to be described still as an enfant terrible? The enfant terrible is getting very old now, so I don't think it's very relevant now. It's just a term used by people who don't really understand what I do... —— How do you describe yourself? That is difficult. I think I am not very interested in myself, as my job is to see to other people. So I don't know. I think I am a little open... —— The people who wear your clothes always look very trendy, but how do you view them? I feel bad if they are too trendy rich people, because I would like people with less money to wear them. But sometimes people can put together their own Gaultier look from buying at a market. They can take a fox fur from their mother, and put it around their neck and have the Gaultier look. —— So you think that you have influenced the way that people dress even if they don't buy your clothes? Yes, I think that is a vicious circle. Some of my ideas come from seeing people in the street, and then they interpret my ideas of them. —— Do you find it annoying that your clothes are so expensive? I don't lose sleep at night over it, no. But it is a problem, and I'm trying to find a solution. Anything that is made of good quality fabric is expensive. I try to make a less expensive collection, Public, but it is still not less expensive. So I try then to design to a minimum, but that is difficult. I would have to work for another company that makes more mass-produced garments. I do feel sad though seeing my clothes on old rich people... —— What do you find stylish? It's more an attitude than clothes. It's how you are with people and your position. —— Which designers not involved with fashion do you find stylish? Oh, I don't know all the names, so if I say some the others will be very frustrated. —— What's your opinion of what is happening with fashion? I think that it is more and more international, and not just French, which is very good. It's great that different people are coming to Paris. I hope that more London designers will come and show what they are doing. Amsterdam and Belgium are also interesting. —— Have you seen any shows in London? No, never. They always come at the same time as my shows, so I can't go. I'm preparing mine and I don't want to be influenced! —— Would you say there is more immediate culture in London? Yes. In Paris we are between England and Italy. We are between the extreme and the elegant, which is a pity because it means we are just medium. We are more snobbish too. —— What is your favourite place to be? It depends on what mood I'm in. If I'm alone I prefer to be in London because very soon I'm no longer alone ... I find some nice person ... more than in Paris. —— Are you happy doing what you do? Of course, I must say yes, because it is exactly what I wanted in the beginning. —— Thank you. Thank you. Now, you don't want a little cake, no...?

███████

BLITZ #41
May 1986

VIVIENNE WESTWOOD
FIRST LADY

The first time I ever heard about Vivienne Westwood, her designs were being described as 'costumes of provocation'. Vivienne was delighted by the phrase. "It's wonderful that someone says that, because my profession is just to cause as much trouble as possible... 'Trouble maker!' "

Vivienne Westwood's personal conception of FASHION has always ensured that she would be surrounded by controversy – whether it's with the nation's law enforcers or its style councillors. Her work first appeared in a flurry of headlines, when the Sex Pistols were Public Enemy Number One and Vivienne dressed them accordingly. Every newspaper was full of grainy, black and white photographs of highly decorated punks, and headlines screamed 'The Filth and The Fury'. Johnny Rotten proclaimed, "We're not into the music, we're into chaos," and Vivienne echoed this with "The clothes are more interesting anyway!" Already the store she ran at 420 Kings Road with music biz entrepreneur Malcolm McLaren had gone through several incarnations. As 'Let It Rock' and 'Too Fast To Live Too Young To Die' the walls were racked with Rock 'n' Roll paraphernalia; and 'SEX' took all the dirty raincoat, brown envelope brigade merchandise and filled the shelves with it. It was this love of the obscure which developed into the punk ethic.

Vivienne stitched two squares of muslin together, stencilled on obscene literature and called them T-shirts; she knitted uneven shapes in mohair, missing stitches here and there, and called them sweaters; she sewed zips into the backs of baggy strides, tied the two legs together with a restrictive strap and called them Bondage Trousers. These were described aptly as 'Clothes For Heroes'.

If 'Seditionaries' and punk had been harsh reality, then her next step into uncharted waters was pure pantomime. A huge clock face now fronted the store, ticking backwards as the hands revolved anti-clockwise. The clock face mirrored Vivienne's progress, travelling back in time, with piratical ponces parading themselves up and down the King's Road. All the time Vivienne smiled a golden smile – her gold teeth came courtesy of the wrapping paper from packets of Benson and Hedges. (Another chance to upset the status quo – you don't need to be rich to look it.) It is the lady's disrespect for convention and her quest for knowledge which proves her driving force. It is so strong as to have a definitely noticeable effect on those around her. When *Vogue* featured the clothes, they were photographed on girls and boys wearing colourful curlers in their hair.

A leap forward onto dry land had her wandering around as yet undiscovered territory. Her fashion shows became the liveliest and most uncontrollable yet seen. The fashion press were stunned. When her 'Nostalgia of Mud' store took her uptown in 1982, she also travelled to Paris, and took the place by storm. She bundled up her Buffalo girls and boys and set them loose in the quaint Angelina Tea Rooms. The catwalk, which eventually collapsed under the strain alongside several international journalists, was no wider than a Buffalo boy's shoulders, but even so they danced on. Designer Issey Miyake sat sipping tea, smiling throughout. On his lapel as he left was pinned a distressed-looking badge, depicting a man's arm holding a cutlass – Vivienne's 'Born in England' trademark.

Soon Punk resurfaced in a more colourful disguise, renamed Punkature, and safety pins returned holding everything together. Tin lids became buttons and patchwork samplers were used as pockets. Seams were askew, jackets fell from shoulders and hemlines dipped, unbelievably at times. Once again Anarchy ruled.

By the time her next collections were presented on the huge runways in Paris – she was the first British designer to show in Paris for ten years – her relationship with Malcolm McLaren was being debated and dissected in the press. It was rumoured that Vivienne longed for international stardom, and money. People whispered that she had signed a contract with a large Italian corporation and that there were 'Made in Italy' labels sewn inside the brighter, crispier, racier garments. Even when out of the public eye she continued to be talked about.

For the last few seasons, Vivienne has always been around during fashion week, whether showing her 'Witches', or 'Mini Crinnies' in Paris, or simply hanging out at the London shows, wearing a hammer head Oxford Street tourist hat.

Vivienne Westwood is undoubtedly one of our major talents and always has something to say. Here she states her intentions and hopes, and reaffirms in my heart her zest for living...

——

Do you still consider yourself to be a punk designer? Punk is definitely part of my history. I'll never get rid of that, but let me tell you what I think street clothes are. They presume that there is an Establishment, and that they are therefore anti-establishment. Typical street clothes have been around since the time of the French Revolution, when the Aristocrats wore their wigs and coats back to front. Now in magazines you see someone with a sweater on their legs, or around their head. This is an anti-establishment motif, because it is counter to the normal way of doing things. Other images include looking dull, sick, dead. It's something which occurs on the presumption that there is an establishment, and therefore there's a door to kick down. But to be honest I don't believe there is such a thing. —— Did you believe there was an establishment when you were doing the Seditionaries store and the Sex Pistols? I used to believe that there was a door to kick down, yes, but now I know it's not all there at all. There are just jumps along the way. —— Is that the result of experience and age? It was going to Italy. Living in England, I still had this island mentality. In Italy I began at last to feel like a member of the world. People imagine in England that they are at the central point of culture – they really think they are at the centre of the world, but what they mean is the rock and roll world. That's the only culture they think is valid. As I got older I realised that punk rock wasn't kicking any doors, and that if there is an establishment it's there just to use the energy of the people who call themselves anti-establishment. I once said that a good idea is a perfect surprise. My idea is that if you do a really good thing, you've already kicked down the door, and you're not excluding anyone from it. It's a generous thing you're doing, for them to look at and be interested in, or to get some kind of joy from. —— **Is what you're doing aimed at anyone in particular?** I think it's good enough to be for everyone eventually. At first, though, it's always for a certain avant garde minority that pick up on it. What I really don't like about that is the set of exclusive credentials that a lot of those who consider themselves to be avant garde think they have. It doesn't exclude anybody. —— **Your name has been linked with Armani. What happened?** I think I should always have control of my main collection. What I am doing at the moment is trying to construct some kind of pyramid, with the Vivienne Westwood name label at the head, and financed by an economic base. I'm trying to do what I should have done before, what every other designer does. They came up through the business and worked for other designers like Karl Lagerfeld, or Dior, or whoever. Then they take on other projects and build up a broader financial base. With the rewards from that they can control their own thing. However, I don't exclude the possibility of working in the way I intended to work with Armani, which was to give somebody else control of what you do – but not artistic control. But we never got to that stage with Armani. I had made a contract with the head of Armani, who died, and he had no other delegates to deal with me. They all closed ranks and my collection rather floundered really.

—— **Was that the collection you showed in Paris?** No, I never did show it. I've been waiting to do that collection. I'm still waiting... **What stage did you get to with it?** Well, it was all worked out and I knew exactly what I wanted to do. —— **Will it ever be seen or shown?** Well, it should be my next winter collection, but I'll probably show that collection in July at the same time as the couture shows, simply because I don't have a big situation to back me up to produce a collection. I want a small situation which I can control. I'm looking at different ways to exploit ... no, to present what I do. At the moment I don't want to do another fashion show. I might do a small one, but I was talking to Jasper Conran the other day and he made a point which I feel to be true: when you do a collection a lot of your energy really gets dissipated in doing the variations and all kinds of other things that flesh out the collection. What I actually want to do is something in the music business. I've written some songs and I want to present them with a video. In that way I could really control everything from the outer wear, the hats, shoes, and everything, right down to the underwear, fewer models with more perfect things. It would be a different project because you'd be looking at different things. You wouldn't be concentrating on the quantity but on the quality. I'm opening my shop anyway, and this collection will go into that. —— **Where's that going to be?** The World's End store, and then I'll definitely do this winter collection to sell in that shop. —— **I suppose that video is a way of bringing out all the detailing of your clothes that tends to get lost when seen on the catwalk...** Yes, I'm really interested in the idea of collaboration. Especially across media. I'm interested in working with other designers as well. I don't want to be snobby. I actually want to do a little knitwear thing and ask others to take part in it, because one thing England does well is knitwear. I'm doing a jeans collection at the moment as a part of the base of this pyramid and I've just done something for a mail order

company. I feel more secure about myself than for a long time, mostly because I think I've got my head straight. I think I've got my thinking clear. It's a question of harmony. It's difficulty for someone avant garde like myself – and I don't use that word to be snobby, just to state a fact – it's very difficult to find people who have the faith in you to let you do what you want. They'd always want to push you into some commercial channel, and it's absolutely impossible because you will never fulfill their kind of quotas. A lot of designers don't make money out of their name collection, but it enables them to do other things – their perfume, their luggage, things like that. That collection doesn't pay, but I think mine will pay, because when I make something so much goes into it. The bondage trousers. The squiggle T-shirt. A friend of my son's sold a ripped squiggle T-shirt the other day for £100. I know that my things will make money. —— **How did you find showing in Paris?** I have never enjoyed it, because I've never really been in control for one reason or another. I've always got to that tent without any kind of plan for the show, never possible to do rehearsal, hardly time to speak to the models.

—— **What do you think of the international fashion situation?** As you know, I've never set much store by English designers, but I think John Galliano is very good. I really do think he's good, because he's got an aesthetic or whatever. That's not to say I like his clothes, or I'd wear them, because to me they are actually old fashioned. They're themes that I was concerned with two or three years ago. —— **A lot of people have said that his things are very close to your original designs.** Yes, somebody said he's like my child. He has got an intensity. He's in touch with the muse. He's incorruptible. He knows in his head what he's after. He won't be corrupted or seduced. You have to research into all the things you care about, and out of the techniques you build up, you produce original things. They come out of the technique and the culture. They don't come from the street. Even if you wanted to copy something, you'd copy it with your own perspective, and that's what makes it individual. John Galliano doing his Merveilleuse dresses is bound to be something individual. —— **So what about the rest of the scene?** I think that Karl Lagerfeld is good. He's one person who goes out on a limb every now and then. He's always trying something exotic. The main boy is Yves Saint Laurent. If you look at Yves Saint Laurent's work, there's not a thing that anyone's ever done that isn't there. Look at his African look. I mean, I did some breast interest things, and so did Jean Paul Gaultier, but he did better than either. He's just fabulous. I think Giorgio Armani is good in Italy. He's the only Italian designer who has influenced international fashion. Claude Montana – he's good, but I don't like him, he's not my thing. I've never liked that big shoulder look, and witchy women look. Even when Thierry Mugler first did those big shoulders I never liked it, because I never thought it was modern. —— **What about the Japanese?** I haven't liked Yohji or Comme for the last few years. There was an article in the *Sunday Times* about good taste, how everyone is conversant with the idea of good taste and everybody's buying it and how sterile it is. Like those terrible black watches. It said that the good taste boy would wear Yohji Yamamoto, and I agree with that. It stands for everything that's sterile. I've never liked Yohji, because he's predictable, no surprises at all. I don't see any kind of generosity in his things. I like Issey Miyake. He's different. I don't particularly think

his things are fashionable at the moment, but there's a warmth about them. —— **After all you've been through, don't you get tired of the fashion world? Do you never get fed up with it?** No, and I never will, because it's so hard. Call it a challenge. At one time I didn't want to get into it, and it was only after helping Malcolm that I realised that I'd always had a talent for making things. I've always had spatial awareness. I could have made a pair of shoes at the age of four. That's my talent. But what has happened is that I always analyse the specific thing I do, which is designing, on a broader cultural base; I use my specific vocabulary as part of the wider vocabulary, which is about living. But I've never had the ability financially to balance my creativity. My friend is a painter, and I can talk about his painting in the same way I talk about my fashion because what I like in his painting is the same thing that I like in my fashion. I'm looking at twentieth century culture. Where it's going wrong, and what it ought to be doing.

—— **Do you still work without sketches?** No. Another thing that I've found is that I should have been doing them all along. I'd have saved an awful lot of time. When I start something new I must work with the fabric, I must go after the form I want, and I do that on my own body. I used to do little diagrams, just linear dresses without arms and legs or a head, to pin down my ideas. Now I find that to put a look on a body with a sketch is going to save me an awful lot more time, but I have to do my shape first with the cloth, otherwise I can't draw it. —— **Do you see yourself as stylish?** Yeah. I do, yeah. I just think the thing that I'm wearing now is the... I couldn't wear anything else. I think it's the only thing that's fashionable. I saw the most beautiful dress the other day by Karl Lagerfeld, I could probably wear that. —— **Does your look change from day to day?** No it doesn't. In fact, when I do a collection I keep hardly anything from it. I take something that will suit me. If I have an outfit I really like, I wouldn't want to wear something that I don't like so much. I have very few clothes, and I don't mix up clothes from other collections. I would like to see people buy not so many clothes. I really do like that 'quality rather than quantity' thing. —— **Do you research quite heavily yourself?** Yes, I do. If I had time I'd like to copy Queen Elizabeth's dress with all the padding and all the sub-structure. I'd love to go out and work with a tailor for six months. Dior used to go to old museums and people would find him underneath all these dresses looking exactly how they are done. When I did the Pirate collection I'd seen a picture of a man whose trousers were too big and they were all kind of rumpled around the crutch and all the pockets were baggy. I wanted to do that, but I couldn't pull that trouser off until I found a book which showed how people made breeches in those days, and I found that the shape of the trousers was quite, quite different. Once I realised that, I got my look. I wanted that rakish look of clothes which didn't fit, and I was into that for a long time, and I splurged off a whole thing of English terrible cutting. —— **Have you ever been offended by anything anyone has ever written about you?** No, I don't read my own interviews usually.

—— **Have you ever considered becoming a fashion editor?** When I've been stranded in an economic desert at least I've thought I could do something else: this, that or whatever. No, I haven't thought of that specifically, but I'd like to write. I like writing. I've been writing songs. I have done some styling for Malcolm. I enjoyed that. When he was doing his *Chicken* magazine.

I was very pleased with that. —— **What do you enjoy most about what you're doing?** I expect really that I'm very encouraged because there is such an interest in it. This is my angle for getting involved in the music business. If the public's interest in music is 100% they get back about 120% because there are some good pop singers around. But if the public's interest in fashion is, say, another 100% they only get 30% back. There's only what you get in magazines, or an event twice a year which has a restricted, elitist audience actually, and a fashion event can be terribly exciting. The first fashion show I ever did, the Pirate collection, was more exciting than any rock show I've seen. I was quite amazed, actually. It was almost like I hadn't done it. —— **Is there a way of making it less elitist?** I think there's a lot of scope. Video and so on. Fashion should be exciting because there's good people in fashion, and there's been some good ideas, and I'd like to take some credit for that. Fashion is such an immediate form of communication. It does really get its results so quickly. People can take it and feel it. —— **Are you going to be involved in the music business personally?** I'm not going to sing anything. No, no, no. I will probably end up with a musical. Fashion set to stage, a little concept with characters. —— **What else can we expect from you? What more can you give us?** I just need a bit of luck really, whatever it is. Slowly, slowly I shall get to the head of my pyramid, and hopefully that head will be a nucleus for all kinds of things. A patronage for other art forms. One would contribute to the other. I sense people aren't interested in politics anymore, and they're not interested in drugs, I hope. There's always an interest in sex, of course, and that's also very important. But culturally, there's almost an anticipation of a collaboration of cultural forms. I see fashion as a point of focus for a lot of things. —— **You talked of Britain's preoccupation with being an island. Do you think the preoccupation with youth isn't all it's made out to be?** I wouldn't want to be one day younger that I am. I'm even quite pleased to look at wrinkles coming on my face, I think it amuses me slightly. Every wrinkle, every scar, makes me feel more beautiful inside, but it' a question of experience. If you read a book when you are eighteen, you'll see so much more if you read it again when you are twenty-five, because everything that has happened to you gives you perspective. So many more points of reference. So that every time you learn something it's like a snowballing experience. If I'm ever fed up – for example, because I don't have a boyfriend – I think, God, I've got so much to do in this life and I don't even know if I've got time for all that... There are just so many more things I want to do... —— **Do you think you will fulfill everything you want to do?** I will fulfill everything I want to do in fashion, I'm sure about that. But there are so many other things I'd like to do as well. I've no idea whether I've got time for them or not. —— **Do you feel sad about that?** No, I don't. No, no, because, as I say, it's expanding all the time...

DONNA KARAN
TALKING TRANSATLANTIC

In New York designer Donna Karan is HOT! Following the presentation of her first collection under her own label, Donna Karan New York, everyone was trying to touch, kiss and congratulate the lady. With projected sales of 11 million dollars for her company's first year, it would appear that everyone is also buying, and wearing, her simple coordinated designs.

For most of her working life Donna Karan worked as a premier designer with the respected Anne Klein organisation, before her meteoric launch as a new fashion star. Her success has been almost as matter-of-fact as her design statements. The Bodysuit, which is the quintessential piece of her design ethic, was created simply to stop blouses, and turtleneck knit tops, from pulling out of waistbands.

Other pieces of her collection, invariably black, navy or a neutral colour, are cleverly pieced together. A scarf which twists into a skirt (a sculptural exercise for Ms. Karan), a blazer or a perfect sweater are the result of Ms. Karan asking herself, 'What should I wear today? What don't I have in my wardrobe?'

It is this desire to design interchangeable clothes for day or night, profession or pleasure, and to make them available on one single shopping trip (handbags, scarves, jewellery, even tights are provided by Ms. Karan and sold alongside the clothes) which many modern women are obviously welcoming with open chequebooks.

American Express. That'll do nicely, madam.

——

Is there a contemporary woman who encapsulates your collection? Yes, she's the international woman ... an executive, a mother, a housewife and a lover. —— **Can your bodysuit be worn by anyone?** Yes, it's no longer a fashion statement but a functional item which has become a part of modern fashion vocabulary. —— **Do you have favourite designers?** I admire everyone's achievements in this business ... I appreciate the difficulties and I admire individual statements. —— **What influences your work?** The needs of the customer – what I see from watching the women around me, the woman in the street. —— **Which fabrics do you like against your skin?** Anything that's luxurious – cashmere, suede, silk. —— **How has your design developed?** In complete response to customers' needs. —— **What is the most important thing in your life?** Keeping my priorities in order, and my first priority is my family. —— **Are you in love?** Definitely! —— **Who do your designs sell to? Is there a difference across the two continents?** They sell to a woman who wants to look good, but who doesn't want to have to think of it; who loves luxury from top to toe ... that's why my collection is different from other collections. I offer everything she needs beyond clothing, from hats and shoes to jewellery ... my collection is about a lifestyle as much as it is about clothing. My woman is an international woman – she can live anywhere. —— **What is the essence of your work?** Woman ... the female form. —— **Do you see your designs as glamorous or otherwise?** The clothes don't wear the woman, the woman wears the clothes ... that's what glamorous about them.

BLITZ #43
July 1986

CALVIN KLEIN
A LIFE'S OBSESSION

The controversial advertising campaign for Calvin Klein's Obsession perfume has once again drawn attention to America's most consistently successful designer. Klein's jeans and underwear lines are a multi-million dollar business in themselves and his latest collection takes a step towards haute couture.

Fashion folklore would have it that Calvin Klein's sensationally successful career took off completely by accident when an important buyer absentmindedly took a lift to the wrong floor and stumbled upon Klein's tiny studio. Another tale has him pushing an early collection singlehandedly up 5th Avenue on a dress rail. Another describes him as being obsessed with his own appearance.

In the world of fashion, meeting Calvin Klein is like meeting the President of the United States. Klein has been at the forefront of American fashion for many, many seasons. Bright young things like Stephen Sprouse may burn themselves out overnight, and others like Donna Karan may be this year's designer to die for, but Calvin Klein continues to produce unmistakably wearable and uncomplicated clothes year in, year out.

From a business which began with six coats and three dresses, Calvin Klein Industries now retail in excess of $700 million a year. Klein has ten licences to his name and presents over sixty different looks each season. His jeans line was selling 400,000 pairs a week at the height of the ad. campaign and his underwear sold $250,000 worth in the first week it was launched at Bloomingdales. Klein himself was estimated to be worth a cool $12 million in 1984. It would appear that everything he turns his hand to likewise turns to gold.

And there's more....

Calvin Klein has also been almost singlehandedly responsible for the American vogue for minimalist living. It is a lifestyle which is now synonymous with good taste, ultimate chic, and the modern working woman who has no room for fuss in her busy life. It is a new conception of the American way which is personified by Klein's attitude to design.

Even so, Klein himself is everything you don't expect Americans to be. His clothes don't shout at you, and neither does he. He speaks in soft tones which mirror his designs. He is charming (beyond belief), handsome (still), and essentially a jeans and T-shirt man stuffed into a suit.

As I sat ten floors above 39th street at the heart of the vast Calvin Klein organisation, surrounded by so much photographic evidence of his success, I could only marvel at the one glaring mistake he has made: you can't buy Calvin Klein boxer shorts in the same perfect pale grey as the Y-fronts. Other than that he's OK by me.

—

How true are the stories about your early years in the fashion business? These stories are completely true. It's one of those American Dream stories. Quite by accident a merchandise manager of Bonwit Teller in March 1968 got out of the lift on the wrong floor and he saw the clothes – I had a rack of six coats and three dresses, and he looked at them and said that they were definitely for Bonwit and Teller. This was Thursday. He said that on Friday the buyer would come down, and by Saturday I would have been discovered. I had to take the clothes to the store and I was so afraid they would get creased or something might go wrong that I wheeled them myself on a rack, from 7th Avenue on 37th Street to 5th Avenue on 56th Street, and one of the wheels even broke. It was a nightmare. It was horrible. Finally she looked at the clothes and said, 'Mister Klein, just carry on making them this way.' And she told me she would pay me twenty dollars more per style than I was asking. Today it would never happen. Maybe twenty dollars less. —— **Have you always been fascinated by fashion?** My Grandmother was a dressmaker, and my mother used to sketch. She never really did anything with fashion except wear it and spend all my father's money. Whatever he had she managed to spend. I love fashion, I always get excited. I never get bored. —— **How important is what you do?** Well, I just co-hosted a benefit with Elizabeth Taylor (The AIDS benefit), which raised close to three quarters of a million dollars, and in that context then maybe fashion is very important, not only because it makes people feel good, but because I helped raise a lot of money. I'm not a scientist, but the scientists need people like us to get the money for them. —— **Can you describe the ultimate Calvin Klein look?** That's a hard question. It changes. That's why I love fashion so much – because it never is 'ultimate', even though I have a style and I'm always concerned with simplicity and with purity. For instance, I collect a million things – tortoise shell, old books, watches, sketches – but I have to hide them. I can't live with clutter. I feel the same about clothes.
—— **They definitely are 'no fuss' clothes. Where does that come from?** My mother, no question. She would have a coat, but she would have it lined with fur. That sense of simplicity and tailoring I now try and take to another level. A lot of the clothes in my new collection will be exclusive to Bergdorf Goodman because Bergdorfs is the only store in the country that can sell that kind of clothes. They're very expensive – they are made at my workroom and I can only make a few pieces at a time. I'm very excited, I feel like I did in 1968. It's like I'm starting all over again. —— **You talk of quality. Your fabrics are certainly some of the most gorgeous. Are you desperately concerned with the quality of your work?** Yes, I'm desperately concerned, and unfortunately in fashion it's really tough. We don't create art, but we're paid pretty well. However, to control it, to make sure the quality is always there, is really tough. You know, it's not a perfect science. You have ten ladies sitting at sewing machines, each sewing the same dress, and they come out slightly different. It's human beings sewing up these clothes. One person takes a little larger seam, and one takes a smaller one... —— **Does the expense bother you?** I do so many clothes. I do some much for American design at prices that many people can afford though my jeans collections and all the rugged, rough kind of clothes, the real sporty clothes, and now a step above that. Although not exactly couture, which

is not a modern American term, I will be doing things specially if someone wants to order one of these dresses in a colour or special size... and that's as close to couture as you can get in this country. —— **I really loved the shoes in your show.** I have a thing about shoes... —— **Do you have set ideas about what sort of shoes women should wear?** Well I started out by ordering a hundred pairs of alligator pumps, and I never used one of them. I decided to go back to suede because I love suede during the day. The mixture of alligator and lizard. The mixture of textured skins are so important. The shape of the shoes. I've always sketched shoes, even as a kid, and now I go through every sketch. I have great fun with that. I'm crazy about shoes ... and gloves – a major accessory. —— **Ah, my next question. What would you say is the 'must have' accessory this season?** I should say shoes because we have a major shoe business, but shoes are a necessity, not just a luxury. I think gloves are the real major fashion accessory. It's just that all of a sudden I didn't like seeing this white hand sticking out. It looked totally wrong, and suddenly when there was suede, or when a tangerine cashmere jacket had yellow stitched pigskin gloves, or sweaters had gloves in other colours, it looked so much better. I think it's so chic, and it's fun. An easy accessory for a woman to afford. —— **Are you obsessed with women and the way they look?** I'm obsessed. Start with that. That's how I got the name of the perfume. Everyone I know, my friends, they're all obsessive people. They're obsessed with their lovers, their wives, their girlfriends, their work. They're passionate people. I think this is a time when people really want to accomplish something, a time when people care, and they tend to be obsessive. It's not just that I'm obsessed by women, but with trying to give women something that I believe in and that will make them feel good and will be tasteful and sexy, and lots of different things. The obsession is with my work. —— **And what you see around you?** I'm not a completely crazy person. I look at it as a positive word. It's not taken to the point of insanity. I'm obsessed to the extent that I want things to be as perfect as they can be, whether it's the way a flower is arranged or the way we advertise. I choose the photographs and work out the layouts. I can't sleep if I'm not happy with it... —— **Speaking of advertising, two of the TV ads for Obsession were banned for a while in England...** I can't believe that. I was shocked, because the English have a sense of humour, whereas we Americans are pretty uptight, especially on network television, and the censors are really tough. I love taking risks, but I never expected that reaction in England... —— **People have said the adverts don't make sense. Was it your intention to be as obscure as possible?** If you advertise in a magazine, the first thing you want is for people to stop. When I think of the word Obsession and think of the shape of the bottle, I have to try and translate that into a photograph. Well, that can't be a girl running through wheat fields. She's not obsessed, she's too laid back. Well, what is Obsession? I have a girl, Jose, who is the image for Calvin Klein. In the photograph I wanted something that shows that people are obsessed with her, as if she is so incredible that everyone just wants to ravish her... —— **And the TV adverts?** The TV adverts were a whole other thing, because when you do TV you have to think of the words. The dialogue is even more important than tonal qualities because every TV is tuned different, so a pale grey dress appears one shade in your house, another shade in mine, and blue in someone else's. You've got to create excitement in another way. It's creating a story, an involvement, and maybe provoking people a little bit to think what is really going on. A lady came up to me and said, 'I love your commercials, but please don't have that woman slap the other woman.' But I like to be a little bit of a bad boy. I have fun.

—— **You mentioned Jose Borain. Is she your ideal embodiment of woman?** Well, yes she is. Every time I see something I design on Jose I go crazy. I mean, she could sell me anything. I think she represents youth and sophistication. A kind of beauty that's sexual, a little bit man and a lot of woman. A lot mystery and refinement. There's never too much make-up, the body is sensational, and the skin is not to be believed.

—— **Do you have an ideal man as a counterpart to Jose?** Well ... yeah. Sam Shepard. He is brilliant. He's so handsome, such a fine actor, writer. He is an ideal man today ... and his looks? I interviewed Katharine Hepburn once, who is my all time favourite idol, and asked if her style developed by accident. She said, 'Are you kidding?' She'd studied everything that she did on the screen. Sam Shepard doesn't look as good as he looks by accident. No one does! —— **You seem terribly preoccupied with physical fitness – your own appearance and that of your preferred models.** I have this enormous guilt feeling right now because I have gained 10lbs and have not exercised for ten weeks. I am now going to be occupied with physical fitness. I feel great when I exercise mentally. I'm middle-aged, I'm no longer concerned with the body beautiful. I'm concerned whether people care about their bodies. I still love to eat. I love pasta, and in order to eat pasta you have to exercise. It relieves my stress. —— **Are you attracted to people by their physical appearance? Do you think you have to be beautiful to be desirable?** Who isn't? Everyone is attracted to people by their physical appearance. That wears off quickly, then what surfaces is real beauty. —— **A recent article in the New York Sunday Times said that 'a sure fire sign of success is a car and a driver.' Are these things which you equate with success?** No, that's not even ... that was funny. That's not a real sign of success. A real sign is to feel good about yourself, and feel like you've done the best you can possibly do, and that people appreciate it. If one thinks a car and a driver are a sign of success, that's just ridiculous. —— **What's your biggest luxury?** I treat myself well. It's easy for me to pick up the phone and in thirty minutes I can have a plane and go anywhere I want to in the world. For some reason fashion designers have become minor celebrities and so you get a good table at a restaurant, and when there isn't a room at a hotel, you get a room. All those things can happen, but you pay a price. In balance some horrible things, very unpleasant things can happen. —— **Is there anything that you would like to be able to do but can't?** I should be able to do anything that I want to. I think life is too short and I think anyone is an absolute fool if there is something that they really want to do and they don't do it. It is maybe a little annoying to walk down the street and have someone come up to you and say, 'oh look it's...', you know. But when people do come up they say the nicest things. —— **Are you happy about the way your career has developed?** I'm very happy and it's also developed in a way that my career is not the only thing in my life. I have a lot of things that are important in my life, which are nothing to do with fashion ... and I love my

friends. It's very important to have friends, people you can count on who will be there at four in the morning when you are hysterical and panicking about the show... —— **In recent fashion journals you've bought vast, sixteen-page advertising spreads. Does the immense size of your business ever scare you?** Yes, it scares me, and it excites me. I've taken on really big responsibilities, but I've done it because I wanted to do it. I wasn't forced into it. I need excitement in my life. I need a certain amount of glamour in my life. I'm certainly very happy.

—— **Do you think that style is inherent, or can you make someone stylish by dressing them well?** I think real style, like Millicent Rogers or Babe Paley or Gloria Guinness (all prominent social figures of America), you just have. I think the job of fashion designers is to make people look good, to help them. That's the job of magazines, of the press, to guide them, to make things easier for people who have very busy lives. I don't know that I can give someone real style, but what I can do is make them look good in clothes which fit their lifestyle. If I can do that then I'm doing something pretty valid. —— **Who do you admire?** I guess Hepburn is a perfect example, and doing the AIDS Benefit I spent the evening with Elizabeth Taylor. I really admire her a great deal, she is really one of the last real actresses. A great star. Another person I admire who has been an enormous influence on my career and life is Nicky de Guinsberg, Baron von Guinsberg. He worked with Diana Vreeland and he worked at *Vogue* and *[Harper's] Bazaar*, and for some reason he took a special liking to me, and always reminded me, "Be what you are. You're an American. Don't look to what's happening in Europe. Do what you're best at." I have a portrait that Horst photographed of him in the 1930s, and I look at it every so often and wonder what he would be thinking right now about my work. I think he'd be really excited.

—— **You talk of being American, do you think you could have had equal success if you had been designing in Paris or London?** It's two different questions. You have the tailors and dressmakers in London. You have the embroiderers in Paris. You don't have them here. There are people who still sit at sewing machines and make something beautiful, but they are old and dying, because the young do not want to do that – they want to be designers, they don't want to be seamstresses. In many ways it's easier to work in Europe, but as an American working in Paris, I don't think that would be so easy, and as an American working in Milan, I think it would be impossible. As an American in London, I really don't know. I mean, I love London so much, and Grace Coddington at British *Vogue* gave me a good deal of publicity for my clothes, but I don't know whether that means I could be that successful actually working in London. —— **Is what you're doing essentially American, in that you combine the relaxed with the ritzy?** I think that's a good way of saying it. I wish I could have said that. That's pretty good. I hope ritzy doesn't mean flashy, though? —— **No, well dressed and glamourous.** Yes, I think a woman could look really glamourous in some of the clothes that I show. —— **If you could only wear one outfit for the rest of your life, what would it be?** Me personally? If you would have asked me that a few years ago I probably would have said my jeans and T-shirt. Now I would say my grey flannel suit from Anderson and Sheppard, but I would also need my blazer. I couldn't decide if it should be my light grey one, or my medium or dark grey one. That's a problem.

A man doesn't need a lot of clothes. —— **Are you more concerned to have people interested in what you create as opposed to what you look?** Well, yes of course. I'm only going to get worse looking as I get older. If I was focusing on just the way I look I'd be heading for a major depression, so of course I'm more concerned about my work. But I know the way a designer looks, appears and relates to people, even the way he photographs, helps to create an image as to what your clothes are about. What you are about ... people want to know that. —— **Looking to the future, where are things leading you?** Well, I think the thing I'm doing with Bergdorf Goodman is an indication of the immediate future. I'm doing more exclusive clothes. It's another stage of my career and I'm very excited by it. —— **Everything else will continue alongside?** Oh yes, sure. —— **And personally, you intend to continue life as a designer?** Certainly. What else would I do? Of course I just want to keep designing new things, but I can't imagine what else I would do. I get through the times when one is not always received so well. You accept that. After so many years you take the good with the bad, but that doesn't deter from the fact that when I look at new fabrics I get excited all over again, and I think what can I do... —— **If it didn't continue to excite you, would you give it up?** Absolutely.

BLITZ #44
August 1986

WILLI SMITH
WILLI!

Willi Smith designs sportswear, even though the English wouldn't call it that. His clothes are invariably oversized, and as funny as the man himself. Born in Philadelphia, his work reflects his black roots, even though he sometimes imagines his blond ones to be showing through. Willi's name has been linked with a number of familiar artists as a result of several joint projects, primarily a series of Artist T-shirts which emblazoned specially commissioned images across the chests of the world. Willi Smith isn't too keen to grow old, and funnily enough last year *People* magazine in the States chose him as one of this generation's 'Baby Boomers'. Willi Smith has a sense of humour. His cartoon clothes do too.

——

Describe the Williwear look. A good question. In turmoil at the moment... It's basically easy, comfortable, somewhat oversized clothes. They're always a little off centre, even when they appear to be classic, because of fabric or colours. They're either two inches longer or have wider shoulders. I take familiar shapes and silhouettes and twist them around a little. —— **What Americans would call Sportswear...** Oh yes, it's definitely sportswear, and that's something which has been invented by Americans. —— **So the eccentricities are important to the look?** Yeah, I don't use the most expensive fabrics, so I try to work with the proportion and shape and details of the thing. —— **Do you take clothes seriously?** They must have a sense of humour. I'm panicked at the moment by what's going on in fashion because we all seem to be taking it a little too seriously. We think we're not, but the look is serious, based on something so classic. I even called my show 'Totally Classic', and for my girls to be wearing navy blue blazers, that's wild for them ... and I put on my black jacket and my white shorts and my beige pants, and I love that, but I have to ask myself, 'Am I in fashion? Did I drop out of fashion somewhere?' I try not to take it too seriously, it's only clothes. —— **You've worked with many artists. What is your fascination with Art?** Designers have the clothing disease, that's just all we talk about, but artists do what comes from within. Regardless of how creative I want to be, I still have to make a tangible product and get it to the stores, and make sure that people buy it. They can be freer, and that attracts me. —— **Tell me about the Christo connection.** Christo is one of my best friends. It's amazing for someone who is so minuscule to have such a huge idea as wrapping the world. It's like you think, 'This little man? Oh forget it. You say boo to him and he's under a chair...' But he's someone who dreams of wrapping the world. We did the Artists T-shirts, and most people were pleased to have their art on the front of a T-shirt, and he was one. So we did a T-shirt for his 'Surrounded Islands' project in Florida. Then he wanted to wrap Paris, and I designed a uniform for everyone involved... —— **Why did you make the video, 'The Expedition?'** I was bored with fashion shows, and I want to get into film. Of course I was trying to star all

the way through it. —— **Why did you decide to make it funny?** It was getting so serious. I thought I was Cecil B. DeMille, looking at all these esoteric scenes of sunsets and all that, and then I thought I'd make it crazy. Most fashion videos are so boring. People watch the film expecting me to appear at the end and say, 'This is our basic shirt'. It was a whole new venture, and we won two awards. —— **How has the reaction been?** People love it. They aren't quite sure what it has to do with the collection, and why they should watch it, and why they should have it in their stores, but with me they're never sure anyway... —— **Do you think wearing clothes should be an event?** No. Well it shouldn't be an event for everyone else and I don't think that you should walk around looking like a statement either, but I think they should do something to your spirit. I like that. What I hate is when what someone is wearing shouts, 'Clothes, clothes, clothes! Here I am wearing my new look!' I hate that. —— **Do you dress up much?** I'm trying to get back into it...because I've got to get out of this black and beige. When we sit down at Williwear to talk about colour everyone panics – they say, 'Oh no, this guy thinks he's Japanese'... —— **Do different places inspire you to dress differently?** Absolutely. When I'm in India, even though they don't like it, I try to experiment with their little looks. They'll wear a baggy shirt, and take a piece of fabric and make like a skirt, and it's great. It's the only time I feel free to do it. Then I get back to New York, and I think I'll try that there, and I have to say to myself, 'Willi, where are you going? The drag show's not here.' Like here in Claridges I feel a little grown up, and I want to dress up a little bit. In Paris they're so chic I never know what to wear. But I never change my feeling. I have to feel comfortable. —— **Do you have a favourite piece of clothing?** At the moment, khaki pants. They're like my jeans; and I have a passion for a jacket which isn't mine. It's by Comme des Garçons, it's black and shiny and it's on my back every five minutes. —— **Is there an item you would like to own?** Yes, and one year I'll get it right for myself. I would like a trench coat that is right; long enough, roomy enough. I've tried them all and I've tried to make them myself. The ones I make come out looking a little too 'designer trench'. Then one time I got a classic Burberry, and I got it in extra, extra, extra large, and it just made me look as though I had on a fat man's coat. That's what I want, and also a terry cloth robe in the same proportion. Those things are just not around but you think they are. I got one from a classic mail order catalogue, and I don't know what the guy in the picture is wearing, but it's not what they sent me... —— **What's next?** More film, and I'd like to do a line in house wear. Just try looking for plain bed sheets in America. When I go to bed I don't want a religious experience; I do not want clouds, and plaids, and prints and flowers. Things like that are impossible. I want blankets and sheets in nice colours, and not expensive. Conran in concept, but Conran is like Benetton – 'I have no mind. Tell me what to do.' But the idea is good. Williwear is ten years old, and I am looking for outlets outside of clothes, something that will enhance the clothing, and broaden my collection. Also, there's a distinction now between how men and women want to dress, and that's for me. Maybe I'll design a good dress, because I'm the worst dress designer in the world. I fired my assistants and I'm going back to doing my own work. I got too removed. My own little pencil is again hitting the sketch pad, because when I don't do

my own work I lose customers. They just know, those girls – especially the black girls – I cannot fool them. Last season we did a whole series of pastel co-ordinates with plaids, and my brother said, 'Willi, you're getting too blond. Get back to Africa.' When those girls lose the spirit, when it doesn't have my touch, it just doesn't happen. —— **And a store?** Yes, one here and one in New York. I'm doing that because I've had it with big stores, they're too confusing. It's the only way I can show my thoughts about subtlety. I'm sick of the superstore, and the statement store. I think maybe I'd like to have some kind of fashion video gallery, where you could play those games or have a coffee. Something in the '60s boutique vein where you knew it was a store so you didn't bring your overnight bag. I'd like a funky designer shop, almost with the designer in the back, and you know you're going into the atmosphere of the person who is designing the clothes. —— **So it would be like a funky version of the Ralph Lauren Polo shop which has opened in New York?** It's hard to imagine a funky version of that, but it is a designer's dream, and it should happen to us all. Yeah, I'd like that. It would be like saying, 'Come on my house', but not with just my things, so that if I don't end up making that robe, but I find it, I'll stock it. It would be like, 'Come to Willi's house', and it's going to be – and don't get nervous – very black. I don't know how to express it other than that. A black nightclub is what I really want. A reggae lounge in London ... and that's something to look forward to!

BLITZ #49
January 1987

ANNA PIAGGI
PIAGGI

There are a number of fashion editors who are as equally stylish as the pages they preside over, women who have become icons, beacons of good looks and personal taste. In New York, the highly worshipped Diana Vreeland dotes over dresses, her earth-spanning career built on a neat patchwork of half-truths (always much more interesting than the whole truth) and heaven sent vision. London has more than its fair share, but one lady in particular, Grace Coddington at *Vogue*, is as much known for her grace and beauty as for her innate sense of pared-down-to-the-bone styling. Italy has but one of these grandes dames, one who screams blue murder to be noticed. Anna Piaggi. Her work took her first to the offices of the grand Italian *Vogue* as freelance fashion editor, and then onto one of its more avant garde sister magazines, *Vanity*, where she became editor-in-chief. Her dress sense has always ensured her a front row seat at international shows, where, more often than not she appears eclectically dressed in a bizarre combination of thrift shop rags and designer gowns. She has been known to wear a horse harness or gardening gloves over a dress by Lagerfeld or something by Chanel.

Her resolute sense of style has been recorded for many years by her close friend, the designer Karl Lagerfeld, who took to sketching Anna's costumes at every opportunity. These sketches began in a restaurant over ten years ago, and follow not just her changing fashions (Anna 'forgets fashion, she knows only her fashion', says Karl Lagerfeld in the elaborate introduction to her book, *Karl Lagerfeld: A Fashion Journal*) but also the way in which someone with a true sense of her own self changes from day to day, dressing by adding and subtracting other pieces of clothing.

When we met, Anna Piaggi was warm and enthusiastic. Before I'd even taken off my coat, she was showing off her travelling wardrobe, piling dresses, coats and hats onto the sofa beside me. She took great pleasure in showing off her latest find, a McDonald's waistcoat which she picked up in a flea market in Paris. "I will probably wear it over some Gaultier," she announced proudly.

I thought I might ask her a few questions, but Anna thought she would ask me some instead. Where could she find Martin Degville? (She was wearing one of his old dresses, bought at YaYa in Kensington Market years earlier.) Was he really a pop star? Who was good at doing hair? What did I think of Kay Montana? What should she wear to the Karl Lagerfeld book signing the next day? We went through a number of hats before I settled on a late-thirties Schiaparelli design with elongated purple feather attached. (She wore it.) Finally I managed to pose a few questions.

As we started to talk she casually patted the Pompeiian powdered wig she had entered the room wearing. Only minutes into the conversation, she adroitly lifted it from her head and placed it on the table beside her, and continued talking without missing a word...

——

Were you always interested in clothes? Yes, I always liked clothes, but for many years I was in uniform in college. Maybe this prepared me to react. I rebelled, which I think is a good thing for anyone to do. To be ready to step out, to be ready to do your own thing, and not to be drawn into the system too much. I was fascinated by movies and movie stars. I was very fond of movies. Then at twenty I began to dress differently, particularly because of the trips, and the people I was meeting who were involved in fashion... —— **Is that when the world opened up to you?** Exactly. Then I began playing the part of a visual editor, I began to do styling and I did it well, and began to have more and more material to shape and to put together and some kind of spontaneity. It is a matter of exercise, you must do it all the time. My way of dressing continued alongside my ability to see things. The possibility of finding things everywhere, that is the great facility which a fashion editor is to always have – a mine of information and treasure. For example, I love prototypes, the first dress off the racks, things which are not in the shops. I don't know why, but I always pick the odd pieces ... quite often when I go into a shop, I pick up the things which belong to the sales girl... —— **What is it then that excites you about clothes in particular?** It was first an attraction, but then it became work, and then more and more a kind of habit, a part of life, like food. Almost a necessity. I have a rapport with clothes. I like to try out a lot of clothes, I am a catalyst with clothes. —— **Is it a matter of fact for you to dress up? It isn't ritual or performance?** No, no, it comes naturally, it's not a production. Totally natural, because I've never meant really to impress. People think I dress to impress but it's not that. It is an attitude which has become quite natural. If I don't dress well I don't think well, I don't feel well, I feel unhappy. —— **Does it follow that if you dress in a different way you feel a different way?** I dress in different styles if they suit me. I also dress differently to integrate into a mood. My styles are never detached. My surroundings, music, the street, give me a certain balance. I don't dress to just play a role. I'm not an actress. One observes and puts it down. It also depends on what I find, what is attracting me. Sometimes I think that if I don't find something I like, I should have something specially made, but I think this way less and less. I like to transform things. I do this quite a lot. I was never a designer, but I am someone who selects. A visualiser. I like to look through lots of things and choose just one thing. When I worked on magazines I never tired of looking through contact sheets. This attitude was mainly born through my work. —— **What was your first step into fashion?** I started by substituting for a fashion editor, and went to the collections in Paris instead of her. This was just by chance. Then I became the fashion editor of a monthly magazine, and I was there for seven years, in charge of all the fashion. This gave me the opportunity to start travelling a lot, and I developed a sense for faces. The magazine had a lot of possibilities, financial possibilities. It was never a problem to call models from different countries. Now it is more difficult. I always seemed to choose girls who went on to be actresses. I was always searching for particular faces. —— **Was it the chance to put all these things together which interested you?** Definitely. Absolutely. That's always been the case. When I was very active doing editorial I even had things made specially for the pictures, or asked an accessory designer to bring materials to the session and create on the spot, and adapt to the mood. Sometimes an accessory can be an imposition, it can destroy the mood of the photograph. I never force. I never impose fashion. It is always spontaneous, not too evident or visible. —— **Have you always found editors and publishers would allow you to do what you wanted to do?** No, not always. I had some disagreements from time to time. I had my first serious crisis after seven years with a magazine, at a political moment in 1968. I did a story in Prague in the Spring, at the time that people were looking forward and I was accused of being too nostalgic. I used 1940s clothes in context, which was considered to be absolutely outrageous, and not at all rational. So I left, because they didn't want any red lipstick, they didn't want any curly hair, they didn't like long skirts or wedges. So I just got up out of my chair, and left. I wanted to go all the way and make a point to the public. —— **So with *Vanity* magazine, did that mean that you had the chance to do exactly as you pleased?** It was a chance to step out of photography, and just work with illustrators. At that time, 1981 to 1984, it was probably a good idea. I wanted to express a little more the idea of fantasies, but I still had to work with banal clothes. The clothes were all tied up with advertising, so to give the clothes a new spirit I commissioned illustrators. It was very relieving. The English clothes could be photographed, but the Italian really need interpretation. —— **How did you choose the illustrators?** Antonio Lopez is one of the greatest fashion illustrators, and we established a rapport, a partnership in work which I have always been in favour of. I would not change too much. Once I establish a team, it matures into a sort of chemistry, but the magazines prefer to change every time. I'm not in favour of that... —— **Ideally, if you say to a photographer that you want a picture to look a certain way, they will know what you mean...** Yes, yes, yes. This was my point. After three years at *Vanity* they said, 'Why do you keep using the same illustrator?', but he was always changing his techniques according to the mood. It was always done as a photographic sitting. Always posed, always with make-up, always a dresser. It was more like movies than photography. It was a great exercise. I like it very, very much. Then photography came back. Again. —— **Do you miss not being with a magazine now?** I don't really know now. I think that there is so much else going on in the media. I am attracted to other fields like television or video, but maybe I am only a paper person. I do not know yet but I have the temptation to try other possibilities. Working for magazines like Italian *Vogue*, they are so much taken up with the advertising, which is the majority of the magazine, and then a little editorial. How do you express so much in so few pages? It is overpowered by advertising. It's much better to find a magazine which has free expression. It is difficult for inspiration if you are suffocated by the commercial side, it's like occupying a space and having to share it with people you don't like. This is what I have been doing with magazines. I have been squatting. Truly. Occupying space, and keeping it. —— **Making it all your own?** Yes. Once I did a column full of information and trends. Very complicated. Two to four pages. It was a very good experience to synthesise into a small space trends, or a concept. That is something which has always interested me very much, and having to express that. —— **What do you**

consider most important, your work or the way you look? At the moment I must say I see myself completely from the outside. Today I went to Bond Street and saw my book for the first time in the shop window. Hundreds of copies. I thought, 'My God', I really got a shock because I had been so cool about the whole thing, because I did not treat the book as nostalgic or geographic, I treated it as a magazine. But today was quite an experience to see myself, on the pages, sitting in the shop. —— **How would you describe yourself?** I don't know how. I never think too much. I'm not a person who thinks a lot. I'm rather superficial. I'm completely superficial. I don't have any particular characteristics. It is difficult to describe myself. I can see the improvement or the contrary by looking at photographs. —— **When I've seen you at shows, you have been photographed almost as much as the things on the catwalk. Don't you ever get fed up of people taking your picture?** Most of the time I don't see the point. But I have great sympathy for the photographers. We have very good rapport. I know them, and I respect what they do. —— **So do you give them what they want?** Yes. No, I don't mind. The fact that I go out like that, I shouldn't mind. Only once I got a little upset, about two years ago. An editor decided to shoot me and my hats, which made me absolutely nervous, and it was to such an extent that I would arrive at this show and this photographer would say, 'Hey, where is your hat?' So then I stopped wearing hats! I think photographers who do the runway shots always tend to get pictures of the audience, and if you are there it is best to look photogenic. When it started, my husband, who is also a photographer, said to me that when they took photos of me they were really just testing the light. —— **Can you imagine life without clothes?** Ah no, no, no. Certainly not, but I wish sometimes to get rid of them. There are moments [when] they don't give me any more interest. I like to change all the time. —— **Surely you don't throw any of them away!?** Ah no, no, no. I don't want to throw away, but sometimes there are too many. Space is getting more and more difficult to find. —— **Where do you keep everything?** I have a big apartment, and an attic where I keep things. In my husband's photographic studio I have two enormous wardrobes ... full. I now have to become more disciplined and decide what to do. I don't throw things away unless they have become so banal. —— **You obviously like people as well as clothes. Are you attracted to people by the way they look?** By their appearance? No, not necessarily. I am attracted by a certain quality, or strength. I like people who have a marvellous manner, or marvellous conversation. —— **What do you like to do with your friends?** One thing, I like to do a lot, very much, which unfortunately, I have not done for a while, is to go to dance. And of course going to restaurants. Milan is very different from London. They go to the movies, but more often to restaurants. But I wish I could go to the dance all the time... Where do you go to dance? (There followed a discussion about London's trendier clubs, which led rather neatly onto the subject of Steve Strange, and then on to the subject of press, publicity and believing one's own press...) One has to be self-critical, to see things from the outside. Then if the reaction of people is good or bad it doesn't really matter because you know what you are doing. This kind of work – styling – is not like anything else, it is all based on the fantasy.

—— Do you enjoy styling other people as much as you do dressing yourself up? Yes I do. I've always liked dressing personalities or young actresses, especially if I have a certain knowledge of them. I like to do portraits, what were once called beauty shots, or even covers. This I like to do very, very much. —— **Do you think that people have become overly obsessed with style?** They are rather obsessed. —— **Do you think it's a good thing?** Within the fashion circle, yes, but I don't like people to be too right, to have all the right clothes on. This is a bit of an obsession. It also makes me dislike certain designers, for example Yohji Yamamoto, because they have become such a fad. He does beautiful things, but sometimes you see people, particularly some men, and all they do is exploit the names or labels. —— **The right name to wear at the right time?** Very much the right name. Milan is very conscious of this, and I hear it is breaking into London. —— **The way you mix clothes, is that very important to you? That kind of disrespect for clothes?** I have respect, but at the same time there has to be a good mixture. There has to be a touch of humour, to send up what one is wearing. —— **So that it doesn't look as though you are paying homage to the clothes by wearing them?** Yes, it looks more natural: simply a good find, or a pun. —— **So it has a freshness?** A freshness, yes. No I don't take myself seriously. One should always have good inventive pieces in the wardrobe, because they break the ice. They establish the thing on a personal level. There always has to be a kind of ironic style of humour. **Amongst all the things you have, is there one dress or one piece of clothing you could never do without?** More than clothes, little pieces of affection. This is a very tiny African bracelet which I could not live without. Things which I am totally fond of. More things that make a dress look different. An underskirt or a panier (a type of bustle), but dresses? I do repeat quite a lot. I don't dress differently every day. I do wear the same dress, as shown in the book, but I wear them in a different way. I have quiet a few old friends amongst my clothes. I almost never wear a thing which I have just bought. I always let them mature. I don't immediately put them on. Then all the time it is like making a new discovery in your wardrobe, which is very good. —— **When do you feel most comfortable?** At ease? Now more and more I am very happy early in the morning. Waking up and staying in bed and taking notes to re-establish myself, or making lists of things I have to do. Programming. On my own. It's very important to me to have these moments of deep concentration. —— **Do you think the fashion images being produced are still able to push barriers as you did? Constantly reassessing?** It is not very, very usual to see something really striking. In photographs, certain looks lose their impact because they have gone on too long. They become comfortable, they become classic, even. It is not usual to see something totally innovative. But it is always extremely refreshing. —— **Is there anything about yourself which you would like to change?** Physically? No, not at all. I've never been thinking this way. —— **Is there anything you would like to do which you have not done?** I don't think so. Honestly not. I am quite happy in my total abstraction. I am so abstract that I am happy.

BLITZ #52
April 1987

ANTONY PRICE
PRICE

The first time I saw Antony Price's name was on the credits of the first Roxy Music album. 'Clothes, hair and make-up – Antony Price.' From that moment I took passionate interest in plastic leopardskin (as worn by Bryan Ferry), Plaza (his futuristic King's Road store) and anything he designed.

The first time I saw Antony Price was over the petits pois in my local Waitrose. I followed him past the dairy products, through cereals, and right up to the check-out, but I didn't dare speak to him. Maybe he'd turn out to be real and it would spoil everything. Instead I hurried home and played *The In Crowd* over and over.

Antony Price put 'satin'n'tat' (as it was then known) on the cover of the first Roxy album and dressed Amanda Lear in a black satin sheath, pillbox and fishnets for the second one. He persuaded tens of thousands of aspiring matinée idols to dye their hair blue/black, and he it was who sold me my very first pair of 'Arsepants' – a peculiar pair of trousers which, by ingenious seaming, made your bottom look small and your balls look BIG.

In conversation, Antony Price is as dynamic as his designs. He is larger than life and lives in a world of theatrically draped curtains and blank venetian blinds which shut out reality along with the light. Price is extremely talkative, although a question is not always met with a straight answer, but instead a succession of thoughts which lead logically, if a little untidily, from one to the other. "Oh, I do go on", he will eventually say. And on and on. I hope.

——

Knowing that I was going to be talking with you, I dug out my old Roxy Music Fan Club newsletters, and in one there was a description of one of the tours, and I quote, 'So over to the adjacent Guildhall to see Antony Price running about with a mouthful of pins.' I can remember thinking when I first read that, 'Wow, this sounds so wonderful'. Was it really like that? Running around with a mouthful of pins? What was I doing? —— **It was when the Sirens joined Roxy.** Oh, that was great, because I was very much involved from day one. Bryan (Ferry) believes very much in his own ideas, and then allows embellishments by other people. I had been allowed to be pretty free with the women and how they looked. To have backing singers seemed to us very right. Casting people who could sing and look good was a nightmare because they were actually going on stage, and every night they didn't have a clue what to do with themselves, so I had to do make-up, their hair, and whatever. So I had to be there. So yes, I was there running around with a mouthful of pins, and yes, it was fun, and they were one of the first bands to insist on a non-squalid tour." —— **Were the cover girls like Amanda Lear and Jerry Hall your ideal women?** None of those things was ever exactly as I wanted to do it. I was much more over the top. Bryan has an eye for what is commercial, which is usually to add a gallon of water to whatever I want to do.

Well, you know we all refuse to add that gallon of water, and insist on the concentrated neat stuff, but to be commercial out there you need to add that gallon, and he would say, 'Tone, it's too over the top', or 'they're not going to get it'. He knew how much water to add. But I was allowed to do my military uniforms with the padded tits, they were real construction jobs. Real uniforms are really quite hideous. —— **Was it necessary to have those girls?** Yes, because he was already associated with that image. Bryan was always much more into fashion, and I was along with him. We were met with horror from the music business, who saw us as prissy, and horror from the fashion business, who saw us as sweaty rock, yet we get to the stage now where the best video is Robert Palmer's, which is purely Yvonne Gold make-up on model girls. So it's girls with our look doing their kind of dancing in the kind of dresses they would like, and the two things finally fuse together. Music is the one international message amongst young people. But fashion was very slow to accept that, and we fell very foul of it, it did us no favours. It's now there, and we blazed that bloody trail and it killed us to do it. It cost me a helluva lot of time and money, and the bed is now made for others to steam in. You were not around when we needed you. *BLITZ, The Face* and *i-D* were not there. You were all at college knowing that you wanted it, but where was it? How long has it taken? How far is television behind? How long before they have a television equivalent of your magazine? They do fashion now but it's all tongue in cheek, and let's have a laugh at it. It's almost Kenny Everett. But it's that good old English idea that design is something to laugh at – design is poofs with pencils and bits of fabric, and you laugh. In England you either get people who understand absolutely everything about design, and are the best on the face of the earth, or you get the most ignorant people. If you get ignorant British, you get really ignorant. The equivalent of ignorant English in Europe can at least speak four other languages. —— **Have you ever been tempted to go abroad?** To go abroad? Yes, we all know people who go abroad, and most are photographers and make-up artists and they carry their worldly goods in a case measuring three by four. How do you get six machinists, four cutting tables, 25,000 square feet of cutting space and whatever else you need on a Jumbo? It's very difficult to move your business if you want to stay in control. Otherwise you have to backed by somebody. All this crap about being backed, they are just giving you a wage. So what you actually do is sell your entire design rights for £300 a week. Big deal, and everybody reads in magazines how fab you are, and they've tied you down because the contract is so vile to get out of. —— **What happened with Plaza, was it a success?** An incredible success. The strong idea was this T-shirt which came out of a bag, and was the shape of a guy. It was that stretch fabric which always works. How do you think Azzedine did it? That's what made the money to finance the shop. I did this T-shirt which looked fabulous on the table, which is the way people buy them, like knickers. They don't try them on. So I put these flocked designs on the back and that's when they added the gallon of water, by not putting the flocking on. I had made the T-shirt purely as a thing on which to put the flocked designs, but for them the T-shirt was enough. And they sold absolutely millions. No magazine would photograph them because they were everywhere. The entire office staff at magazines were wearing them. In fact a lot of my clothes have been snubbed because of that, because they've been so horribly commercial. No one wanted to photograph them because, as you know, fashion magazines are incredibly snobby, and they want things that nobody else has got. —— **The Plaza shop was pretty uncommercial too.** I made it like a hamburger joint, where you point to a picture, then someone measures you, goes down, gets one, brings it up and you try it on in the changing room. It was perfect, they couldn't nick it. But again it was too early. They came in and asked, 'Where's the stock?' and would just leave. By the time they understood what a good idea it was, we'd closed. —— **What made you decide to open a shop on the corner of South Molton Street?** It's the position of it. It's right on the corner where all the cabs stop, and the one way system just gutters them in with all their money. I've had plenty of experience with the right stuff, wrong place, now I may venture to say right stuff, right place, wrong city, because everybody with any money is now spending a year abroad for tax reasons. —— **What do you think of your clothes?** I think everyone who buys my clothes has got a strange eye to notice things. My business manager says to me, 'Tone, you've done all the seaming and all they're buying is the bow on the back.' They could just as well buy any black dress with that bow on it and they wouldn't really know the difference. The trouble is that I know people who would know the difference, and I care about their opinions and we all end up in those clubs bitching to each other about those opinions, and that's what we all have in common because we all know we do notice those things. That's what ties us together, and I do care about their respect. But caring is a very expensive business, it costs you a lot of money. —— **Do you think you can sell glamour by the yard?** I don't think so, there's more to it than just putting the dress on, you've got to get the right shoes, and the rest of it. They've got to stand right in it. It's terrifying really, because we get little girls who come in who know exactly how to wear that dress, and would never dance around in it with their legs wide apart or would never get pissed, and would look fabulous, but they don't have the money! What can you do? —— **You haven't been taken that seriously by the grander ladies of the press. Do you think it's because of your rock and roll associations?** That's right, but I would like to say we're going to win in the end, aren't we, because I always knew that magazines like yours would come along, and that you would be the *Vogue* for young people. But the name *Vogue* still does mean everything. People who work in your business probably still do aspire to work for those magazines, which I find quite frightening, but then their power is so established. I think it would have been nice if they'd used my clothes, because I think they're incredibly photogenic, and photographers would love to take pictures of them but are not asked. —— **So have the associations been a bit of a cross to bear?** Absolutely. The Bryan Ferry thing lasted a long time. Everyone who could afford my clothes didn't want to be seen copying him. Then literally overnight every guy in every band was in the shop buying one of these suits because it was either that or Savile Row, because I was the young people's Savile Row. —— **Does press help?** Not really. When people see a picture in a magazine they don't notice it. OK, I hear stories from America of how they come running into a store holding a picture saying, 'I want this', but forget it in this country. I don't think we've ever sold a dress from something somebody saw in a magazine. What you really care about is if it's going to be a nice picture you can keep for yourself. They always get it wrong with me, it's always 'over the top, sexy clothes', and yet with Azzedine they got it right, they put the sexy clothes on great looking girls from Paris, instead of a Page Three horror. —— **Are the shows a necessity to you as a designer?** You will never be taken seriously by magazines unless they can come in and be part of that thing. It's part of the magazine snobbery, they like to be asked, and now that we've got back to little salon shows, they're actually thrilled to bits with it. I thought that when I did my Camden Palace show they'd enjoy being with the rest of the world but they hated it. With a show, at least you can style it up with the hats, the shoes and the music, but they're still probably not going to like it anyway, because it doesn't fit in with the look that they've decided to do. 'I'm doing sailor suits,' they say. 'Do you have any sailor suits?' No, nobody is doing sailor suits at all, but that's what she wants to do, and that's the way it is, and she's going to put it with anchors and guys in hats, and that's it, that's set in her mind, and 'sailor' it is. In the end she'll just take it in navy and white, so your whole look and everything is a complete waste of time. I've always said fashion shows should be for everybody, but now the smaller the shows are, the more honoured they feel and the more they'll kill to get in to see it. They feel ultimately exclusive and privileged to see it. I did the exact opposite by staging a show at the Camden Palace, invited the whole world, and made them pay... —— **What do you think of the way English fashion magazines are changing, the clean-machine Americanisation?** I see it as being hideously advantageous towards people like myself. I've heard stories of models being pulled off the front page and someone famous being put in their place in the same dress. Well, what can I say? If the picture is as good, and it's just another face and she's still in the same coat, why not? England is a very strange place. Snobbery here is on an unbelievable level. If you've got money in America and you're famous, nobody cares how you got it, even if you were a porn star, but here they can still throw it at you years later – 'Yes, but look what you did to get it'. Breeding and connections matter more here, but we've lost every single industry we had, and soon we'll lose the fashion industry as well. —— **Is there anyone you'd rather be?** It's that usual dreadful thing, which is I'd like to jump inside some great-looking 18-year old boy's body and take my mind with it. Who wouldn't? —— **Accepting that we're all going to age, do you think you have to become a character to retain people's attention?** We're living in London with all these fab people and mixing with all these fab people, and we are all a bit over the top. I mean, we've now got to the stage where most people we know are dressed in clothes that the public would never actually wear, and the public are putting on clothes to look like we used to look. And then there's me in my yellow thing with the shoulders, and I'm much resented by certain people for daring to look like that, but I think it's better that I look like that than to look like people like Ray Petri. They get annoyed that nobody recognises them, but it's difficult to recognise them when they are wearing clothes they've deliberately put on to hide themselves, in which they look like a slightly sophisticated football hooligan except for the minuscule detailing which you are meant to spot. But then that's the game isn't it? Spotting the things, and that's a look in itself.

There is an immense snobbery in obscurity. —— **So what makes you smile?** Having done loads of things first. I've got them there on video, but they all looked at it and ignored it. I believe you would have seen it, I believe you were there and saw it, but you weren't working on a magazine at the time. But they sat there and ignored it. Most of them didn't even go. They didn't even go...

BLITZ #52
April 1987

JASPER CONRAN
CONRAN

A couple of years ago, when international fashion was being turned upside down and inside out by the new stars of the British fashion circuit, one young man sent straightforward sheepskin jackets, classically striped wool shifts and sequins aplenty down his catwalk. Only a few seasons later those new stars seem to have burnt themselves out, whereas Jasper Conran is still dressing his models with a restraint (of cut and colour) which last season earned him the title Designer of the Year. Conran is only 27, and his snappy clothes and blonde mop of hair make him seem much younger. And yet it is his remarkably grown-up attitude to design which has pushed him to the forefront of British fashion, and which makes his clothes some of the most desirable, and saleable, on the market. Only recently an article in *Vogue* pronounced that he could well be our very own Calvin Klein or Karl Lagerfeld. Such praise is further reinforced by the endless list of high profile women who wear his designs, from the Princess of Wales to TV personalities like Paula Yates and Selina Scott. As a child, Conran had always drawn dresses and at sixteen he ran away to New York and enrolled himself on the fashion design course at the prestigious Parsons art school. Whilst in the United States he spent a time working for the flashy fashion company Fiorucci, but soon returned to England and designed a 'Special Label' collection for the more conservative Wallis company. In 1978 he presented his first independent label collection to press and buyers. They were unanimously impressed. Alongside the womenswear which had started to earn him a tremendous reputation for a quality and cool professionalism far beyond his years, he began to produce successful menswear and shoe ranges, to be joined later by a Jasper Conran line of lingerie. Last year he opened his own retail outlet in a smart Beauchamp Place which not only stocks the menswear and womenswear collections, but also furbishes the Conran fan with knitwear, shoes, tights and a whole host of accessories. This season, fearing overkill, Jasper Conran has taken a step backwards and will unveil his newest collection away from the spotlights in the calm of his elegant West End showroom. His own habitat, if you like...

——

How difficult is it having the name, the inherited 'Conran' tag? Do you know what's most difficult about it? The reason that I had to do this, had to design, was to get out of the situation of being the son of somebody. Because otherwise I'd just have been somebody's son for the rest of my life. So I had to be good, and I had to sell, and I had to make it, but my father didn't want me to do it so there was no money or anything forthcoming, and I didn't really want it. But the most difficult thing still is people's reaction to me, because there is still a general hate or loathing. I suppose it's a good excuse for other people, I don't know, I never did anybody any harm."

When you first appeared in the press you were sent up madly as Superboy, son of Superwoman Shirley. Yeah, how would you like that...? Even so, I've lived most of my life in adverse circumstances. I haven't lived this supposedly privileged life. So I think I'm very thick-skinned to ignore it. It's not that criticism doesn't hurt, it's just not going to do me in. Over the years I've seen a lot of people come and a lot of people go. I'm not going to allow myself to go with them as a result of that kind of criticism. —— **It's a bit like the sins of the father being visited on the son.** Well I don't believe that it has anything to do with a sin being perpetrated. I make clothes which sell, and I've never liked overly costumey clothes. I mean, when I first started I was one of the only day-wear designers. I don't like all that kind of kitschy business, I like real clothes, and I think I deal with reality. —— **Do you think your period in New York had anything to do with that, the American ideal of simplistic dressing?** No, I don't. I used to look at the Americans and loathe Calvin Klein's clothes. I loathed them. I thought they had nothing. The real reason why I did those clothes was because I wasn't going to fuel the fires by doing anything too outrageous, and that's how I've kept it for a long time. You know, I'm 27, I've got a few collections in front of me. I don't really care what people say because I've built up out of basically nothing, and that's exactly the way I wanted it to be. —— **So how did you find New York back then? And how did New York find you?** You wouldn't believe I was the same person. I think I'm the complete opposite now. I was quite bizarre, anybody would tell you that. I used to wear amazing outfits, I had some stunning ensembles. For me it was lovely because I'd been locked in boarding school since I was 7. I was working for Fiorucci, I was 16, a virgin, and for the first time in my life I could walk down the street and be totally myself, and free to do whatever I liked. It was a heady sensation, and it did indeed go to my head. They found me quite bizarre. —— **Did the work you were doing at the time echo what you were wearing?** It was much younger, what I was up to then, but I always looked at these fabulous outfits which had been so wild and fabulous last week and they would be defunct the next week. Fiorucci in New York at that time was like what Gaultier is today. It was fabulous, but, as I say, it was in and out, and I think that might have defined it all. All those rows of ruined disco boots... —— **And gold plastic trousers?** Oh God, I had the works. Yes, I used to stop traffic in my gold plastic trousers. —— **Was it always your intention to design?** Oh always, always, always. That's the only thing I've ever wanted to do. —— **How did your family react to that?** I didn't tell them until I went to New York, and then I got myself into Parsons and told my mother I wasn't coming back. I was always impressed by the designer image, as it were. You know, that thing that's fed to you, the glamourous lifestyle. I think it was that that appealed to me. Of course, had I known the truth... It's also a good form of mental torture, but yes, it's all I ever wanted to do. —— **Has it turned out the way you hoped it might?** I haven't finished yet. Let's wait and see. The trouble with being successful, especially at the moment, is that everybody is waiting for me to start getting grand on them. They're dying for it so they can tear me down. But there is only one way to combat venom, and that's to be better. It's my aim to do good work, and I think what I do, and the way the collection is perceived, is good, is done. —— **It must be difficult though,**

waiting for the press to turn on you like that. It's life. If you think, 'Fine, that's the way it's going to be', then it's a lot easier to deal with. Of course it's offensive, because it has no basis, but you put up with it. —— **In that case, would it be easier not to be quite so popular with the press as you are at the moment?** You've got to understand. There are three parts. The beginning, the middle and the end. The journalists are only the middle. The end is the person who puts the dosh on the table and buys the stuff. You can get very confused as to where you go. It's where Katharine (Hamnett) knows her business and Jean (Muir) knows her. You've got to keep the people who buy the clothes in mind because it's very easy to get hyped up in the direction of the press and go off. I work, I go home, I go to sleep, I go to work... I don't really give a toss what the press think as long as the whole process is working. People have been very nice to me, but I do have the feeling that they're going to stick their daggers in without me even having to give them a reason. I find that pretty wicked because it's only a journalistic ploy. —— **In that case, what importance do you give to the shows which are for the press of course as much as the buyers? I read that you sob 'real tears' backstage after a show...** Yes, you build up tension that you can't relieve. It's an involuntary act, you don't know why you're doing it. I think shows do bizarre things to you, which is why I don't really like that whole show thing because it blows everything up out of proportion. There may be three hundred important fashion people – press and buyers – in the world, and I don't see why I should do a show for a thousand. For what? I much prefer to do it here in my showroom where it can be controlled. I get a lot of 'Oh, the British Fashion Designer of the Year is not doing this', or 'So that's the way it is, is it?' Forget it, I almost wish they hadn't given the bloody thing to me.

—— **Does the title change anything?** Well, it's very pleasant. But I have never said I was the be all and end all of all creation. I'm working you know, and I learn every day. It's very nice, but it's just a statue. It doesn't have an international relevance, and what I am interested in is international relevance. —— **Do people perceive you differently because of it?** I can only see that they give me a really hard time because of it, that's all. I don't think anybody really intelligent does. —— **Don't you ever get scared?** Yes, I'm in a permanently scared situation. I've got thirty people's livelihoods to think about, apart from my own, and my dog's.

—— **Do you think it helps being scared? Do you use it to positively?** I do get incredibly wound up by whether something is the right thing to do. Doing a collection isn't sitting down and doing sixty drawings. There's the commercial side and there's the poetic. The two have to marry. If you only have the poetic, then however fabulous it is you're going to be bankrupt. I'm only just getting to the point where I'm allowing myself to indulge, and I only do that after I've done the hard-core selling part. It is a business. When I get really frightened, and I think I can't do this anymore, for about five minutes my courage fails. Then I think, 'Oh yes, fine, but what are you going to do instead?' And then I paint a life of grey misery for myself, and I decide it's not quite as bad as it could be. I think the problem is that I set myself a higher standard all the time. It's difficult to get objective about it because I'm on top of it all and have no perspective. You can only do that if you go away and come back to it. —— **Do you travel?** Yes, but I can't really be

away from here for too long, otherwise all sorts of things happen. —— **Does your travelling usually relate to work?** I don't like to travel for work anymore. It ruins the rest of the world for you. I think you have to be very careful of that. You start to think, 'Oh yeah, I'll go to Japan, and then I'll go to New York, and then I'll go to Tokyo and stopover in Paris on the way back, then I'll have five minutes back home, then I'll go off again'. It sounds glamorous but it's a horrible thing to do, really ugly. So now I'll only travel for pleasure. I haven't been away for a year, so after the collection I'll try and go somewhere new. I want to go to Jamaica. —— **Does the fact that you are constantly considering how to dress other people make you look at yourself in a different way?** I don't think of dressing others at all, I think of clothes as a 3D object and I also think 'Would I wear that? Would I spend that kind of money on it?' It's got to be something you'd wear again and again and again. I like clothes that work and are going to last you a long time. Because that's where I come from. I would never buy some designers' clothes. Katharine Hamnett's are working designer's clothes. I've never said I make 'Fashion'. For me, there's a strong differentiation between what I do, and Fashion. Fashion is something which is here today and gone tomorrow, by definition. That's not what I want to do. —— **Do you have a specific design ethic?** I think I'm working on an ethic. I don't think I've necessarily got it yet. I'm not rigid enough, probably. I wouldn't say never to an idea or an approach because, the next thing you know, you find yourself suddenly doing it, doing everything you thought you'd never do. I use unnatural fibres. I use zips. I even use buttons... —— **So anything's possible?** Well, I've never used velcro yet. But why not?

—— **People talk of your work having a consistency. Where do you think that came from?** My work should follow on from what I've done before. Consistent implies that it doesn't get better, and I think it does get better. I just want to do my business and work and get on with it. I think there is too much of that 'I'm the most wonderful designer, you must watch my show.' People can come and watch my show if they want, but if they don't want to they don't have to. There's never enough time to get everything you want done. There's so much work in getting a collection together, it's outrageous. But I'd hate to be a little dressmaker, working to one-off commissions.

—— **Don't you think that by making your show more exclusive...** You said that. I didn't. You said that. —— **...Anyway, don't you think it will make people want to get it even more?** Would they? No, of course I'm not doing it for those reasons. I've always been absolutely terrified of doing those big shows and I wake up in the middle of the night, and I get so wound up. I don't want to live that kind of life, there's more to it than that. Not a lot, but there is more. —— **So how long is your day?** I'm here at nine and I work till eight. Sometimes till eleven. —— **Do you ever shut off when you're not here?** There is a continual questioning of yourself. —— **So when do you know when to stop? When do you know when a collection is finished?** It somehow has its natural ending. I work very differently to most people. I just make clothes and then I put them together, that's another reason I found those big shows vile to do because they didn't have a natural flow. You know, you'd send out eight blue dresses at once for effect. Ridiculous rubbish. It's fine as theatre, but it has no relevance. Watching the Saint Laurent show in Paris was really good because I saw a different

way of doing things. One person at a time, which is what we did for the end of our show last season, and that's how you perceive a person walking down the street. —— **You mentioned to me that you've bought a dog. What was the reason?** I found that I was going home to nothing after a life here where I must answer ninety questions a minute, and then I'd go home and there was zero. —— **Isn't there anyone to go home to?** I don't know that I want anyone else to go home to. No, it's not that I don't want anybody, but I get so wound up that it's not really fair to ask someone to understand that. I'm in another world and I can't give of myself. I can't, it's not possible, so I thought a nice dumb animal, doesn't answer back, doesn't eat lots ... but it's so much fucking work.

—— **Whether you like it or not, people compare you with Calvin Klein in America and Armani in Italy. What do you think of that comparison?** I think saying that is a journalistic easy solution. I don't think it's looking at the thing at all. I very much avoided marketing myself, as it were. I kept myself open. I don't do Russian collections, or Hawaiian grass skirt collections, I make clothes. I think there's cheap thrill clothes and there's the other. I think it's too simple to say, 'Oh he's the so-and-so of England'. Listen, Calvin Klein is a very rich man, so's Armani. I'm saying nothing. I don't think there is any real comparison to be made, because it assumes that I am making a statement. I haven't made any statements. I put things into the collection which are not serious at all. There are little messages in the collection, you know. It's not dry or as well thought-out as Calvin Klein. —— **Are you forced financially to include things you would rather not?** Sometimes. Not particularly, but it's difficult because you do have to make money. If I told you how many frilled bubble skirts sold against how many crepe de chine dresses... —— **With hindsight, seeing what does and does not sell, would you still develop something which doesn't sell if you thought it was right?** Oh, yes, a great deal of thought does go into what I do. I don't just do a collection. I really, *really* think it out, and everything on the catwalk you can buy, which is not really the case with most people. It's just that there are those which are definitely going to sell – and I could tell you which ones, and tell you how many they will sell – and those that won't. But doing both is the right thing to do, because one will pay for the other, and that's how I approach everything. —— **While we're talking dirty, how much are you worth?** What I am worth is totally academic as to what I will be worth. —— **And will you go into licensing your name?** We're talking Italian. I will drop a bomb on this country like you won't believe.

—— **What do you think of the British Fashion Industry?** I wish it would regard itself as a real fucking industry. It still has its bar mitzvah side, which I can't bear. I won't say who, and I won't say what, but the trouble is, anyone can go out there and say 'I'm a fashion designer', and it's not good for how we are perceived in general as a country, which is still as a nice little cottage knitwear industry because there is no base of manufacture. —— **We tend to go in and out of fashion as a country.** That's because we let it happen. We offer a diversion whilst their palates are jaded with Milan and Paris. We offer somewhere for them to pick up ideas. This is what I've been trying to fight for a long time. People thought they were going to be international stars overnight and they weren't. There's no such thing. It's ridiculous to assume that's going to happen – it's easy come, easy go. —— **When all is said and done, do you think you're the same Jasper Conran who used to make dresses for his friends and relatives?** Mmm, I think so. I'm a lot more distracted now than I used to be. Yes, I am definitely, I'm possibly a nicer person. —— **So are you happy?** Not necessarily, but I should be so lucky. Who's happy? What is happy? —— **Do you stand by what you have done, instead of wishing you'd taken a different route?** Yes, yes. I've never directly worked for my father. —— **Has it ever occurred to you over the years to change your name?** It's a fucking good name. A really good name. I wouldn't dream of changing my name because that would be more hypocritical than anything. That would be being beaten.

BLITZ #56
August 1987

FRANCO MOSCHINO
IL CATTIVO

Franco Moschino is the 'bad boy' of Italian Fashion

—

When did your career in fashion begin? Almost ten, twelve years ago. Maybe fifteen. I'm getting old. Yeah, I think fifteen years ago. The main reason I started designing was because I'd always been interested in becoming a painter or designer – mostly an illustrator or painter. So I went to the painting academy in Milan, the Brera, for three, four years, because I was interested in learning how to design the body, which is my favourite object to design. The fastest and easiest way to make money was to try with fashion. I had a lot of friends – models or pattern makers, you know, technicians in fashion – who introduced me into the fashion business, and I worked for different little designers. Then, Gianni Versace saw my sketches, by accident, and he asked me to illustrate his collection. This was 1972 or '73. The only thing was that my way of designing was very academic – you know, big woman, Michelangelo – so I had to change it, to transform it into the fashion approach – tall, skinny, lots of attitude. So I went to a little fashion school for a month, and changed my way of designing. Gianni liked it and he gave me all his publicity to advertise instead of taking pictures. But I never wanted to become a couturier at all. I think I would be a better photographer than a fashion designer, because I don't really care about the fabric. This is cashmere, wool, acrylic – it's fine! Of course, it's fun creating, but creating doesn't mean anything anymore. Issey Miyake may be a great creator, or perhaps Balenciaga or somebody in the past. But I don't think we have creators now because we can't create anything. The only thing we can do is to make little commercial changes on very usual, normal clothes. I mean, if I had to change that jacket, I might design the pocket a little lower, but this is not creation, only alteration. —— **So your philosophy of fashion very strongly guides what you do?** Yeah, in fact, you can tell very easily that I'm not a fashion designer because my fashion philosophy is not commercial. I say you can wear whatever you want. If you want to go to the theatre like that, well, go – it's up to you. If you want to go in tuxedo with black tie, and that's how you feel comfortable, then that's the best outfit. Of course I have to give suggestions, but they are merely suggestions, nothing more. —— **Has there been more freedom in fashion recently, or has it been developing gradually?** I think that fashion is the slowest element in our society to evolve. It cannot be compared with anything. Compare fashion with music, which has really evolved. Look at a fashion magazine today and one from ten to twenty years ago and you'll notice a lot of changes but with music, it differs from yesterday, last month, last year. I mean, it's changing so much, where fashion is not. Also, fashion is directed by couturiers who are only regular tailors. They don't have intellectual minds. They are very good at choosing and working with most delicate and

sophisticated fabrics but most of them don't use their brains that much. That's why fashion is so slow to develop. —— **You have been called the Italian 'bad boy'. What do you think of Gaultier?** I'm often compared with Gaultier in Italy, but I think that it's a most absurd comparison because the only thing Gaultier and I have in common is we both make jokes about fashion. About Gaultier, I say thank God we have Gaultier. I would have had such a hard time if he hadn't been that strong and powerful, even if he is in Paris. He helped me a lot, giving people a more relaxed, more funny, more ironic point of view in fashion – like his last show, for instance. He creates fashion in a very avant garde way, very new, very now, so I like him. It doesn't mean I like 100 percent of what he does, but the things I like, I adore. —— **What was it like to work for Versace?** I have to be very careful here. Versace is ... well, let me give you an example. Once he told me, 'I have this fabric to use, what would you do with it?' You see, during the last two years of our four-year collaboration, Gianni kept encouraging me to become an accomplice in the designer aspect of the job, not only the illustrator, and I accepted because, you know, he was there, he was already very well known at that period, so I was kind of safe. So, when he asked me once what I'd do with this fabric – a piece of white jersey – I took it home, and the first thing I thought about was to look at the way old Roman or Grecian ladies were dressed. So I designed using my knowledge of art history, which I had learned at the painting academy, and I kept at it until I had designed lots of these kind of things. I brought all the sketches to him and he said, 'Oh, this is great, but I will never sell one of these.' I said, 'I'm sorry, but this is the only thing that came to mind.' Well, he used those sketches and really killed them. He deformed them, he made them very easy, very commercial. He took a very uncommercial style and was clever enough to make it extremely commercial. —— **Did they sell?** Oh, yeah, like hell. I mean he has been working on that style for years. My suggestion would have been a real nothing if he hadn't used that knowledge about what is or is not commercial. He's not a fashion designer, no – he's more a house designer, a commercial designer. But he's not a creator, he's not an Issey Miyake. That's God, for me. Gianni still has this big power, he really knows very well what women want, how they want to look, as much as Valentino. For me, it's boring, it's all the same stuff, but this is what they want. So, congratulations. —— **Besides Miyake and Gaultier, are there other designers you admire? Do you get inspiration from other sources?** Well, Miyake is really over the top, in a good sense. There are many designers I like a lot: Lagerfeld, sometimes; Vivienne Westwood is very close to Miyake for me; in America, I think Zoran is the last designer to create strong emotions in fashion. Stephen Sprouse has been very, very exciting and interesting. Thinking about Paris, I think that Christain Lacroix is really extremely good – he has such a deep knowledge about fabrics, you know, the technical aspects of building a dress, which is very important. I think my favourites are not fashion designers. Levi's is my favourite designer in the world. —— **What gave you the idea to design ballroom gowns in denim?** Evening gowns have been designed for centuries, and I'd say the last most exciting, modern ones were from the fifties, so I took a very classic, basic Rita Hayworth gown from Gilda and instead of doing it in silky taffeta,

I used denim. A basic fabric with a basic shape. The only thing was the way it was put together and this made it weird, interesting, commercial, whatever. People said it was odd. All this belongs to my concept of fashion, it all seems to be very logical and it is, but I have to include another aspect, which is the mysticism of fashion. I think that people need to have a little part of a dream or hope about a dress. We've all, maybe without realising, searched for something different through a garment that we don't own or have the money for. So it's a dream. I don't condemn a woman who wishes for a Valentino evening dress or an Oscar de la Renta full of ruffles and gold embroidery. Sometime in her life she probably has the right to wish to be a princess. —— **Do the people who have the money to buy Valentino or de la Renta see fashion as a mystique?** More money, less mysticism. No money, lots of mysticism. That's very banal I know, and I'm not the first person to say that. But I don't think the rich lady from Milano walking down via della Spiga, going inside of every store to see what's new, has an ounce of mysticism in her brain. But this woman walking down via della Spiga, rue Faubourg St Honoré or Madison Avenue, she does have her way of dreaming – for instance, if she goes inside of Gaultier's store and say's, 'I want to look like one of those tall, hard, sexy models of Gaultier' and she's fat, she's dreaming ... except she can buy it, so it's not a dream. —— **How much do you get involved with you advertising?** I do it all. I'm very proud of it. That's why, as I said earlier, I think, I'd make a better fashion editor or photographer or movie director than designer. When all the clothes arrive in this room and we put them together for a fashion show, I don't see the clothes anymore, I see the way the show has to be, as a theatre director. So I am more into choosing the right actress, if you like, for making those objects live. This is the fun aspect, this is what I like to do. —— **The fashion shows are a lot of fun. Are they a good selling point for you?** Yeah. We really build an image completely from nothing. The Moschino campaigns and the other ones from Cadette have all been done with a regular photographer, not Meisel, Avedon or whoever. This is because I was trying to build with Babic, my photographer – I love him, he's one of my friends, but he knows very well I'll be sitting on his shoulder and saying 'That's the wrong light, no, she has to move...' I always make the picture, the only thing is I can't hold a camera – I always break it. But the trademark has been designed, the whole visual aspect and image has been chosen, designed, thought out and so on by me. —— **I remember an article from 1983, when you started Moschino, and of the designers mentioned you are the only one still around. How favourable has the press been to you?** Well to tell you the truth, Italian and international opinion of us is not terribly high and the press has not been Moschino's friend, but they are probably right. Fashion does not have to be intellectual – clothing can be fun, nice, expensive, I don't care, I look great. Gaultier? Buy, buy, buy. They like that aspect of fashion, but I am less interested in that. I think it's very stupid to think about fashion in that way, so I insist very much on being very intellectual on the social aspect. And journalists, even newspaper journalists who should be more intellectual ones – the ones who know what is going to be news all over the world – become very stupid when they work in fashion. So we're not very good friends. Sometimes they've written good things about me, but it's like little

drops here, little drops there. —— **Are you gaining more acceptance or are you retaining your 'bad boy' image?** In the beginning, when they call me 'bad boy' I was a bad boy. At this point we were selling more, we were more popular. It became fashionable – our label sells because I'm a bad boy. So if I wear a regualar suit, they say, "what are you doing like that? Wear your leather jacket. Are you a bad boy or what?" So I play bad boy. I go dancing with my friends, I go to parties. I've always had the same uniform – sometimes I should change it, but at this point I can't change it anymore. The bourgeois of fashion, they want me a bad boy – it makes money, it makes news, they find a name for me. It's good for me, but I don't think I'm a bad boy in a real sense. I think I cry very easily ... sensitive is such a horrible word. Human, yeah. I'm very human. I hate violence and all that stuff. Leather jackets, things like this – I like to play it because it's fun, and it's very comfortable. You can do anything you want. —— **How do you relax?** I stay at home, smoke a cigarette, watch my cat. But I don't have any hobbies; I don't have a particular kind of music, I don't go to the movies, I can't concentrate on reading. I used to like dancing very much. I hate sports. I'm fat. I've belonged to a gym for ten years and every year I keep renewing it – I go for a couple of weeks and then I stop because I'm always away. I'm really not lazy, just very busy. I would like to go to the gym, not because I want to look like Arnold Schwarzenegger, but at the moment if I took my clothes off and compared myself with a model, I would kill myself. —— **The Americanisation of fashion is a recent trend that has been developing. Do you feel you have had anything to do with getting Italian people to use more denim and leather?** Yeah, I think I have. But I also think it is because Italians have been like that since the Roman Empire. For its geographic position in Europe, Italy is right in the middle of everything, so that's why Italians are so different, so crazy. There are many different aspects. You can't compare an Italian with another, in the good or the bad sense. So of course the food, the music, the architecture, everything has always been mixed. And the same thing happens with fashion now. You see how many burgers there are around here? It's ridiculous! The food in Italy is amongst the best in the world, and we are eating hamburgers? And then they are horrible! Hamburgers are great in New York, but here they are horrible! That's Italy. But I think America is involved in every nation, even Russia is trying to be American. It's the way of being right now. It is the modernisation of everything, so of course Italy, which is very sensitive to absorbing foreign new stuff, especially since the last war, is easy to Americanise. —— **Would you think of doing anything else besides fashion designing?** As much as I mature, as much as I go on, I realise this is more and more impossible. But I want to. Fortunately I found this social human aspect of fashion that makes it living. But yeah, I would like to be a movie director – in fact, that's the only thing I've tried, editing the videos of my shows. And I like to do it, watch it, to do them again. I think that would be a job for me. However, I don't know if I will ever be able to find people good enough to run the company by themselves. —— **Are there any Italian designers who are going to follow in your footsteps, pushing things even further than Moschino?** No. Fortunately or unfortunately, no. I think it would shock me less to see people on the street going much further than fashion designers. The fashion designers, they think

fashion – they're not open at all. Even the young ones, they try to be Yamamoto, they try to be Romeo Gigli, Armani, whatever. They don't realise why people wear, buy, need clothes. They don't think about it. And that's why they don't follow me. They say, 'Fashion? OK, black, that's been done last year. Let's do ... pink.' That's it. It's too bad. I mean, to understand what I just told you, you don't have to be so intense. It's easy. It's obvious.

* This interview was originally credited to Iain R. Webb/Wong.

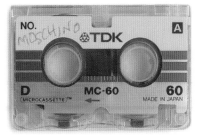

CONTRIBUTORS

MARC ASCOLI — still continues to be one of fashion's most influential art directors. His work with Yohji Yamamoto in the 1980s changed the visual/marketing landscape. He has also collaborated with Jil Sander, Chloé, Cerruti and Hugo Boss. He is married to Martine Sitbon and is image director for her Rue du Mail label.

PETER ASHWORTH — achieved notoriety when Mari Wilson sang that, 'an Ashworth snap' was all she ever wanted. Having snapped pop royalty – Eurythmics, Soft Cell, Visage, Bananarama, Grace Jones, Tina Turner, Adam Ant – he still delights in taking photographs. Latest projects include exhibitions of style icons Annie Lennox, Stephen Jones and Leigh Bowery. He is currently shooting fashion editorial and compiling his archive online.

RACHEL AUBURN — went on to become a 'hard house' DJ and dance music producer right through the nineties. She has one lovely son, Jack, and now lives in west London, teaching yoga and generally being arty.

MARTINE BARONTI — is an art director. She loves to write. She is looking for editors to publish her Mooks (magazine meets book). She now lives in Sète, South of France, where she designs costumes for theatre, festival and musical shows.

ERIC BERGÈRE — left Hermès to work for a variety of fashion labels in Italy and Japan. Today he is a fashion consultant for a range of brands in Italy, Japan and France.

PAUL BERNSTOCK — continues to work with Thelma Speirs at Bernstock Speirs. 2012 marks the label's 30th anniversary. He still lives and works in Shoreditch, east London.

DARRYL BLACK — is still creating OOAK up-cycled clothing eighteen years after setting up business at Portobello Market. Her clothing is available at www.etsy.com She lives in Brighton with her teenage son.

MANOLO BLAHNIK — has earned the reputation as premier shoemaker; his magical shoes known simply as 'Manolos'. His influence and inspiration has captivated fans worldwide. He has been the focus of a solo exhibition at the Design Museum and a storyline in *Sex & The City*. In 2007 he was awarded a CBE. He lives between London and Bath.

ALISTAIR BLAIR — has worked in the fashion industry since leaving St Martins in 1978. Alongside his own label and stints at Laura Ashley and Louis Féraud he has assisted all the glamorous greats including Valentino Garavani, Karl Lagerfeld, Hubert de Givenchy, Nino Cerruti

and Marc Bohan at Dior. He is still creating gorgeous couture gowns.

JUDY BLAME — is still the troublemaker, sewing and styling his way in and out of fashion. Always inspired and individual. No job big enough, no task too small!

SALLY BOON MATTHEWS — is a mixed media artist living in New York City. Her love of photography remains unabated and she teaches at The City University of New York. In her spare time she drinks High Mountain Oolong tea, writes a food blog and plans her next trip to Asia.

HAMISH BOWLES — is American *Vogue's* peripatetic International Editor at large, curator, professor, Best Dressed Hall of Famer, and collector of haute couture. He lives in Manhattan but travels the world reporting on all things stylish. Other assignments have included Outdoor Survival School in Southern Utah, auditioning for *X Factor* and playing basketball with New York Knicks' Amare Stoudemire.

DEAN BRIGHT — has designed for David Bowie, Boy George, Grace Jones and Erasure. He has collaborated with Barbara Hulanicki and Donald Urquhart and created costumes for Glenn Close. He is still taking private commissions.

CAROL BROWN (LANGBRIDGE) — is happily and successfully still working as a make-up artist, living in London, married to Sam.

PETER WESLEY BROWN – moved to Beverly Hills, California in the early 1990s. He is still taking photographs although the emphasis has shifted to the luxury travel and lifestyle market. Brown can now be found, dry Martini in hand, on glorious beaches, resorts and private homes around the globe.

SAM BROWN — still lives in London; no longer working as a photographer, he makes bespoke furniture and is developing a range of gentlemen's valets in the hope of making that elusive first million.

DEBBIE BUNN — launched the vintage inspired kids clothing label Bunny London in 1999, which she ran for seven years. She is currently involved in restoring her beloved Datsun 280ZX, is volunteer PR for the UK Z Club and is a recently appointed media spokesperson for Alzheimer's Research UK. She lives in Battersea with her small hairy dog, Archie.

GILLIAN CAMPBELL — lives in the mountains of Southern Portugal with Bert her Great Dane. She continues to work in the photography industry, working with three friends producing large, archival giclée prints. (www.gicleeportugal.com) and has an online shop selling giclée images (theimagelocker.com)

SCARLETT CANNON — is a glamorous gardener. She lives in London, where she grows vegetables, takes photographs, wears lipstick and bakes bread. With an innate understanding of the healing power of the earth, she works as a horticultural tutor, food-growing consultant, garden writer and healing therapist.

AMANDA CAZALET — now lives with her husband Chris as a member of a community offering education in sustainability and nature connection in north east Scotland.

PALLAS CITROEN — lives in Islington with her rather gorgeous thirteen-year-old daughter India Bluebell. She is an artist specialising in sculpture, installation and performance. Her latest aim is to walk to Rio de Janeiro by 2016, get a studio on the beach and a pet horse, and live happily ever after.

JASPER CONRAN — *still* designs collections twice a year as well as working with Wedgwood, Waterford and Debenhams. He is now also the chairman and chief creative director of the Conran shops. He lives in London and Wiltshire with several dogs.

LOUISE CONSTAD — works as a fashion make-up artist in film, TV and editorial. She consults with make-up companies like MAX FACTOR and clients including Tina Turner, Kristin Scott Thomas and Helena Bonham Carter. She runs her own make-up school and lectures at top London colleges. She lives happily in Paddington, London, with her artist boyfriend.

DAVID CONVY — moved to Hamburg at the end of the '80s and carved out a career as a DJ. He returned to London and the modelling industry in the mid-90s, this time as an agent with Models 1, and has been there ever since. He lives in South London.

STEPHANIE COOPER — worked in Italy and Japan before setting up a design studio in Shoreditch, before it became trendy. She now works on Design Consultancy projects, custom-made clothing and lectures at Central Saint Martins. She recently fulfilled two lifelong ambitions: designing for music icon Annie Lennox and exhibiting the frock at the V&A. She lives in Notting Hill borders, before it becomes trendy, with her astonishing fourteen-year-old daughter.

MICHAEL COSTIFF — has lived in the same flat in west London since 1972. He now has three shops in Beijing, Tokyo and Dover Street Market. 'It's much the same vibe but just more expensive.' He has been a muse for Rei Kawakubo.

MARIA CORNEJO — lives in Brooklyn. She is creative director of Zero+ Maria Cornejo NY, founded in 1998 and has three stores in New York. In 2006 she won the prestigious Cooper Hewit National Design Award. She is married to artist/photographer Mark Borthwick and is mother of Bibi, twenty-one, and Joey, fifteen.

PAUL COSTER — is still modelling at Select Model Management, although acting is starting to become his main job and love. He is not married but hopes to be very soon to his sweetheart girlfriend.

RICHARD CROFT — lives in France and continues adding to the list of destinations he has photographed. Combining his passion for both photography and travel has presented many exciting challenges, not least of which is the ongoing desire for a better understanding of composition light and colour.

MONICA CURTIN — is still taking pictures, and has had solo shows in London and Portugal. 'Commentaries on Living' at the Centro de Artes in Sines, Portugal, also included other work using textiles, paper and found stuff. She has a twenty-two-year-old daughter and a garden where she would spend all her time pottering if she could.

MICHAEL DAKS — is now Senior Lecturer in Fashion Photography at Southampton Solent University. He is also Director of Photography for 5thcharacter.com, a new online fashion and fine art magazine, and a Contributing Director for xxxxmagazine.com. He is currently working on two book projects: *Just Good Friends*, photographs of his friends naked, and *In Hindsight*, a 30-year retrospective of his landscape photographs.

DEBBIE DANNELL — has toured with music artists including Dusty Springfield, Morrissey and Elton John. She now works mostly in television as a make-up designer but still gets booked for 'odd' jobs like the sports presentation for the 2012 Olympics and collaborating with performance artist Linder Sterling and photographer Tim Walker on *The Dark Town Cakewalk*.

GREGORY DAVIS — spent the tail end of the '80s and early '90s in Barcelona living as a make-up artist. In 1991 he returned to London. After working as an art director he joined Models 1 in 1996, where he is now head booker of women. He lives in stylish Dalston.

TAMZIN DAVIS — lives in East London with her partner and son. On finishing school, she escaped to agricultural college in Devon and has since been managing nature reserves in London, Essex and Hertfordshire. More recently, she has been working in Ecology Consultancy.

ANN DEMEULEMEESTER — is still married, still lives in Antwerp and still designs six collections a year.

RONALD DILTOER — lives in Norwich. He is still a photographer, concentrating mainly on real people photography (family and children's portraiture), the occasional wedding (friends only) and in truth anything that people want him to photograph.

CHRISTIAN DINH — moved to Los Angeles after twenty years in NYC. Although he feels fashion photography has changed considerably during the last fifteen years, and is now an over crowded industry, he still does a gig from time to time. Today he focuses on writing, producing, directing TV shows, movie and documentaries (reality and scripted).

SIMON DOONAN — is a writer and the Creative Ambassador for Barneys New York. During his long career in fashion he is best known for his innovative window displays. He has written five books and regularly pens a column for SLATE.com.

ANITA EVAGORA — spent 28 years running Fred Bare (the headwear company). She has now returned to her first love, and 'mucks around with clay' — before the arthritis sets in'. She lives in York, Yorkshire, with her painter husband and two teenagers whom she frequently orders to 'turn that music up!'

NICK FERRAND — moved to Milan and worked for Condé Nast. He returned to London in 1993 with wife Margherita Gardella and started an interior and architectural design company, Domusnova, which developed into a real estate company in Notting Hill. In 2004 he sold everything and returned to Italy. He now lives in Umbria and restores beautiful Italian villas and castles for beautiful people.

KEN FLANAGAN — has been married twice and is now separated. He has a wonderful eleven-year-old daughter, Edie, and lives in west London. He now works in documentaries and information art as a director, producer, editor and composer.

PRINCESS JULIA (FODOR) — lists her 'expressive outlets' as *GQ Style* (Senior Contributing Editor) and *i-D* (Music Editor). Writing, interviewing and getting involved with facets that cross over into fashion, personal style, music and art. She has been part of London's creative scene for over 30 years. She continues to DJ at various events and parties around the world.

SIMON FOXTON — lives in west London with his long-time partner, Donald. He is still working as a stylist/art director/creative consultant. In 2009 he had a solo exhibition of work, 'When You're A Boy' at The Photographers' Gallery. He is Visiting Professor in Menswear at the RCA and an allotment holder.

CARYN FRANKLIN — went from Fashion Editor and Co-editor of i-D to prime-time TV fashion expert, writer, educator and activist. She has co-chaired the award-winning 'Fashion Targets Breast Cancer' for seventeen years and co-founded the award winning 'All Walks Beyond the Catwalk' to broaden body and beauty ideals. She still writes for *i-D* and still wears her Westwood bondage strides from time to time.

LYNNE FRANKS — has spent the last twenty years working on the empowerment of women, founding SEED learning programmes teaching women how to do business using the feminine principles, based on her book *The SEED Handbook*. She opened a group of women's business clubs called B.Hive with Regus. She lives between Sussex, Mallorca and London and has four beautiful grandchildren.

JEAN PAUL GAULTIER — still designs in Paris. In 1997 he opened an haute couture atelier and shocked the world with ballgowns made from denim and plastic. He has designed for film and opera and been a TV presenter. In 1988 he recorded a rap song, *How To Do That*, and his exhibition, 'The Fashion World of Jean Paul Gaultier: From Sidewalk to the Catwalk' pushes the boundaries of museum display.

GEORGINA GODLEY — has worked as a creative director in fashion, interiors, home accessories and luxury branding, in that order. She is now Director of Creative Enterprise at Higher and Higher, London and Sao Paulo, a creative agency founded by Mario Testino. She is divorced, and has two sons living at home in north London.

ZIGGI GOLDING — is a photographers' agent representing a small group of brilliant photographers within the art and commercial world, each with their own career. In the 1990s and early 2000s she lived in New York with her husband and two children, experiencing September 11th first hand. Now divorced, she lives and works in Berkshire.

KATHARINE HAMNETT — is still creative director of her label. In 1985 she launched *TOMORROW*, the short-lived magazine that mixed fashion and politics. She was awarded a CBE in 2011 and continues to use her iconic slogan T-shirts as placards for her political and ethical principles.

RICK HAYLOR — is an extrovert photographer and former creative director of Vidal Sassoon. He now lives in Brooklyn, married to a drop-dead gorgeous wife, a father of two artsy daughters and a gay fox terrier. When not taking pictures he loves to cycle, watch films, and dance to reggae.

JANE HILTON — works as a documentary filmmaker and photographer. She spends a lot of time in the American West, has published a book on cowboys, and another on working girls in Nevada is due next year. She lives in London, happily married to Nick and they have an eighteen-month-old little cowboy.

DAVID HISCOCK — turned his back on the UK commercial photographic and art scene, where he was a stalwart for the last 25 years, to take his wife and son to tropical climes, having heard the siren call from his early days spent in the Sculpture Department at St Martin's School of Art. He has been creating a series of commissioned monumental sculptural works in South East Asia ever since.

PAM HOGG — is a designer, rockstar, DJ and artist who infiltrated the elitist ranks of the conventional fashion world in the 1980s with her self-taught wild brand of outrageous fashion. In 1991, she appeared on Terry Wogan's BBC chat show as 'one of the most original, inventive, creative designers in Britain'. In 2009 she received a lifetime achievement award from the Scottish Fashion Council. Today she continues to excite and inspire with clients who include Siouxsie Sioux, Kate Moss, Kylie and Rihanna.

DAVID HOLAH — went back to Art College and in 2006 obtained an MA in printmaking at Camberwell Colege of Art. He now makes art prints using traditional printmaking methods. Along with Stevie Stewart, he is curating the Bodymap archive. In 2011 the pair were invited by the Museo de Moda in Santiago Chile to exhibit in a show called 'Volver a las '80s' and more recently were part of 'SPORT & FASHION' at Fashion Museum, Bath. A Bodymap book is planned.

BARBARA HORSPOOL — is still obsessed with fashion after varied design roles across the industry. Currently she is creative director for Jigsaw and continues to be inspired by her teams of passionate designers and stylists, who paint the future and envy her past. She lives in Camden with three amazing children who only want to write, dance, model and design.

MARTINE HOUGHTON — went on to study photography, working with Michael Roberts, Mario Testino, Paolo Roversi and Lucien Hervé. Following a brief flirtation with fashion photography, she now lives and works as a photographer of interiors and still life in Paris with her cellist boyfriend and twin sons.

KIM JACOB — has been married for nineteen years to Simon Godfrey who she met while nightclubbing in the '80s. They have two children, Oliver (eighteen years) and Alice (thirteen years). She has just launched a cosmetic range, Wild About Beauty, with business partner Louise Redknapp and is still working as a make-up artist in London and still loving it.

MARC JACOBS — is one of fashion's most influential practioners. In 1997 he joined Louis Vuitton as Artistic Director. His collaborations with artists are legendary. During his career he has won nine prestigious CDFA awards, including the Geoffrey Beene Lifetime Achievement Award in 2011. He lives between New York and Paris.

STEPHEN JONES — is a milliner who makes fancy hats for even fancier clients. Based in Covent Garden he travels the world to create his own and other designer collections. He has many other part time jobs, such as curating at the V&A, Headonism, mentoring other milliners, and working as a Professor at Central Saint Martins.

BARRY KAMEN – artist, stylist, maker of images, continues to live and work in London in a beautiful house, with a beautiful wife.

CHAZZ KHAN — is a tennis coach at the Chelsea Harbour Club. As a nationally ranked player he reached #20 GB. He still plays at the Wimbledon Seniors event. He has written a book, *The Divorced Man's Survival Manual*, lives in London and collects interesting old mobile phones. He is still modelling but is now on the classic board at Nevs.

MOOSE ALI KHAN (MASOOD ALI KHAN) — continues a respected career as a full time model. He lives in Los Angeles with his yoga teacher wife and son, and is pursuing acting with one movie, *The Italian Key*, under his belt. As his life's mission to help humanity, he has taught yoga, meditation and energy healing to anyone that wants to learn. He has a PhD in Universal Energy Healing and a Diploma in Acupuncture. As an eclectic musician, stretching from dance music to New Age, he has released two music albums as 'The Yoga Sessions' series.

NICK KNIGHT — is acknowledged as one of the most influential photographers of his generation. His collaborations with Yohji Yamamoto, Christian Dior and Alexander McQueen are the stuff of fashion legend. He is director of SHOWstudio.com, an online platform for fashion and art practitioners. He lives in London with his wife and three children.

SHERRY (SHERALD) **LAMDEN** — is a freelance creative consultant in the fashion industry, most recently on Alexander McQueen's McQ line. She resides very happily in Brighton with her partner Pablo and their two children Shay and Sky.

JEREMY LESLIE — has tried to escape the grasp of magazines but always returns to them. He now runs magCulture, a design and editorial consultancy working with clients in print and online. He writes the magCulture blog, celebrating creative magazine publishing, and regularly speaks at conferences. He has just finished his third book about editorial design, to be published autumn 2013.

MARK LEWIS — lives between Johannesburg (South Africa) and Mbabane (Swaziland). His photographic work enables him to travel throughout the continent working with an Africa correspondent on social, political and economic stories for magazines.

STEPHEN LINARD — changed careers from fashion design to textile design twenty-two years ago. He has worked continuously as designer for Drakes of London. He spends his spare time sailing and fishing in the Thames estuary, near to where he now lives.

MATT LIPSEY — found love, happiness and comedy. Love in the form of Susie, followed by two daughters Sophie and Tallulah. Happiness from them is followed by comedy in the form of TV shows which he directs when they'll have him. Highlights include *Psychoville*, *Human Remains* and *Catterick*.

DAVID MCINTYRE — now lives in New York with a family. He still shoots fashion although mostly on a video camera.

MISSY (MIXON) — became a photographic agent in London and New York representing Juergen Teller, Jamil GS and Donald Christie at Z Photographic, as well as stylists and art directors including Lee Swillingham and Venetia Scott. She still reads Italian and American *Vogue*, and holds memories of her friends and time in the fashion industry close to her heart.

KUMARS MOGHTADER — moved to the US and worked with *Star Wars* consumer products as Director of Product Development at Lucasfilm and later became Director of Branding for Barbie at Mattel. He has gone on to work as a creative director for a variety of industries, from interior design to beauty products. He is currently developing a new project: personal interviewed biographies.

MARK MOORE — is founder of chart-topping, sampling and dance music pioneers, S'Express. He is still DJ-ing around the globe, plus producing and remixing. He does 'a bit of writing for various magazines' and has a weekly music column in *QX International* magazine. He lives in west London.

JAMIE MORGAN — is still a maverick working on the fringes of the industry, shooting for art fashion magazines like *POP* and *AH+*, and the new CR with Carine Roitfeld, He also shoots fashion advertising. He has always stayed true to the Buffalo fashion portrait aesthetic which has been his major inspiration.

PAUL MORLEY — is a writer, cultural theorist, composer and broadcaster who has written books about interviewing pop stars, suicide, Kylie Minogue, the Moog synthesiser and Joy Division. His latest books are a history of the Bakerloo tube line filtered through the music of Can and a history of the north of England filtered through his own memories. He lives in north London with his partner, Elizabeth.

PETE MOSS — is a photographer, shooting mainly portraiture, and Managing Director of Waddington Studios in Stoke Newington London. He lives with his partner, artist Jasmina Cibic, and daughter Una, in Stoke Newington.

CHRISTIAN NGUYEN — currently works as a visual merchandising stylist for Renaissance Corporation in Mayfair. He spends his time between London, Singapore and the South of France.

WILLEM ODENDAAL — is a professional horse trainer, nowadays. He has currently finished writing on his book about training cow horses in the tradition of Californian Vaqueros. His passion for picture-making has never lessened. Most of his spare time is spent working on photographic portraits of cattle, titled 'Curious Critters'.

ROBERT OGILVIE — funded medical training from '80s photography and set up as an acupuncturist and herbalist in 1991. A proud father, he works from his London clinic, with monthly visits to treat patients in downtown Beirut. He found his calling and has never been happier.

MIKE OWEN — is happily married to Patty. He has two sons and lives at the seaside. He lectures and still continues to take pictures, a job he loves.

RIFAT OZBEK — was acclaimed Designer of the Year in 1988 and '92. He continued to show eponymous collections before becoming creative director at Pollini in Milan. He retired from the fashion business in 2009 and launched Yastik, designing cushions and interior decor. He lives between London, Istanbul and Bodrum.

ANNA PAOLOZZI — lives in Primrose Hill, London, and has been a make-up artist for the last twenty-four years, working on magazine shoots, TV and videos. She is working on a make-up book, a range of make-up products and has a make-up website www.annapaolozzi.co.uk

MICHELE PARADISE — has always been fascinated by human behaviour so studied it properly and is now a therapist/hypnotherapist, enabling people to move forward with their lives. She has two fabulous children who keep her excited and involved. She still loves the London life.

ADRIAN PEACOCK — continues to work as a photographer. He had his first solo show in 2011, and has been selected for the 2011 National Portrait Gallery – Taylor Wessing Photographic Portrait Prize. He lives in St Leonard's on Sea with his wife and children.

SIMON RINGROSE — left London and the world of fashion in 1986, returning to his passion, trees. He attended Arboricultural college 1988–89 and then worked in Australia climbing the biggest trees he had ever seen. There he met a fantastic Australian girl, Megan. They set up a small Arboricultural contracting and consultancy business in Oxfordshire in 1991, married in 1995 and have two fantastic daughters, Mati and Georgia. The business now employs ten people, and is going strong.

LUIVEN RIVAS-SANCHEZ — continues to be creative. He is the director of Bougainvillea Couture, a company dedicated to the endorsement of ethical and sustainable practices in fashion and textiles. He has travelled extensively in order to be inspired and remain connected with professionals who share his vision.

MIKEL ROSEN — learnt the meaning of life. He now lives in San Francisco, USA. Apart from opening a store and working with food, he continues to be a consultant about his first loves, fashion and style, in many parts of the world.

JOHNNY ROZSA — left England to try his luck as a photographer in the USA. In the nineties he lived and worked in Los Angeles, moving to New York in 2000. In 2010 he published a book of celebrity portraits called *UNTOUCHED*. He has exhibited his photographs in museums and galleries worldwide, including MOCA in Sydney, the TNC in New York and the Kunsthalle in Vienna. At present he is writing an illustrated biography about his grandmother.

PAUL RUTHERFORD — lives in New Zealand on Waiheke Island with husband Perry and babes Lucy and Macy (dog and cat), sun, sea but no piracy. He has still got a hand in music (for his sins), taking lots of photographs (who knows maybe one day you'll get to see them?) and eternally missing Blighty.

PIERRE RUTSCHI — lives In Paris and travels the world for pleasure as often as possible. Still passionate about photography, he now takes a more personal, intimate and sensual approach with a focus on black beauty, selling fine art prints to private collectors, as well as trading rare first-edition books on photography and Africa from his collection.

SIBYLLE DE SAINT PHALLE — is a casting director and a stylist. She has been married and is now separated, has a wonderful ten-year-old son, Shaun, and lives in Paris, France.

VICKI SARGE — is still one half of the iconic design brand Erickson Beamon, which has kept its status as one of the most sought after jewellery brands for 30 years! She is living in London and has a twenty-four-year-old daughter called Beatrice, who is now making her mark in the Soho Scene.

LEAH SERESIN — trained as an actress, worked in the film industry as director, writer, and script editor. She has a seven-year-old son, Finbar, and is currently involved with making perfume and the wine industry.

BEN SHAUL — is a photographer and artist, living in NYC. He occasionally misses England. He has two sons and set the world record for being unable to remember much of his past. It is his aim to remember more in the next twenty-five years.

MARTINE SITBON — reinvented the Chloé label at the end of the '80s. Her Rue du Mail label, launched in 2006, continues to combine French allure and rock 'n' roll attitude. Her stylish clients include Cate Blanchett, Tilda Swinton, Zoe Cassavetes and Gwyneth Paltrow. She still lives in Paris with Marc Ascoli; her heart in fashion, her head in the clouds and her feet on the ground.

PAUL SMITH — is one of British fashion's best loved characters. Knighted in 2000 for services to the menswear industry, his label is coveted the world over and embodies the individual style and eccentric playfulness that defines the designer. He is married to Pauline.

THELMA SPEIRS — continues to work with Paul Bernstock at Bernstock Speirs. She is still fashion-obsessed and also works part time as a DJ.

STEVIE STEWART — now works as a costume, set and production designer and fashion stylist. Clients include Michael Clark Dance Company, Russell Maliphant Dance Company, Leona Lewis, Cheryl Cole, Westlife and Kylie Minogue. Film credits include Baillie Walsh's *Flashbacks of a Fool* and Jan Dunn's *The Calling*. Theatre credits include Jan Willem van den Bosch's *Mother Courage*, David Fielding's *The Importance of Being Earnest* and William Baker's *The Hurly Burly Burlesque Musical*.

CHRISTOS TOLERA — has followed his heart as an artist, regularly exhibiting, whilst also eking out a living through painting commissions, designing wallpapers, interiors or anything that comes his way. He continues to act in the occasional commercial, loves having his picture taken and is never far from a spotlight.

MARCUS TOMLINSON — is a respected fine art filmmaker who has collaborated with Hussein Chalayan, Issey Miyake, Gareth Pugh and Hermès, exhibiting at Tate Modern, MOCA Los Angeles and MUDAM Luxembourg. He also heads up MTStudio, a network of creative talent that facilitates projects, events and installations focused on fashion film. He has two beautiful daughters who enjoy his work and keep him driving forward in his beliefs.

STEFANO TONCHI — has continued his life-long love affair with magazines being Creative/Fashion Director of *L'Uomo Vogue*, *Self* and *Esquire*. In 2004 he conceived and edited *T*, the *New York Times* style magazine. He is currently Editor-in-Chief at *W* magazine. He lives in New York and just published a new book *W: The First 40 Years*, following the success of *Uniform* and *Excess*.

JAIME TRAVEZAN — returned to London, which he identifies as his city, after living for many years around Europe working as a fashion photographer. He now lives happily with his boyfriend and still works in the same field, combining fashion and portraiture with social projects, mainly linked to his native country, Peru.

ALEX TURNBULL (LIM) — recently finished his first film *Beyond Time* and is working on his next, a history of street wear. While playing with 23 Skidoo he has rediscovered his love of drumming. He is now trying to concentrate on the important things in life – his wife Maya, his children Kim and Jackson, surfing and 'being present'.

DICK TYSON — worked as an art director in advertising agencies, most recently as a Creative Group Head at Publicist in Baker Street. He gave it all up four years ago to write (and design) books about rugby and football. His fourth rugby book was published in 2012.

ANDRE VAN NOORD — is still modelling in catwalk shows, editorial and advertising campaigns, including Trussardi, Lee, Esprit, Auben & Wills, that also featured his landscape photography. He was featured in The Kooples advert with his wife Marisca, who shares his life along with three kids and a pig in the country just outside Amsterdam.

BAILLIE WALSH — has moved behind the camera and has been directing music videos, commercials, documentaries and feature films since 1990. He has worked with Kate Moss, Kylie Minogue, Boy George and Daniel Craig.

JAN WELTERS — currently lives in Paris with his wife and two beautiful children. He is still shooting with a big body of work behind him. Recent career highs include French, Dutch, Spanish and German *Vogue* editorials, numerous high-end advertising campaigns and the 'icons' book and exhibition for *Antidote* magazine at Joyce Gallery in the Palais Royale in Paris.

VIVIENNE WESTWOOD — is Britain's best known fashion designer. Her provocative fashion statements that meld her fascination for the historical with her political agendas have won her international acclaim. In 2006 she was made a Dame of the British Empire. She lives in London with her husband Andreas Kronthaler.

CAROLE WHITE — continues to be a voice of authority and experience in fashion, with over 30 years in the industry. Having co-founded Premier Model Management in 1981, she has been instrumental in discovering, nurturing and building the international careers of some of the world's greatest modelling names. She lives in London with her family.

HELEN WHITING — worked as a make-up artist for the music, film and commercial industries for twenty years before retraining as a therapist in 2000. She continues to live in west London near her much-loved Portobello Road market.

DAVID WOOLLEY — still travels the world snapping away and after three exhibitions and living in Australia with his wife and two children, has returned to the UK and settled in Brighton. He is the co-founder of limitlesspictures.com and continues to indulge his dual passions of surfing and cycling.

MICHAEL WOOLLEY — has returned to London after ten years in Paris and is balancing a new family with fashion editorial and advertising photography.

MARYSIA WORONIECKA — moved to New York in the nineties to work in the then brave new world of the internet, but ten years later she missed the fashion business, so joined forces with designer Maria Cornejo. They now have three stores for their brand Zero + Maria Cornejo and sell all over the world. She is married to artist Kenseth Armstead and lives in Brooklyn.

CERITH WYN EVANS — has earned a reputation as a flamboyant auteur. His artworks in a variety of media including film, sculpture and installation have been exhibited globally. In 2003 he represented Wales at the Venice Biennale. Celestial Bonnet is a recent collaboration with Stephen Jones for Britain Creates. He is represented by White Cube.

—

CAREY LABOVITCH & SIMON TESLER — closed *BLITZ* magazine in 1991. Following the closure they built up a business publishing group which became part of Pearson plc in 1996. In 1998, Simon launched Adbrands.net, the business information service for the advertising industry, which he still runs. Carey founded and runs the event company ExtravOrganza Events. They are married with seventeen-year-old triplet daughters.

IAIN R. WEBB — is an award-winning writer and Professor of Fashion at the Royal College of Art and Central Saint Martins. He now lives in Bath, where he consults for the Fashion Museum and muses over his life in frocks.

EIRE (' 33 (inc VAT) USA $2.95 AUSTRALIA A$2.50 GERMANY 6DM FRANCE Fr 22 ITALY L3800 SWITZERLAND SFr 4.50

DECEMBER 85/JANUARY 86 No.37   80p

BLITZ

Raise your spirits

IMMACULATE!

P e t e r   M u r p h y: *f r o m   G l a m   t o   G l u m*
M i c k e y   R o u r k e: *H o l l y w o o d   B a d   B o y*

~Dexys Midnight Runners and David Owen and John Lithgow and
Hermes' Eric Bergere and Float Up CP and The Fabulous Pop Tarts